Research Meth
and Health Psychology

Research Methods in Stress and Health Psychology

Edited by

Stan V. Kasl
Yale University School of Medicine

and

Cary L. Cooper
The University of Manchester Institute of Science and Technology

JOHN WILEY & SONS
Chichester · New York · Brisbane · Toronto · Singapore

Baffins Lane, Chichester
West Sussex PO19 1UD, England

National 01243 779777
International (+44) 1243 779777

First published in 1987 as *Stress and Health: Issues in Research Methodology.*
Reprinted in paperback January 1995 as *Research Methods in Stress and Health Psychology.*
Reprinted October 1995

Other Wiley Editorial Offices

John Wiley and Sons, Inc., 605 Third Avenue,
New York, NY 10158-0012, USA

Jacaranda Wiley Ltd, 33 Park Road, Milton,
Queensland 4064, Australia

John Wiley & Sons (Canada) Ltd, 22 Worcester Road,
Rexdale, Ontario M9W 1L1, Canada

John Wiley & Sons (SEA) Pte Ltd, 37 Jalan Pemimpin #05-04,
Block B, Union Industrial Building, Singapore 2057

British Library Cataloguing in Publication Data:
A catalogue for this book is available from the British Library

ISBN 0-471-95493-4

Printed and bound in Great Britain by Antony Rowe Ltd, Chippenham, Wiltshire

Contents

Contributors

John M. Bailey	*University of Texas at Dallas, USA*
Terry A. Beehr	*Central Michigan University, Mt. Pleasant, USA*
Rabi S. Bhagat	*University of Texas at Dallas, USA*
Richard J. Contrada	*Rutgers University, New Brunswick, USA*
Frances Cohen	*University of California, San Francisco, USA*
Cary L. Cooper	*University of Manchester, England*
J. Graham Jones	*MRC/ESRC Social and Applied Psychology Unit, Sheffield, England*
Stan V. Kasl	*Yale University School of Medicine, New Haven, USA*
Ronald C. Kessler	*University of Michigan, Ann Arbor, USA*
David S. Krantz	*Uniformed Services University of the Health Sciences, Bethesda, USA*
Howard Leventhal	*University of Wisconsin, Madison, USA*
Nicola Madge	*St. Mary's Hospital Medical School, London, England*
Michael G. Marmot	*Middlesex Hospital Medical School, London, England*
Kirk O'Hara	*Central Michigan University, Mt. Pleasant, USA*

ROY L. PAYNE — *MRC/ESRC Social and Applied Psychology Unit, Sheffield, England*

LEONARD I. PEARLIN — *University of California, San Francisco, USA*

LYNDA H. POWELL — *Yale University School of Medicine, New Haven, USA*

ANDREW TOMARKEN — *University of Wisconsin, Madison, USA*

HEATHER A. TURNER — *University of California, San Francisco, USA*

Introduction

Research into stress is growing by leaps and bounds (Cooper and Payne, 1988). This applies to the occupational (Cartwright and Cooper, 1994) as well as the health psychology (Cooper and Watson, 1991) fields. The studies are multiplying at such a rate that there has been little attempt to reflect on the variety of research methodologies employed and the future direction of the research generally. Many of the areas of concern or the methodological focal points are similar, but the specific measures, research designs, and methods of analysis are as diverse as the populations they focus on. The purpose of this volume is to correct this imbalance and begin the slow process of assessing what is being used, its usefulness, and where research methodology should be going in the future.

The first part of the book will examine disciplinary perspectives (e.g. epidemiology, health psychology) and more general methodological issues, such as measurement bias in stress and health research, stress reduction intervention designs, data analysis and research design strategies in the field generally.

The second part of the book will focus on several important specific topic areas, which seem to predominate in the stress literature. The intention here is to deal with several issues for each of these topics: (a) the measures that are available and measures still lacking or needed; (b) if comparisons are possible, to highlight the better and inferior measures (and why): (c) special problems typically encountered when these measures are utilized in stress and health studies; (d) a review of some of the main studies and results. Our contributors explore the areas of the family as a context of the stress process, social support, stressors at work, Type A behaviour, and coping.

Finally, we conclude the volume with brief chapter on salient issues in stress research methodology, highlighted by the previous chapters. We hope that this work will make a contribution to the ever burgeoning research literature on stress and health.

CLC and SVK

References

Cartwright, S. and Cooper, C.L. (1994). *No Hassle! Taking the stress out of work.* London: Century Business Books.

Cooper, C.L. and Payne, R. (1988). *Causes, Coping and Consequences of Stress at Work.* New York & London: John Wiley & Sons.

Cooper, C.L. and Watson, M. (1991). *Cancer and Stress: Psychological, Biological and Coping Studies.* Chichester & New York: John Wiley & Sons.

PART ONE

Methodology of Stress Research

Chapter 1

An Epidemiological Perspective on Stress and Health

Michael G. Marmot

Department of Community Medicine, University College London and The Middlesex Hospital Medical School, London

Nicola Madge

Academic Department of Community Medicine, St Mary's Hospital Medical School, London

INTRODUCTION

Epidemiological approach

Epidemiology has made significant contributions to our knowledge of the aetiology of disease and premature death. The crucial role of environmental factors in disease has been emphasized and many of the ways in which physical and biological factors affect health have been teased out. It is largely from epidemiological investigations that we appreciate how well-being and longevity are affected by lifestyle, e.g. diet, smoking, levels of hygiene, physical activity.

Despite these advances in our knowledge about the development of disease at the population level, our ability to predict an individual's health status remains limited. Partly this is inevitable. The necessary crudity of measurement techniques in population studies cannot take account of the full range of an individual's characteristics and circumstances. In part, however, it may stem from a narrower view of factors affecting health. In particular, it has increasingly been stressed that our powers of explanation are due to a failure to take the role of the psychosocial environment properly into account. A growing view is that many forms of psychosocial stress—at work, in personal relationships, following from life events and so on—predispose towards disease and warrant more study than they have been accorded in the past. The call for investigation in this area has been widely answered by researchers in many fields, including epidemiologists who have now provided a proliferation of research evidence.

Research Methods in Stress and Health Psychology. Edited by S. V. Kasl and C. L. Cooper.

The aim of this chapter is to examine some of the achievements, limitations, and potential of epidemiology in examining the links between psychosocial stress and health. We do not attempt to present a comprehensive overview of knowledge across the breadth of the area—this is done in many other chapters in this volume—but rather focus on methodological issues, using empirical findings only selectively by way of illustration.

Stress must be studied epidemiologically

Within epidemiology there have been two poles of opinion on stress research (Marmot, 1986). One has it that the concept is too vague and general to be useful: stress cannot be defined or measured or measured adequately and cannot therefore be studied. The other appears to believe that standard psychosocial instruments can be administered and their results entered into multivariate analyses and causal inferences thereby derived. In our view, the first has not taken account of the detailed work attempting to define and measure specific aspects of the psychosocial environment. The second pole perhaps has a tendency to err in the other direction and treat 'stress' variables as if they were like height or vital capacity.

To study stress epidemiologically one must recognize that it is more difficult than and different in important ways from, say, studying smoking. On a spectrum of difficulty of measurement, smoking would be at the relatively easy end, stress at the other, with physical activity and diet somewhere in-between. What has made smoking accessible to study is the relative ease of quantification, the now ready availability of data that allow the charting of time trends and international comparisons, and the ease of interpreting what smoking 'means' biologically in different cultures and social sub-groups. All of these are more problematic in the study of psychosocial factors. Lack of attempts to solve these problems may, in part, account for the widespread scepticism with which stress research is greeted by researchers in other fields. It is our contention that stress can, and must, be studied epidemiologically—but these problems must be addressed.

CHARACTERISTICS OF EPIDEMIOLOGICAL INVESTIGATIONS

Traditionally the epidemiologist, from a medical perspective, is concerned with establishing the incidence and prevalence of disease both within and across populations. Comparisons are made between populations in different places, or in the same places at different times. An important variant is to study the effects of migration by, say, comparing two stable population groups with the mobile members who have moved from one of the groups to the other. The epidemiological strategy has usually been to collect extensive information on large numbers of people using vital statistics, and other readily available population data, data from special surveys, and clinical data collected on individuals. The business of epidemiology is to generate, test—and, if necessary, reject and regenerate—hypotheses of the causes of specific diseases.

These methods clearly have implications for the type of information that can be collected. It is easy to see how vital statistics lend themselves to the study of smoking and disease, or social class and disease, in countries such as England and Wales where such data are regularly reported. The type of psychosocial data that can be gathered from such sources is, of course, limited. Nevertheless, some such approaches are possible. For example, in England and Wales, nationally collected data have been used to look at the impact of the death of a spouse on the mortality of the surviving partner (Jones, 1986). Marital status has similarly been studied. In Sweden, disease rates by occupation have been used to test hypotheses on job stress (Karasek et al., 1982). These data cannot be used to look at individual differences in response to social class membership, occupation, bereavement, or marital status but they are useful in indicating general patterns.

Sample surveys conducted for a specific purpose are in a position to gather more detailed data on individuals. However, if they are conducted to determine prevalence or incidence of disease they must be very large. This, of course, limits the complexity of data that can be collected. More detailed data on individuals can come from more clinically orientated studies. These have other drawbacks.

The strength of epidemiology is that it studies diseases where they occur—in populations. It is difficult to see how conclusions about aetiology can be drawn without some form of epidemiological investigation complementing other types of research. But epidemiology must accept the relative crudity of measurement of psychosocial data. This will lead to imprecision in classifying individuals, and has implications for study design. For example, if comparisons are made between individuals within a population, misclassifying them will reduce apparent associations between the characteristic and the disease under study. By contrast, if groups are characterized and compared, such imprecision may not seriously bias the comparison.

The major limitation of epidemiology in the study of stress and disease is inherent in the above. The need for mass information necessitates standardized, reproducible measures of both psychosocial factors and health. This limits the subtlety of detail that can be collected and hence the insight that is possible into the human processes involved in links between putative causal and outcome measures.

STUDYING STRESS AND HEALTH EPIDEMIOLOGICALLY

Defining and measuring stress

How has the epidemiologist dealt with stress, and how well equipped is he to investigate a variable which has little in common with the more physical or biological characteristics to which he is accustomed? Stress does present very different measurement challenges from diet or blood pressure or serum cholesterol. The latter are not always straightforward to investigate, but they are on the whole easy to conceptualize, they are somewhat easier to measure, and there are established routes whereby a specified cause can lead to a specified outcome. The case of stress is quite different. There is disagreement about the meaning of the term, there is disagreement about how it should be measured, and there is a lack of understanding about quite how aspects of the psychosocial environment might actually make a person ill.

The absence of a consensual definition of psychosocial stress provides a fundamental empirical difficulty. At one level, there is some confusion about whether stress refers to a 'stressor' or to 'perceived stress'. Some investigators have assumed that stress means environmental circumstances which affect health directly or indirectly, whereas others have emphasized the individual's state of being stressed. Selye (1956) and Wolff (1953), who were among the first to examine stress in a social context, regarded the bodily reaction to unpleasant external stimulations as critical. Some subsequent research—for instance investigations of personality or Type A behaviour—has followed in this tradition, but other forms of enquiry—as in most studies of social networks and social support—have focused almost exclusively on situational factors. In some cases there have been attempts to take both processes into account. Holmes and Rahe (1967) did this to some extent in their early work on stressful life events as, although it was the presence or absence of a variety of life events which were in the end related to health, the stress rating of these events followed from the testimonies of large numbers of individuals. A parallel strategy is found in work on the effects of stress and work reported by Karasek and colleagues (1982). The strategy adopted to identify stressors in the work environment was to ask individual employees to report on aspects which increased their perceived stress, and then to amalgamate responses to provide population measures.

Brown and Harris (1978) have argued that taking self-reports of stress is leaving the job of measurement up to the subject. It belongs more properly with the investigator. Their stress measures are therefore neither the simple 'bereaved', 'divorced', 'unemployed', of the usual epidemiological approach that assumes that, on average, these will be stressful for individuals. Nor are they the individual responses to environmental circumstances, but something in-between. The investigator assesses the context and makes a judgement as to whether a life event is stressful for the individual concerned. This has the advantage of having individual based measures of stress that have meaning to the individual. The major drawback is logistical. These contextual measures are based on several hours of interviewing, rating recordings and transcriptions of interviews.

Measurement and study design

Measurement needs to be good enough for the purpose at hand. If the purpose of a study is to identify features of the social environment that may increase the risk of disease, then measuring individual differences in response may be less important than adequate characterization of the environmental factor: poverty, unemployment, social isolation. A different type of question might be the reason for the individual differences in response to the environment. It is then crucial to study individual responses and search for factors relating to differential vulnerability.

It may be possible to provide at least a partial solution to a measurement problem by appropriate study design. The difficulties in studying stressful life events can, to some extent, be bypassed by examining the impact of loss of a spouse or unemployment, the assumption being, as stated, that these will be stressful for most individuals concerned. While this loses the richness of studying more idiosyncratic events, it has the advantage of generalizability.

Conversely, a particular approach to measurement may be dictated by the study design. Take the example of stress at work in relation to health. It is important to ask if the higher rates of illness consistently observed in some occupations result from higher rates of stress. How does the epidemiologist deal with the measurement of stress at work across a wide range of occupations? There seem to be two main ways in which this problem might be tackled. One approach is to go for comparability in terms of perceived stress and the other is to try to develop ways of measuring the common dimensions of stressors, e.g. time, pressures, physical effort. The drawback of the first approach is that quite different things will be measured in each case, and the limitation of the second is that there may not be much overlap between certain types of jobs (and the crucial stresses in particular jobs may not be included in comparisons) and different things may still be being measured.

The latter approach would seem to be the best strategy for the epidemiologist in that there is at least some means of comparing and contrasting workplaces, but its success depends very critically on identifying the significant dimensions of stress and translating the details of a specific workplace into these concepts. A good example of a successful attempt of this kind is reported by Karasek and colleagues (1982). Their strategy to identify stressors in the work environment was to make use of a survey that asked individual employees to report on the things they found stressful and then to amalgamate their responses. They then rated stress on two main dimensions—job demands and decision latitude. In this way they were able to compare very different occupational settings, and from several studies employing different methodologies found consistently that low decision latitude—especially if combined with high demands—was associated with increased coronary heart disease, morbidity, or mortality.

Even with social supports, where much of the debate has been about the relative importance of availability and adequacy of supports (Henderson and Byrne, 1981) it is important to match methodology to the empirical issue and the disciplinary approach. This is illustrated by the longitudinal study of the Alamada County Human Population Laboratory which provides the most convincing evidence of a link with mortality (Berkman and Syme, 1979), but which used only simple measures of social networks. Had measures of adequacy of support been available, perhaps the relationship with mortality would have been even stronger but it seems unlikely. The measures used were adequate to the task at hand.

Studying the appropriate level of social organization

We have been arguing that different types of study require different types of measurement. From a public health perspective an appropriate level of concern is with the social environment. Just as the epidemiologist enquires into the quality of the chemical, physical, and biological environment, so is it appropriate to enquire into the health effects of the social environment. It may be argued that the appropriate level to study social effects is at the social level.

Going back to Durkheim, even so individual an act as suicide was studied using social characteristics derived from a social level of analysis (Durkheim, 1966). More recent studies of suicide have continued in that tradition. For example, Kreitman and Platt (1984) have studied trends in suicide mortality in Britain. They show fairly convincingly that although unemployment has an effect on suicide rates, the availability of methods of suicide has an effect on the rate. The detoxification of domestic gas in Britain after 1963 led to a drop in the suicide rate while the unemployment rate rose. This was in contrast to earlier British experience and trends in other countries. Similarly, a social level of analysis was used to assess whether organized support systems (the Samaritans) have an effect in lowering the suicide rate. Jennings et al. (1978) conclude that there is no evidence that the presence of a branch of the Samaritans in a town leads to lower suicide rates.

Assessment of ill health

In studies of psychosocial factors it seems, too often, that any health 'outcome' will do. Too little attempt is made to specify whether stress affects health, or the occurrence of specific physical and mental diseases, or something in-between such as symptoms.

Mortality rates are the stock-in-trade of epidemiology. They are widely available, lend themselves easily to comparisons by time, place and personal characteristics, and the fact of death is subject to less misclassification than most indicators—although even deaths may be miscounted and cause-specific mortality is subject to vagaries in classification. The criticism of mortality rates is what they leave out: morbidity, particularly mental illness, and vaguer concepts such as ill health and well-being.

Problems arise where investigators wish to examine not death or clinically-defined disease but ill health more generally within the population. The use of physiological and biological indicators such as tissue damage, blood composition, protein in the urine, have the advantage of objectivity but there are uncertainties about their relation to ill health. Administrative definitions of ill health have been used—people hospitalized or undergoing treatment—but these raise problems of comparability and completeness, and may not reflect health in the population at large.

Alternatively, self reports on health may be used. These have both strengths and weaknesses. It is easier to administer a questionnaire than provide clinical examinations where large numbers of people are involved. However, there are problems in interpreting findings. The precise wording of questions will affect the apparent prevalence of ill health: for example, a change in the British General Household Survey questions on chronic ill health between 1976 and 1978 presumably accounted for a change in reported complaints. In addition, what people say about their health may be affected by their personality and the extent to which they adopt a 'sick role' (Scheff, 1966). There is a concern that a person with a certain type of personality might be more likely to report both illness and dissatisfaction with social supports or conditions at work, thus producing a spurious association.

The contamination of health measures and independent variables such as personality can only be overcome by ensuring that the mode of assessment of one is not influenced by the other. In principle, if stress is subjectively determined, ill health should not be. There may be exceptions, but these need to be determined empirically. For example Kaplan and Camacho (1983) discovered a strong association between perceived health ratings ('excellent', 'good', 'fair', and 'poor') and mortality over the subsequent nine years among almost 7,000 Californians. This association remained even when age, sex, health at the beginning of the study, health practices, social networks, income, education, health for age, anomie, morale, depression, and happiness were taken into account. It is possible that original self-perceived health in some way caused higher mortality but the fact that depression and other personality variables were controlled for makes this interpretation less likely. All the same the limitations of subject-reported health should be recognized. One significant point is that it may reflect age and expectations—Maddox and Douglas (1974) found that elderly people frequently said their health was good even when they had clear clinical signs of pathology.

However ill health is assessed, a number of prior decisions might be made. If people are to be classified as 'ill' or 'not ill', where is the cut-off point to be? What is the duration of ill health? What are the practical implications of illness and how does it interfere with day-to-day life? It is rarely possible to collect 'ideal' data but matching the definition and measurement of health to the purpose for which the information is required—whether this be to provide treatment, to examine thc aetiology of disease, or to plan and/or evaluate medical services—is evidently an important precondition for successful data gathering.

Models of association between stress and health

It is important that research proceed on some theoretical basis and test a particular model of association. Unfortunately, however, in the field of stress and health there are more data than hypotheses to be tested, as evident from Hopkins and Williams' (1981) report that at least 246 factors have been found to be associated with an increased risk of coronary heart disease. Moreover where research does set out to test hypotheses they are often too general and insufficiently specified.

It is helpful for a true understanding of links between psychosocial factors and health to have an informed view on what the mechanisms involved may be. The problem in specifying testable hypotheses is that too many possible pathways have been proposed. There has been little attempt to marshall the evidence linking particular stressors to particular pathways. Perhaps psychosocial stressors lead directly to physiological reactions, such as excessive secretion of corticosteroids, or catecholamines, elevated blood pressure, raised plasma lipids, which in turn increase the risk of clinical conditions such as ulcers, heart disease and so on. Perhaps they lead to these associations via psychological reactions such as misery, anxiety, and depression, or perhaps the links are more indirect. It is possible that links between environmental stresses and health act via changes in behaviour, such as a stressful work situation or a lack of social contacts encouraging a person to smoke and drink heavily.

In cases where it remains unclear what processes are involved, it seems crucial to consider not only sociological and psychological factors on the one hand and medical data on the other—but also variables that are likely to intervene. It is here that much epidemiological research has demonstrated its shortcomings in not taking biological and physiological mechanisms sufficiently into account. Largely this is because the role of such variables, and their interaction with psychological factors, are not sufficiently well specified in models of the aetiology of cancer, or coronary heart disease, or other diseases, to point to appropriate research strategies. For example, our theoretical understanding does not lead us to know whether variations in social supports are better able than smoking and diet to explain cultural variations in disease rates, nor does it give any clues about the manner in which these two sets of variables reinforce or oppose each other.

It is important to determine whether psychosocial factors directly affect the risk of morbidity and mortality, or whether they have an impact only in the presence of some additional stressor. To take the case of social networks, do these in and of themselves affect health ('main effects'), or is their influence only that, if present, they protect against the impact of other psychosocial stressors? There has been much support for the latter view (e.g. Cassel, 1976; Cobb, 1976; Dean and Linn, 1977; Brown and Harris, 1978) as well as some empirical demonstration that unemployment, stress at work, bereavement and so on have a lesser impact on health when social support is available (e.g. Gore, 1978; House and Wells, 1978; McKinlay, 1980). Nonetheless some well conducted studies have indicated main effects by showing that social networks have a fairly constant impact at all levels of risk and that the risk of mortality decreases consistently with the degree of social support (Berkman and Syme, 1979; Joseph, 1980; Reed et al., 1981).

Many further question marks remain in attempts to specify a model of the association between psychosocial stress and health. One issue of especial interest to the epidemiologist concerns the possibility of a 'dose–response' relationship. In other words, does the risk of disease increase with degree of exposure to the appropriate stressor? With many biological mechanisms this relationship holds, as, for example, with smoking and disease, the effects of drugs, and alcohol and liver disease. Is the same true, however, for the effects of psychosocial factors? If it is not the epidemiologist loses one of the main tools available to assess whether an association is likely to be causal.

An understanding of biological processes involved is important not only to determine the mechanisms of action of psychosocial factors on health, but also to assess potential confounding. Too often studies of diet, smoking, and physical activity neglect the social environment. Unfortunately the converse is also true. For example, do people in certain jobs have higher rates of disease because of occupational stress or is it because they belong to a particular social class and share life-style characteristics with other members of that class, perhaps being more likely to smoke, have worse diets, or become exposed to other noxious influences? It may not be the job that predisposes to these characteristics but other aspects of the wider social environment. Sorting out these interrelationships entails a very careful specification of causal models. 'Controlling' for social class may be inappropriate. The argument for controlling for social class is that it controls out other sources of variation. It may however control out the factor of interest. If the link between social class and disease is occupational stress characteristics of lower status jobs, controlling for social class will, inappropriately, remove the factor of interest from analysis. This emphasizes again the importance of following a particular model when gathering and analysing data.

It is not up to the epidemiologist alone to develop models of psychosocial stress and the mechanisms by which health may be imparted or promoted, but it is essential that efforts are made in this direction and that empirical research proceeds accordingly. Such models almost certainly need to take a multi-disciplinary perspective since behavioural, psychological, and physiological processes, as well as individual differences, may all be operating. It is time to stop collecting data for its own sake and to ask why it is being collected and whether or not it might be better to exercise some shift in focus.

TYPES OF EPIDEMIOLOGICAL STUDY

The study of subcultures

Clinical thinking relates characteristics of individuals to individual risks of disease. The epidemiological approach uses this but, in addition, it explores similarities and differences between populations to look for causes. Although, as mentioned below, investigations are sometimes cross-cultural or cross-national, more often they are between sub-groups in a particular cultural and national context. Within this classification comes much of the work on the effects of social networks, life events, stress at work, and unemployment and so on.

By analogy with smoking and lung cancer, it may be thought that for causation to be established, a factor should correlate with disease rates both when the level of analysis is individuals and when the level of analysis is groups or populations. But smoking/lung cancer may be atypical. We would not, for example, expect an environmental characteristic that affects all individuals within a community to a similar extent to be related to disease risk of the individual; we would expect communities that differ in their exposure level to have different disease rates. Conversely, we might expect genetic characteristics to play a part in determining individual risks of disease but they are likely to play very little part in determining community rates of disease. As Rose (1985) observed, the determinants of population risks of disease may be very different from the determinants of the risks of individuals within those populations.

Much depends on the range of variation of the independent variable between populations and within populations. Where the range of variation is small, the chances of detecting an association between characteristic and disease become correspondingly reduced. This is especially true in studies of individuals within relatively homogeneous populations if intra-individual variability is large. In such a case, the group level of analysis may be the most appropriate. To illustrate, an approach employing both group and individual level of analysis has been taken in exploration of the factors underlying socio-economic differences in mortality.

A major health problem facing industrialized countries is the persisting social class differences in the incidence and prevalence of the major chronic diseases (Townsend and Davidson, 1982). From the epidemiologist's point of view, the important thing is to establish the precise nature of these contrasting patterns of mortality and morbidity and to seek explanations for them.

Our own data illustrate an epidemiological investigation in this area. The Whitehall Study of British civil servants examined mortality among men in different grades of employment, working in central government offices in London and demonstrated remarkably clear gradients of age-adjusted mortality by occupational status classified as administrative (the highest), professional, executive, clerical, and 'other' (mainly messengers and unskilled manual workers Marmot et al., 1984). These findings are shown in Table 1. For every cause of death (except genito-urinary disease causing eighteen deaths), the lower two grades have higher mortality risk than the two higher grades of employment, and for nearly every cause there is a stepwise relation between grade of employment and mortality—the steepest gradients are for lung cancer, chronic bronchitis, and other respiratory diseases.

These striking differences, even among men working in the same offices, highlight the power of the social class factor and indicate a fruitful area for further investigation. An explanation of these remarkably robust patterns is likely to shed light on the reasons for social class differences observed in national figures as well as, more generally, the causes of morbidity and mortality among office workers.

Two types of explanation might account for these grade differences in mortality. Perhaps life-style and behaviour associated with social class membership are important and the risk of disease is greater in the lower social classes because people are particularly likely to smoke, eat foods rich in saturated fats and carbohydrates and low in fruit and vegetables, take little exercise, and so on. Or it may be something about the work that a person does that make a particularly marked impact on his health.

The Whitehall Study indicates that both types of factor are likely to play a role. For example, twice as many men in the lowest grade as in the administrative grade smoked. Hence smoking must be of importance in determining the grade difference in some diseases. However, the mortality gradients were found in non-smokers, smokers, and ex-smokers. Similarly, there was an inverse association between grade and obesity, leisure-time physical activity, blood pressure and blood sugar (although not plasma cholesterol)—but as Figure 1 shows, all these risk factors accounted for only 40 per cent of the risk of CHD associated with grade.

Might these social differences in disease rates be psychosocial in origin? Psychosocial stress might stem from the nature and quality of social relationships and networks, or from contrasting levels of stress at work. To pursue this possibility, we conducted a small cross-sectional study in the civil service. New samples of men and women (not included in the original Whitehall Study) from the four grades of employment in one civil service department, the Department of the Environment, were chosen at random and questioned closely in relation to various areas of their life. Our preliminary analyses did show differences in reported psychosocial factors by occupational grade. Table 2 shows that the

Table 1: Age-adjusted mortality in 10 years (and number of deaths) by civil service grade and cause of death

	10 Years Mortality % (no of deaths)				Relative Mortality*				X test for trend (1 df)
	Adminis-trators	Professional & Executive	Clerical	Other	Admin	Professional & Executive	Clerical	Other	
LUNG CANCER	0.35(3)	0.73(79)	1.47(53)	2.33(59)	0.5	1	2.2	3.6	54.62
OTHER CANCER	1.30(12)	1.70(195)	2.20(73)	2.20(46)	0.8	1	1.4	1.4	7.08
CHD	2.20(17)	3.60(399)	4.90(160)	6.60(128)	0.5	1	1.4	1.7	38.24
CEREBRO-VASCULAR DISEASE	0.13(1)	0.49(51)	0.64(23)	0.58(14)	0.3	1	1.4	1.2	1.70
CHRONIC BRONCHITIS	0.00(0)	0.08(8)	0.43(15)	0.65(13)	0.0	1	6.0	7.3	21.01
OTHER RESPIRATORY	0.21(2)	0.22(24)	0.52(18)	0.87(15)	1.1	1	2.6	3.1	11.99
GASTRO-INTESTINAL DISEASES	0.00(0)	0.13(15)	0.20(7)	0.45(15)	0.0	1	1.6	2.8	6.26
GENITO-URINARY DISEASES	0.09(1)	0.09(10)	0.07(2)	0.24(5)	1.3	1	0.7	3.1	2.46
ACCIDENTS AND HOMICIDE	0.00(0)	0.14(17)	0.18(5)	0.18(5)	0.0	1	1.4	1.5	1.36
SUICIDE	0.1(1)	0.15(18)	0.15(4)	0.25(4)	0.7	1	1.0	1.9	0.97
NON-SMOKING RELATED CAUSES									
CANCER	0.90(9)	1.2(145)	1.50(50)	1.60(33)	0.8	1	1.3	1.4	4.70
NON-CANCER	1.00(10)	1.9(216)	2.80(93)	4.20(82)	0.6	1	1.5	2.0	31.83
ALL CAUSES	4.70(41)	8.0(892)	11.70(393)	15.60(326)	0.6	1	1.6	2.1	144.05

**Calculated from logistic equation adjusting for age*

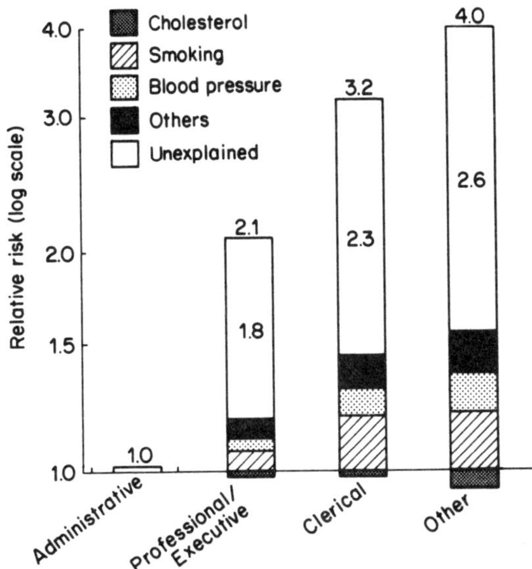

Figure 1: Relative risk of CHD death in different grades 'explained' by risk factors (age-standardized)

lower the grade, the lesser the degree of social support apparently available (Marmot, 1983). The questions used to assess social support were similar to the network questions in the Alameda County Study as well as questions on availability of a confidant.

These civil servants also revealed contrasting reactions to their work environment and content. Not surprisingly, we found Type A behaviour to show a positive association with grade (higher grade, more Type A). This may be a reflection of bias both in the conceptualization and measurement of Type A behaviour. This illustrates both the problem and the value of comparisons across groups. If Type A behaviour is typical of a certain social class/culture/occupational group, the methods of assessment may not be class/culture free. For example, 'taking work home' may characterize a Type A administrator, but it is not a relevant question to a clerical officer or a doorman. Thus the problem of comparison across groups. The value of attempting such comparison is the pointer it gives to potential inadequacies in the Type A concept. If indeed Type A behaviour is manifested by a particular social class when under stress, it is not an appropriate way of attempting to compare stress across classes. We need a concept and a measure that are more generalizable. Work characteristics provide one approach.

In the civil servants' study men in lower status positions reported their jobs to be more monotonous, to provide less opportunity for control and for use of skills (Table 2).

To complete the picture, it emerged that men in the higher status grades were most likely to participate in a variety of leisure time activities outside work. If recreation of this kind can validly be seen as a relief from work pressures, or as an additional means to gain fulfilment or of social supports, this may be an extra way in which social class differences in health arise.

Table 2: Per cent of men reported selected psychosocial characteristics according to grade of employment in the British civil service

Characteristic	Administrative	Professional & Executive	Clerical Officers	Others
Social Supports				
See confidant daily	92	86	82	80
No contact with relatives	15	17	20	22
No contact with neighbours	37	40	55	69
No social contact with people at work	55	66	72	82
No contact with other friends	20	22	20	40
Job attitudes				
Underuse of skills	50	58	68	67
Little or no control	7	14	18	33
Not fair treatment	11	16	16	33
No variety	0	4	21	37
Job of little value	2	2	6	9
Activities outside work				
Involved hobbies—solitary	46	36	26	20
Organised social—sedentary	45	39	30	29
Active—not vigorous exercise	85	86	62	40
Active sports	39	32	24	33

These data are group data. It is fashionable to criticize such data as subject to potential ecological fallacy. It is worth re-emphasizing, however, that if a factor does not correlate with group differences in disease rates, i.e. does not follow the distribution of disease in the population, it cannot *per se* be the explanation of those differences among groups in disease rates—whether or not it is related to disease in individuals. In addition, if occupational groups, such as civil service grades are relatively homogeneous with respect to work characteristics, searching for correlations in individuals within a grade between work stress and disease may be the wrong approach. (In fact we believe there is enough individual variation to make such a search worthwhile.)

Cross-cultural comparisons

There are two reasons for wishing to carry out international studies of psychosocial factors and health: (a) to test the degree to which international variations in disease occurrence correlate with international variations in psychosocial factors; and (b) to test the reproducibility of research findings, and thereby their generalizability under different conditions.

The comments on problems and value of making sub-group comparisons within a population, referred to in the previous section, apply similarly when making international comparisons.

International studies are an important part of the epidemiological method. Occasional attempts have been made to use them in the study of psychosocial factors. For example, Henry and Cassel (1969) furthered the hypotheses about the relation of acculturation to hypertension, by examining the rise of blood pressure with age in societies undergoing varying degrees of contact with western, urban life style. But in general, there has been little attempt to link international differences in disease rates with international differences in psychosocial factors. The difficulties are obvious: developing methods of assessment that are applicable in different cultures. However, if it is not to be tried, an important part of the epidemiological method is lost and one can never determine, for example, whether the marked international differences in CHD mortality rates could be ascribed to psychosocial factors. As illustrated below, one way of approaching the question is through the study of migrants.

The other benefit to be derived from international studies is testing the robustness of psychosocial concepts and measures. Kittel et al., (1986) have reviewed studies of Type A behaviour and CHD. The results from Europe have not fulfilled the promise of the earlier American studies. This provides the stimulus to rethink what it is about Type A behaviour that led to its relationship with CHD in California businessmen and men and women in Framingham, Massachussets, but not in several European populations. Might it be, for example, that hostility is an important component; and that this is better captured by the Type A measures in the USA than in Europe?

Similarly with social supports, Berkman (1985) has reviewed the various studies linking social supports and social networks to morbidity and mortality. There is enough in the studies from different cultures (those of California, North Carolina, Massachussets, Japanese Americans in Hawaii, Israel, as well as more recently Finland and London) to suggest some general applicability of the concept that social supports protect against the development of physical disease. There are, however, inconsistencies. The relation with incidence of CHD was only with angina in Israel, non-fatal myocardial infarction in Hawaii, and mortality in California; and supports seem more protective for men than for women. By exploring these inconsistencies and searching for dimensions of the social support measures that may cross cultures, more is likely to be learnt.

Within one culture, the various dimensions of support are likely to be highly correlated. Crossing cultures holds more prospect of distinguishing one from another.

Migrant studies

Migrants provide an opportunity to examine the impact of culture from an epidemiological perspective which minimizes some of the measurement problems involved in cross-cultural studies. Moreover, by looking at the similarities and differences with populations of origin and destination, some light is thrown on the relative importance of the two influences and hence some hints are gained about the aetiology of disease or other characteristic under study.

The rate of disease among migrants is influenced by: genes; persistent effects of the old environment, including aspects of lifestyle that persist; effects of the new environment; and the process of migration, including both the selection of who migrates and the effects of arriving and resettling in new surroundings. Complex as this appears, by comparing the rates of disease of migrants with that of residents of the old country and of the new country, by examining the effect of length of stay and age at migration, by analysing the experience of the second generation, and finally by examining characteristics of the migrants themselves, it is possible to separate out the factors affecting health and disease in migrants.

Cassel (1975), reviewing studies of hypertension in migrants, concluded that the increase in blood pressure, and rise of blood pressure with age, that occurs with urbanization, is more likely to result from psychosocial factors than from dietary or other changes. Some direct evidence comes from the Tokelau island migrant study. Migrants to New Zealand from these coral atolls in the Pacific have higher blood pressure than their compatriots remaining on the islands. The 'selection' effect is shown to be unlikely, because persons who subsequently migrated, when studied on the islands prior to migration, were found to have similar blood pressure to non-migrants. Further study within New Zealand linked social ties with blood pressure level (Beaglehole et al., 1977). Tokelauans who 'interacted' mainly with other Tokelauans, and who were therefore presumably less acculturated and more supported by traditional social networks, had lower blood pressure than those who were more in contact with white New Zealanders.

A similar combination of between and within population comparisons was used in exploring the reasons for the six-fold higher CHD mortality in the USA compared to Japan. Many factors vary between Japan and the USA, among them ethnicity, cultural practices and diet. Migrants from Japan to Hawaii and California have progressively higher CHD rates (Syme et al., 1975). Japanese-Americans have higher levels of plasma cholesterol and blood pressure, but these differences do not account for their higher disease rates (Marmot et al., 1975). This study, therefore, provided the opportunity to test the hypothesis that the group orientation and socially supportive nature of Japanese culture provided partial protection against the occurrence of CHD. This was borne out in a study within the Japanese population in California. More traditional Japanese men measured on a scale of culture of upbringing and social assimilation had lower CHD prevalence than more westernised men, independent of differences in diet or established coronary risk factors (Marmot and Syme, 1976).

The problem with pursuing such studies further is that measures of social support or acculturation are not readily available. They must be developed specifically for the group under study. For example, Indian migrants to England and Wales have a high CHD mortality—higher than the England and Wales average (Marmot et al., 1984). Might this be related to psychosocial factors? Anecdotal evidence suggests the persistence of the extended family among Indians in Britain. Should this not provide social supports and buffer stress? Then why the high rate of CHD? A detailed knowledge of the immigrants' culture and culture-specific measures would be needed before this question could be approached. There are no obvious short-cuts.

Unemployment

We close with an extended discussion of the data on unemployment. It is an important social and psychosocial problem. The data are relatively easy to obtain; and a variety of techniques have been used in the study of its health effects. The arguments have been summarized by Marmot and Morris (1984). They are reproduced here because they illustrate many of the methodological problems of epidemiological studies of psychosocial factors.

A specific factor?

As conditions of the social environment change, we might expect health and disease patterns to change. The most dramatic change facing capitalist and 'mixed' economies is chronic high unemployment. There are at least two reasons for speculating *a priori* that unemployment may have an impact on morbidity and mortality. First, it can be an indicator of conditions and standards of living (Morris and Titmuss, 1944). As the level of unemployment rises more and more people have their material conditions markedly worsened. Second, unemployment is a stressful life event that becomes a chronic problem. In a work-oriented society, work has social and psychological meaning that goes beyond its economic import. To become unemployed is to be deprived of a social role and function. The self-image of the unemployed person is changed as is the pattern of social relationships.

The existence of plausible theoretical reasons why unemployment might affect health status is no guarantee that such a relationship can be demonstrated. One difficulty comes in isolating the effects of unemployment from the effects of other social or economic conditions. In a sense, this is an artificial question. If unemployment leads to increased mortality rates for the first of the above reasons—that it increases poverty—then it becomes difficult to separate the effects of unemployment from the effects of poverty: poverty is the effect of unemployment which anyhow is particularly likely to affect the poor. The unemployment question is then seen as part of the general question: does increased poverty lead to increased morbidity and mortality? In the second case, i.e. unemployment as stressful life change, it will again be difficult to isolate the health effects of this particular stress from the other stresses associated with poverty.

One might argue that unemployment is unlikely to have the same effect on all societies at different times. This is theoretically true, but the same argument might be raised about social class. Remarkably, social class, despite the crudity of the measures employed, has been a strong predictor of mortality since it was first measured as such in England and Wales in 1911 and the same is true of other industrialized countries.

Two potentially important distinctions should be made, however. First that between temporary and long-term unemployment (>1 year). These are likely to affect different people by age, skills, social class, and health record and may have different associations with ill health. And secondly, whether only the health of the unemployed is being considered, or whether the health of employed and unemployed people is considered in relation to unemployment rates.

Methods of study

Broadly, two approaches have been taken to studying the impact of unemployment on morbidity and mortality: (a) correlational studies of whole populations or sub-groups thereof, and (b) studies of unemployed people. Each has advantages and limitations as detailed below.

Correlation

Among the earliest of these was the study of Morris and Titmuss (1944) of rheumatic heart disease mortality in young people in the county boroughs of England and Wales, related to the depression of the 1930s. They showed a correlation between increase in overall unemployment rates and change in rheumatic heart disease mortality—the towns worst hit by unemployment had the worst mortality record. The correlations were strongest with a 'lag' period of up to three years and were apparent even after standardizations for an index of poverty and overcrowding.

Best known among recent studies is the series by Brenner (1977, 1979). He has argued that increases in unemployment affect not only the unemployed, but also those still in employment, that is, a rise in unemployment is a general indicator of economic instability, which leads to loss of income, social status, and close personal attachments, and to stress in employees of firms experiencing economic difficulties (Brenner, 1979). In his American studies, Brenner (1977) claimed that peaks in mortality from a variety of causes follows peaks in unemployment with a lag period of between nought and five years. One of his major critics, Eyer (1977), agrees that peaks in mortality rate do correspond with the business cycle, but he comes to the opposite conclusion to Brenner. He argues that troughs in unemployment correspond to peaks in mortality, with no lag period. Eyer did not use the same complex multivariate statistical models as Brenner, who rejected this interpretation.

Brenner (1979) has applied a similar statistical analysis to mortality trends in England and Wales. He analysed mortality for the period 1936–76, that is before current recession and mass unemployment. His statistical model to 'explain' trends in mortality—both the long-term secular decline and short-term fluctuations—includes four components: (a) economic growth trend; (b) rate of unemployment; (c) rapid economic growth (that is, deviations from the long-term exponential trend in real per capita income); and finally (d) government expenditure on 'welfare' as a percentage of total government expenditure. Unemployment is built into the statistical model with a variable lag period.

The results, on the surface remarkable, are very difficult to interpret. The R^2 value (a perfect correlation has an R^2 of 1, no correlation $R^2 = 0$) of his multiple regression equation in 0.97. Interpreted literally, this means these four economic indices 'account for' 97 per cent of the variance in death rates, over the period in England and Wales. Similarly, in a regional analysis of counties in England and Wales, 1971, Brenner finds that economic indices including unemployment 'explain' 95 per cent of the variance in total death rates.

It is not the present purpose to enter a general discussion of regression analyses, but to put these results in perspective, we should note that completely different variables also find high orders of correlation. For example, in England and Wales the mortality rate is higher in winter than in summer and the winter excess is greater in severe winters (defined by weather, not economics), with high rates of influenza, than in mild winters.

For arteriosclerotic heart disease mortality in England and Wales, over the period 1950–62, the correlation between the winter excess in mortality and coldness of the winter is 0.95. Ninety-five per cent of the variance, the year to year fluctuations in winter excess, can be 'explained' by temperature (Rose, 1966). It is similarly possible to show that trends in heart disease mortality are correlated to a high order with consumption of various foods and cigarettes (Armstrong et al., 1975).

Brenner's high order geographical correlation between economic factors, economic growth, unemployment etc. and mortality in England and Wales can also be reproduced with other variables. For example, an analysis of mortality 1969–73 from cardiovascular disease in 253 towns in England, Wales, and Scotland found the following correlation coefficients with mortality (SMR): water hardness −0.67; mean daily maximum temperature −0.70; total annual rainfall 0.58; latitude 0.68; air pollution (mean annual smoke) 0.54; blood group (per cent A-frequency) −0.59 (Pocock et al., 1980).

If economic indices, including unemployment, account for all the variation in mortality over time and place, how can it be true that this same variation is also 'explained' by variations in temperature, longitude, water hardness, air pollution, and consumption of flour and fresh vegetables? There may be several answers. Many of these variables are highly inter-correlated and a multiple regression equation is not the appropriate tool to tell us which of these variables is causally related to mortality. It is too affected by circumstances and quality of measurement to sort out biological hypotheses. Second, by allowing for variable lag periods between unemployment and mortality, as Brenner does, and by selecting some variables (for example, percentage of workers in chemical industries, and farm employment) but not others, it is possible, *post-hoc*, to fit a curve to the data with a high order of precision.

An important test of the statistical model is its ability to predict mortality beyond the period for which it was developed. Gravelle and colleagues (1981) have criticized Brenner's analysis on a number of grounds. For example, the strong correlation between unemployment and mortality seen in the period 1936–76 is no longer evident if the period is extended to include 1926–76. Further lack of 'robustness' is demonstrated by the failure of the model to predict mortality subsequent to the period over which it was developed, better than a simple extrapolation.

The lesson from this exchange is not that unemployment has no relation with general mortality, but that such a relation is difficult to tease out of a number of inter-correlated variables. Certainly, few would find difficulty in accepting that the long-term downward trend in mortality in England and Wales, the US, and other countries, is related to general improvements in standard of living. Whether short-term fluctuations in mortality are related to fluctuations in economic fortunes has not been demonstrated unequivocally by this type of analysis (Kasl, 1979). There are other difficulties apart from methodological ones. For example, unemployment, since the depression of the 1930s, has not been a reflection of general economic decline. Those in employment (close on 90 per cent in England and Wales) have continued to enjoy an increased standard of living, at least until now—although this may change.

Studies of unemployed people

These studies present different problems. It has commonly been found that unemployed people have a higher morbidity rate than those in employment (Stern, 1981). For example, in the General Household Survey (1976) in Britain, the proportion of males reporting a long-standing illness was nearly 40 per cent higher for the unemployed. This finding is consistent with three alternative explanations: (a) the unemployed differ from the employed with respect to other characteristics that account for their ill health; (b) ill health causes unemployment (c) unemployment causes ill health. There is some evidence in support of all three of these.

Several studies in England and Wales have shown that unemployment affects selectively people in low social class and low incomes (Stern, 1981). For example, a 1978 survey showed that half the entrants to unemployment had prior incomes in the bottom 20 per cent of the earning distribution. This makes it difficult to separate the effects of unemployment from the effects of prior poverty and thus to see if unemployment increases further the disadvantage of this high-risk group. A major British study of the 1930s found difficulty in separating the effects of unemployment from the effects of working-class life on a low income, but emphasized the likely ill-effects of the latter (Pilgrim Trust, 1938).

Clearly, ill health can also lead to unemployment. The 'healthy worker' effect is well recognized in epidemiology. People in employment have lower mortality rates than those out of employment. For example, Table 3 from the OPCS longitudinal study (Fox and Goldblatt, 1982) shows that among men aged 15–64 years, those actively in work have an SMR of 86, that is 86 per cent

Table 3: Mortality 1971–75 of men and women in the OPCS Longitudinal Study according to age and economic position at the time of the 1971 census

	Men (15–64 years)			Women (15–59 years)		
Economic position	Observed	Expected*	SMR	Observed	Expected*	SMR
Active						
Employed	3021	35087	8	682	884.4	81
Off work, sick	211	65.3	323	48	11.1	432
Seeking work	165	126	130	20	25.0	80
Inactive						
Retired	91	59.4	153	37	26.2	141
Permanently sick	370	94.5	392	101	20.1	502
Student	26	1.5	83	16	17.5	91
Other inactive	43	410	105	646	605.9	107
Total	3927	3927.3	100	1550	1550.2	100

**Expected deaths are calculated separately for each sex using death rates for 1971–75 (in five-year age groups) for all male/females in the Longitudinal Study 1971 Census sample*

of the average mortality. With the exception of students, all other groups of men have a higher mortality than the average—at least in part because the non-working group includes people off work, sick (SMR = 392). Findings for women were similar. If the definition of 'unemployment' is restricted to people not off sick and seeking work, the SMR is still raised for men (130) but not for women (80). Even this latter group of men could include some people who lost their jobs through ill health.

These national data for England and Wales illustrate the problem. Unemployed men and women have a higher mortality than the employed, but sickness is one reason for being out of work. From a study that examines employment status at one time, it is difficult to distinguish ill health as a cause or effect of unemployment. Longitudinal data on health status before and after jobs are lost are few. One American study of this type reported an increase in blood pressure after unemployment (Kasl and Cobb, 1970).

Recent data from the British OPCS longitudinal data do point to the unemployed having an increased mortality not due to health selection (Moser et al., 1986).

These studies have all been based on relatively 'hard' endpoints. Clearly, unemployment can have a major impact on family life, on general well-being, and on the children of the unemployed, whether or not this is reflected in usual measures of morbidity and mortality.

The difficulty in demonstrating an effect of unemployment on health and disease independent of other factors does not exonerate unemployment. No evidence does not equate with no effect. At the very least, one can conclude that the failure to show clearly such an effect of unemployment is due, in part, to the strong harmful effects of poverty. As Stern (1981) comments: 'The incidence of unemployment is non-random and reflects wider economic inequalities. High unemployment reveals the consequences of low incomes more starkly'.

These studies of unemployment illustrate a major point. Psychosocial factors are part of a broader social context. They should be studied in that context whatever difficulties that makes for study and establishing causal links.

REFERENCES

Armstrong, B. K., Mann, J. J., Adelstein, A. M., and Eskin, F. (1975). Commodity consumption and ischaemic heart disease mortality with special reference to dietary practices, *J. Chronic Dis.*, **28**, 455.

Beaglehole, R., Salmond, C. E., Hooper, A., Huntsman, J., Stanhope, J. M., Cassel, J. C., and Prior, I. A. M. (1977). Blood pressure and social interaction in Tokelauan migrants in New Zealand, *J. Chronic Dis.*, **30**, 803–12.

Berkman, L. (1985). The relationship of social networks and social support to morbidity and mortality. In S. Cohen and S. L. Syme (eds.).

Berkman, L. F., and Syme, S. L. (1979). Social networks, host resistance and mortality:

a nine year follow-up of Alameda County residents, *Am. J. Epidemiol.*, **109**, 186–204.

Brenner, M. H. (1977). Health costs and benefits of economic policy. *Int. J. Health Serv.*, **7**, 581.

Brenner, M. H. (1979). Mortality and the national economy: a review, and the experience of England and Wales 1936–76. *Lancet*, **ii**, 568.

Brown, G. H., and Harris, T. (1978). *The Social Origins of Depression: a Study of Psychiatric Disorder in Women*. London, Tavistock.

Cassel, J. C. (1975). Studies of hypertension in migrants. In Paul, O. (ed.) *Epidemiology and Control of Hypertension*, Symposia Specialists, Miami, 41–62.

Cassel, J. (1976). The contribution of the social environment to host resistance, *Am. J. Epidemiol.*, **104**, 107–23.

Cobb, S. (1976). Social support as a moderator of life stress. *Psychosomatic Medicine*, **38**, 300–14.

Dean, A., and Lin, N. (1977). The stress-buffering role of social support, *Journal of Nervous and Mental disorders*, **165**, 403–17.

Durkheim, E. (1966). *Suicide*, translated by Spauldrig, J. A., and Simpson, G., Free Press, New York.

Eyer, J. (1977). Does unemployment cause the death rate peak in each business cycle? A multifactor model of death rate changes, *Int. J. Health Serv.*, **7**, 625.

Fox, A. J., and Goldblatt, P. O. (1982). *Longitudinal Study* 1971–75, HMSO, London.

Gravelle, H. S. E., Hutchinson, G., and Stern, J. (1981). Mortality and unemployment: A critique of Brenner's time series analysis, *Lancet*, **ii**, 675.

Gore, S. (1978). The effect of social support in moderating the health consequences of unemployment, *Journal of Health and Social Behaviour*, **19**, 157–65.

Henderson, S., Bryne, D. G., and Duncan-Jones, P. (1981). *Neurosis and the Social Environment*, Academic Press, Sydney, London and New York.

Henry, J. P., and Cassel, J. C. (1969). Psychosocial epidemiologic and animal experimental evidence, *Am. J. Epidemiol.*, **90**, 171–200.

Holmes, T. H., and Rahe, R. H. (1967). The social readjustment rating scale. *Journal of Psychosomatic Research*, **11**, 213–18.

Hopkins, P. N., and Williams, R. R. (1981). A survey of 246 suggested coronary risk factors. *Atherosclerosis*, **40**, 1–52.

House, J. S., and Wells, J. A. (1978). Occupational stress, social support and health. In A. McLean, G. Black and M. Colligan (eds.) *Reducing Occupational Stress*, Washington DC, Department of Health, Education and Welfare.

Jennings, C., Barraclough, B. M., and Moss, J. R. (1978). Have the Samaritans lowered the suicide rate? A controlled study. *Psychological Medicine*, **8**, 413–22.

Jones, D. (1986). Mortality following bereavement: some results from the OPCS longitudinal study. *Postgraduate Journal* (in press).

Joseph, J. (1980). Social affiliation, risk factor status, and coronary heart disease: A cross-sectional study of Japanese-American men. Unpublished Ph.D. Thesis, University of California, Berkeley.

Kaplan, G. A., and Camacho, T. (1983). Perceived health and mortality: a nine year follow-up of the human population laboratory cohort. *Am. J. Epidemiol.*, **177**, 293–304.

Karasek, R. A., Theorell, T. G. T., Schwartz, J., Pieper, C., and Alfredsson, L. (1982). Job, psychological factors and coronary heart disease, In H. Denolin (ed.) *Psychological Problems Before and After Myocardial Infarction*, Basel, Karger.

Kasl, S. V. (1979). Mortality and the business cycle: some questions about research strategies when utilising macro-social and ecological data, *Am. J. Public Health*, **69**, 784.

Kasl, S. V., and Cobb, S. (1970). Blood pressure changes in men undergoing job loss: a preliminary report, *Psychom. Med.*, **32**, 19.

Kittel, F., Kornitzer, M., and Dramaix, M. (1986). Stress and the individual evaluation of Type A personality, *Post-grad Med. J.* (in press).

Kreitman, N., and Platt, S. (1984). Suicide, unemployment and domestic gas detoxification in Britain, *J. of Epid., and Comm. Health*, **38**, 1–6.

McKinley, J. (1980). Social network influence in morbid episodes and the career of help seeking. In L. Eisenberg and A. Kleinman (eds.) *The Relevance of Social Science for Medicine*, Dordrecht, Reidel.

Maddox, G. L., and Douglas, E. B. (1974). Ageing and individual differences: a longitudinal analysis of social, psychological and physiological indicators. *Gerontology*, **29**, 555–63.

Marmot, M. G. (1983). Stress, social and cultural variations in heart disease, *Journal of Psychosomatic Research*, **27**, 377–84.

Marmot, M. G. (1986). *Postgraduate Journal* (in press).

Marmot, M. G., Adelstein, A., and Bulusu, L. (1984). Lessons from the study of immigrant mortality, *Lancet*, **i**, 1455–57.

Marmot, M. G., and Morris, J. N. (1984). The social environment. In W. W. Holland, D. Detels, and G. Knox (eds.) *Oxford Text Book of Public Health*, Volume I, Oxford, Oxford University Press.

Marmot, M. G., Shipley, M. J., and Rose, G. (1984). Inequalities in death—specific explanations of a general pattern? *Lancet*, **i**, 1003.

Marmot, M. G., and Syme, S. L. (1976). Acculturation and CHD in Japanese-Americans, *Am. J. Epidemiol.*, **104**, 225–47.

Marmot, M. G., Syme, S. L., Kagan, H., and Rhoads, G. (1975). Epidemiologic studies of CHD and stroke in Japanese men living in Japan, Hawaii and California: Prevalence of coronary and hypertensive heart disease and associated risk factors, *Am. J. Epidemiol.*, **102**, 514–25.

Morris, J. N., and Titmuss, R. M. (1944). Health and social change 1: the recent history of rheumatic heart disease, *Medical Officer*, **9729**, 69.

Moser, K. A., Fox, A. J., Jones, D. R., and Goldblatt, P. O. (1986). Unemployment and mortality: further evidence from the OPCS longitudinal study 1979–81, *The Lancet*, **i**, 365–6.

Pilgrim Trust (1938). *Man Without Work*, Macmillan, London.

Pocock, S. J., Shaper, A. G., and Cook, D. G. et al. (1980). British regional heart study: geographic variations in cardiovascular mortality, and the role of water quality. *Br. Med. J.*, **280**, 1243.

Reed, D., McGee, D., Yano, K., and Feinleib, M. (1983). Social networks and coronary heart disease among Japanese men in Hawaii, *Am. J. Epidemiol.*, **117**, 384–96.

Rose, G. (1966). Cold weather and ischaemic heart disease, *Br. J. Prev. Soc. Med.*, **29**, 97.

Rose, G. (1985). Sick individuals and sick populations, *Int. Journal of Epid.*, **14**, 1.

Scheff, T. J. (1966). *On Being Mentally Ill: a Sociological Theory*. London, Weidenfeld and Nicholson.

Selye, H. (1956). *The Stress of Life*, New York, McGraw-Hill.

Stern, J. (1981). *Unemployment and its impact on morbidity and mortality*. Discussion Paper No 93, Centre for Labour Economics, London School of Economics.

Syme, S. L., Marmot, M. G., Kagan, H., and Rhoads, G. (1975). Epidemiologic studies of CHD and stroke in Japanese men living in Japan, Hawaii and California, Introduction, *Am. J. Epidemiol.*, **102**, 477–80.

Townsend, P., and Davidson, D. (1982). *Inequalities in Health*, Harmondsworth, Middlesex, Penguin Books.

Wolffe, H. G. (1953). *Stress and Disease*, Springfield, Illinois, Thomas.

Chapter 2

Stress and Illness: Perspectives from Health Psychology

Howard Leventhal and Andrew Tomarken

Department of Psychology, University of Wisconsin, Madison

INTRODUCTION

The aim of the present chapter is to present a social-psychological perspective on stress and illness and to use it to identify the key problems in method and theory that have prevented investigators from testing and 'validating' hypotheses about the stress–illness process.

Our problem starts with the stress–illness link: Does stress cause illness? If yes, how does it do so? These questions may seem anachronisms to the majority of lay persons and health practitioners as it is virtually a cultural truism that 'stress causes illness'. The current opinion was foretold by Sir William Osler, the Oxford and Johns Hopkins University distinguished Professor of medicine:

> A man who has early risen and late taken rest, who has eaten the bread of carefulness, striving for success in commercial, professional or political life, after twenty-five or thirty years of incessant toil reaches the point where he can say, perhaps with just satisfaction, 'Soul, thou hast much goods laid up for many years; take thine ease,' all unconscious that the fell sergeant has already issued the warrant.

The belief that stress leads to illness has a long history. During the 1700s and 1800s, many physicians thought emotional trauma a cause of cancer, a belief expressed by Galen centuries before (LeShan, 1959). Widespread, forcefully expressed, cultural norms of this sort played a key role in initiating the study of Type A behaviour. The two critical factors that led Friedman and Rosenman (1974) to undertake these studies were: (a) Reports from the wives of their coronary patients, who pointed out that diet could not be the cause of CHD since their diets failed to differ from those of their ill husbands (Friedman and Rosenman, 1974, p. 56); and (b) Their survey of 150 businessmen and 100 physicians, which indicated that a majority of both groups believed stress to be

Research Methods in Stress and Health Psychology. Edited by S. V. Kasl and C. L. Cooper.

the main cause of coronary disease. While neither piece of evidence could be regarded as a 'scientific' demonstration of the plausibility of the stress–illness hypothesis, they are clear examples of the cultural assumption of such an hypothesis. We would have little difficulty finding other such examples (e.g. Shekelle and Lin, 1978).

It is also relatively easy to find critics of the aetiological role of stress in illness. For example, the opinion of the prominent physician Arnott (1954) was: 'So far as I can see, this hypothesis has no scientifically credible basis whatsoever—in fact most of the evidence adduced in its support is dubious and much of it absurd.'

Indeed, the very concept of stress itself is under attack. Mason (1971; 1975a; 1975b) argues that there is no such thing as a unitary stress state and suggests that extremely complex and varied physiological responses are associated with environmental stressors. Engel (1985), in discussing the meaning of stress, goes one step further by concluding that '... stress is neither a noun, nor a verb, nor an adjective. It is an escape from reality' (Engel 1985, p. 10). If there is no such thing as stress, it would be fruitless indeed, as Arnott claims, either to write a chapter on stress and illness or to study the stress–illness link.

It may help if we begin by making a few basic points respecting stress–illness research. First, to a substantial degree the term stress has served to label a research area that investigates the way in which economic, social, and psychological variables reduce an individual's resistance to disease or serve to precipitate or promote disease (See Syme and Berkman, 1976). This is most apparent in so-called Marxian analyses of the relationship of institutional and economic variables to disease (Schnall and Kern, 1981). However, as Lazarus has pointed out (Lazarus and Folkman, 1984), it is nearly impossible to find the concept stress used in a well wrought or even partially worked out theoretical system. Second, the stress process and/or the responses comprising it can be conceptualized as distinct from the situational stimuli or stressors that initiate it. Thus, it can be conceptualized as distinct from the situational stimuli or stressors that initiate it. Thus, it can be conceptualized and described at the social (e.g. Pearlin, 1983), psychological (Lazarus, 1966; Lazarus and Folkman, 1984; Leventhal and Nerenz, 1983), and biological level (Selye, 1973, 1975, 1976; Mason, 1975a, b; 1971). While the multi-levelled nature of stress is obvious to virtually everyone, theoretical and technological complexities have led to a substantial degree of isolation between researchers at each level. The consequence is that conceptual models at one level may not reflect the latest knowledge at the others.

For example, a large portion of the social and psychological research on the stress–illness link assumes a unitary, underlying biological stress process (Cassel, 1974), such as that popularized by Selye (1976), rather than a complex multivariate system, such as that suggested by Mason (1975a; b). Investigators conceptualizing stress as a unitary system tend to treat stressors as a homogeneous domain, either as demands for change (Holmes and Rahe, 1967; Holmes and Masuda, 1974; Rahe, 1972, 1974), or as negative events (Pearlin, 1983; Pearlin, Lieberman, Menaghan and Mullan, 1981). As a result, they ignore possible differences between various classes of stressors, or between the linkages of particular types of stressors and individual diseases in specific population sub-groups. In short, acceptance of a unitary model of the biology of stress resulted in a unitary model of the social psychology of stress, rather than a complex model of multiple social-psychological stress processes. Our own bias is clearly toward the multiplex side. Thus, we believe that the umbrella term stress will need to be replaced by designations for multiple stress processes. At the phenomenological level, this will mean the proliferation of terms to describe a variety of subjective states, for example, negative emotions such as depression or anxiety. At the behaviour level, this means we should expect different behaviours or coping patterns in response to each of these different emotions. At the physiological level, we need to search for different patterns of response accompanying subjective and behavioural events (e.g. Ekman, Levenson, and Friesen, 1983). Finally, at the social level, we must search for classes of institutional and role relationships that are correlated with these psychological and biological processes. It will be a major challenge to understand how these cross-level associations come into being. Specification of particular situations and specific stress processes linked to particular diseases in particular sub-groups would be the expected outcome of such a differentiated approach (e.g. Depue and Monroe, 1986).

Two other important factors need to be mentioned that are often omitted in discussions of the stress–illness link. The first concerns time: it is clear that stress *operates over time*. This means that one must not only demonstrate that stress is antecedent to illness, but that the time frame of the stress/emotion process under study overlaps the time frame of the physiological processes that initiate or promote disease (Cohen and Wills, 1985; Kasl, 1983). All too often we are presented with data where depression follows an event by four years (Pearlin, Lieberman, Menaghan, and Mullan, 1981), or death and hospitalization fail to follow events a year earlier (Goldberg and Comstock, 1976), with no justification as to the plausibility of finding each disorder in the specified time frame. Second, there is often no effort to distinguish disease outcomes from illness outcomes in analysing the effects of stressors (Kasl, 1983; Mechanic, 1974). 'Disease outcomes' are the impact of stressors and the stress process on biological processes, and are defined in biomedical terms by disease diagnoses. 'Illness outcomes' refer to the total impact of a disease on the activities of an individual in his or her social network.

In elaborating our thesis, we will start with a brief review of selected experimental studies investigating the stress–illness link in laboratory animals. This will allow us to highlight the key factors in theory and method essential for a clear understanding of the stress–illness process. We then contrast the work on animals with stress–illness research on humans, starting with a critical methodological issue, the absence of randomization. The discussion then turns to the central topic of the failure to use sufficiently complex theory to study the mechanisms involved in the stress–illness dynamic. In doing so, we examine various problems and deficiencies subsumed under this issue, such as the non-independence of the operational measures of stressor, stress process and illness, the absence of adequate time frames for plausible causal inferences, etc. We also offer a series of methodological and theoretical elaborations that we believe can help to resolve the above problems and advance stress research.

THE STRESS–ILLNESS LINK: ANIMAL MODELS

The experimental paradigm

As an example of the contributions that can be made by animal models of the stress–illness link, consider studies on the effects of controllability and predictability of a stressor on ulceration in rats (See, e.g. Weiss, 1972). Typically, these investigations have assessed the effects of shock on three groups of animals housed in parallel cages: a group that can 'control' the shock by turning a wheel; a second 'yoked' group that receives the same amount and duration of shock as the control group but that cannot alter its duration or occurrence; and a third 'comparison' group that is not shocked. The 0.2 second duration shocks are delivered every 200 seconds for a defined period of time (e.g. 2 or 24 hours). The results of studies using this paradigm generally show that the animals who can terminate the shock by turning a wheel develop relatively little stomach ulceration while the yoked animals who are unable to respond and control the shock develop extensive ulceration from the identical noxious stimulation. The unshocked animals are also relatively free of ulceration.

A number of variations can be performed on this basic paradigm. For example, shock can be preceded by a single clear warning signal and a signal can follow the response terminating the shock. Both these signals further reduce the rate of ulceration in the animal 'in control' such that the level of ulceration is then below that in the unshocked controls (Weiss, 1971). On the other hand, when the animal who can control the onset of shock is warned with a long series of loud beeps that extends the pre-shock warning time and introduces what may be a noxious signal, an increase in the amount of stomach ulceration is observed (Weiss, 1971). Additionally, if the animal 'in control' is given a very mild shock after making the avoidance response, the level of stomach ulceration for this animal is far in excess of that for its yoked companion (Weiss, 1972). Thus, threatening or conflicting information may not only eliminate the benefits of being 'in control'—it may even make things worse.

Finally, Weiss and his collaborators have examined the potential biological mediators of these effects. Specifically, they have assessed the level of brain norepinephrine in whole brain homoge) and found substantial reductions in those animals that develop the most severe ulceration. They have also directly reduced the level of this neurotransmitter using monoamine oxidase inhibitors and found the same behavioural consequences as those observed under their high 'stress' conditions (Weiss, Glazer, Pohorecky, Bailey, and Schneider, 1979). These converging operations (Garner, Hake and Eriksen, 1951) are persuasive evidence for a biological stress process that is heavily influenced by behavioural outcomes.

Advantages of the experimental paradigm

There are five major reasons why these studies provide a convincing demonstration that stress associated with varying degrees of controllability, predictability, and conflict can cause ulceration of the stomach. First, the experimenter controls *the stressor*: he or she delivers the stressful stimulus (shock). Second, the experimenter can introduce and vary other experimental conditions that *moderate* the stress–illness link. Thus, he or she determines whether wheel turning does or does not terminate and avoid shock, or whether a pre- and/or post-response signal affects ulceration. These manipulations of moderating factors demonstrate that the *clarity of safety information* (objective details versus noxious warnings and/or information conflict) and *behavioural control* are important determinants of stress and illness.

Third, the animal investigator can *randomly assign* subjects to stress and non-stress conditions. This allows a comparison of animal groups with the knowledge that neither prior disease nor any other individual difference factor is sufficient to generate the relationship found between stressor and disease. Fourth, the animal investigator *obtains critical data at the biological level*. This includes a direct measure of disease (millimetres of stomach ulceration) and measures of the physiological changes making up the biological sequence that is disease inducing. Thus, the investigator can detect a variety of biological reactions immediately contingent upon the animal's behaviour and trace the steps from them to subsequent changes directly involved in ulceration or disease generation. Finally, both the independent, mediating, and dependent variables are collected within a *defined and finite time frame* leaving no doubt that the physiological processes induced by the noxious stimulus overlap the chain of mediating events that led to the indicators of disease.

Unanswered questions

The animal data provide convincing evidence for the role of stress in the generation of stomach ulceration in laboratory rats. Other similar data make clear that stress, in combination with various biological factors, can produce other diseases such as elevated blood pressure (Anderson, 1985) and cancer (Riley, Fitzmaurice, and Spackman, 1981; Sklar and Anisman, 1981). Data of this sort provide convincing evidence that stress can be a causal factor in the generation of disease. Moreover, the simplicity and visibility of the experimental operations help us to fully understand the meaning of the variables and allow us to take a major step toward identifying the mediators of the stress response. Finally, the studies provide an initial view of the connections between psychological and biological processes.

However, the animal data create a number of problems for a theory of stress and illness. The very same conditions that prevent illness in certain physiological systems may induce illness in others. For example, the persistent exercise of behavioural control, which, as noted above, can prevent stress-induced illness in monkeys, can also produce prolonged blood pressure elevation in dogs ingesting large quantities of sodium (Anderson, 1985). These differing results appear attributable to the fact that lack of control selectively activates the pituitary-adrenocortical axis, while effortful control produces elevations in sympathetic nervous system activity (Schneiderman and McCabe, 1985; Steptoe, 1980).

Second, there are instances in which it is simply unclear why variations in the stimulus domain cause variations in physiological responses. For example, while relatively short-term electric shock (e.g. a single session on one day) can enhance tumour growth, long-lasting repeated shock (e.g. ten days) does not (Sklar and Anisman, 1981). Effects are also complex over long time spans. For example, stress during an animal's infancy assures a normal stress response later in life; animals lacking early stress experiences show later deficits (Levine, 1971). Third, many stress effects hold within some species but not others. For example, severe emotional disturbance and corticosteroid output produced by separation from the mother is far more intense in the squirrel monkey than the rhesus monkey (Coe, Rosenberg, and Levine, in press). Similarly the increase in cancer mortality following stress is only pronounced for cancer-susceptible strains of rats (Riley, 1982). Species differences may have their analogues in individual differences within the human species, both of which hinder understanding of the stress–illness link in humans. At any rate, the cause of both types of effect need to be better understood.

Fourth, knowledge of precise causal sequences at the biological level is limited; we do not know all of the links in the chain connecting the initial, intermediate, and ultimate physiological reactions that induce or promote disease. Fifth, it is not always clear whether stress initiates or promotes the development of existent disease.

Despite the above problems, the animal work is cumulative. It provides clear evidence of a stress–illness relationship, and a good deal of data pointing to behavioural and biological components of the stress process and to the relationships between the two. As such, it provides an interesting touchstone against which to compare research with humans.

STRESS–ILLNESS: RESEARCH WITH HUMANS

It has proven more difficult to demonstrate unequivocally that stress is a cause of disease for the human animal and it has been far more difficult to spell out the mechanism or sequence of events by which stressors generate disease. Indeed, despite a sizable and rapidly growing literature, as Kasl (1983) has suggested, research on stress and illness in humans has failed to provide the cumulative insights into the stress process that one would expect from a scientific endeavour. Thus, recent research generally fails to provide greater understanding of, or evidence for, the stress–illness process than earlier investigations. For example, approximately twenty years ago, epidemiological data of a quasi-experimental form suggested that social structure and life stress are interactive determinants of cardiovascular disease (Stout, et al., 1964). These studies compared two Italian immigrant communities in Western Pennsylvania, one of which adopted contemporary American values and organization and the other of which retained traditional social structure and support networks. Though the residents emigrated from the same area of Italy, the coronary disease rates in the contemporary community were significantly greater than those in the traditional.

A second example is a study published eighteen years ago by Kasl, Cobb, and Brooks (1968). It compared physiological reactions (cholesterol and uric acid levels) of workers in three factories who expected and then experienced job loss to the reactions of workers in two similar plants that were not closed. The men who lost their jobs were likely to have elevated cholesterol levels (although cholesterol was not elevated in anticipation of job loss) and elevated uric acid levels. These elevations returned to baseline once the men found new employment. In addition to comparing levels of two physiological indicators in a quasi-experimental design, Kasl, Cobb and Brooks (1968) used path analysis to evaluate the impact of loss of self-esteem and time out of work on these disease-like endpoints. They found anxiety and low self-esteem to be associated with higher levels of cholesterol. While equally persuasive evidence of the stress–illness link and its moderators can be found in specific contemporary investigations (see Brown and Harris, 1978; Cohen and Wills, 1985), the increased yield of even the best studies appears relatively modest. We will now turn to several of the major methodological and procedural issues that may help explain this state of affairs.

Shortcomings in human stress–illness research

A comparison of the animal and human research can help us to identify two fundamental shortcomings in the latter: (a) the absence of random assignment to conditions; and (b) the inability to elucidate the components of the stress process and its moderators due to the absence of a comprehensive theory prior to the initiation of data collection. Two points can be subsumed under this second weakness. The first is a failure to appreciate both the complex nature of causality for human disorders and the complexity of the stress processes that interact with disease processes. The second is a failure to take into account the heterogeneity of the population exposed to the stressor and the effects of heterogeneity on the stress process.

Three additional shortcomings in human stress–illness research are noteworthy, all closely related to the two major issues raised above. They are the non-independence of the operations used to assess stressor, stress response, and disease, the inability to control or assess multiple levels of response (e.g. social, psychological, and biological), and the lack of a time frame for plausible inference. We will discuss each of these factors in turn.

Absence of random assignment

Because methods grow out of theory (Conant, 1947; Kuhn, 1962), it might seem appropriate first to discuss the need for a comprehensive theory and then to turn to a discussion of randomization. The absence of random assignment, however, has such a major impact on human studies of stress–illness research that it should be treated first to set the stage for the discussion of theory.

Confounds

When individuals are not randomly assigned to stressor and non-stressor conditions, it is always possible that some third factor correlated both with the stressor and the disease outcome is responsible for the association of stressor to illness. Many types of confounds exist. One of the most serious occurs when the disease antedates and is responsible for the stressor (Kasl, 1983). For example, early, subclinical levels of depression may interfere with interpersonal relationships and performance at work and lead to disruptions in relationships and/or job loss, events that are universally regarded as stressors (Dohrenwend and Dohrenwend 1974; Kasl, 1983; Mechanic, 1974; Thoits, 1983).

This problem is more subtle and serious when the dependent variable is a physical illness that may remain at subclinical levels for many years (Fox, 1978; Lilienfeld and Lilienfeld, 1980; Sklar and Anisman, 1981; Thomas, Duszynski, and Shatfen, 1979). For example, a low level cardiovascular condition may produce mini-haemorrhages that could lead to forgetfulness and irritability and result in job loss before the disease is diagnosed. Lipowski (1975) lists eight ways in which physical illness may cause psychological changes and distress. These include induced cerebral pathology altering the subjective experience of illness and impairing the capacity to cope with needs and role demands, altered sensory inputs, and disturbed sleep patterns. All these effects may occur prior to the clinical manifestation of the underlying disease. When the disease is finally clinically manifest, it may be attributed incorrectly to psychological states that are themselves incorrectly attributed to antecedents such as job loss or marital disruption. In reality, however, these latter changes may be triggered by interactions between disease-induced changes and other social variables.

A second type of confound could involve some individual difference of a psychological or biological nature, (e.g. neuroticism) that accounts for high scores on both the measures of stress and the measures of disease (Brown, 1974; Depue and Monroe, 1986). Socialization may also serve as a third factor generating personal styles that lead to high scores on measures of stressors and disease (Thomas, Duszynski, and Shatfen, 1979). Finally, socio-demographic variables that determine life-styles (e.g. social class (Syme and Berkman, 1976), institutional position and work roles (House, 1974), or life patterns (Kasl, 1983)) could generate high scores on measures of both stressors (life events) and illness. Confounds of this sort may lead to inaccurate identification of the stressor.

Detecting interactions with moderator variables

The animal research not only permitted randomization of individuals to stressor conditions, it also permitted random assignment of subjects to variables crossed with the original stressor (e.g. signalled versus unsignalled shock) and random assignment of subject characteristics (species of cancer-susceptible versus non-cancer-susceptible rats) to both types of conditions. Analogous variables in the human literature, such as variables deemed to create vulnerability to life events or to buffer their impact, are handled with difficulty. Once again, the prime problem introduced by the absence of randomization is the inability to insure independence between stressors, moderators, and illness or to clarify the nature of complex causal relationships. For example, social support, or intimacy, can serve as a buffer to depression in women exposed to a major loss, but the loss itself may reduce social support (Brown and Harris, 1978). Substantial detail, hence lengthy interviewing, is needed to obtain independent estimates of events and support. Findings are less clear where such effort is not expended (see Cohen and Wills, 1985).

The longitudinal design and causation

Investigators of the stress–illness relationship often suggest that longitudinal designs are essential to clarify causal sequences (Hudgens, 1974; Kasl, 1983). While such designs are invaluable in ruling out many of the problems inherent in retrospective case-control designs, their value in unconfounding variables and revealing causal networks is dependent upon a host of other considerations. These include accurate timing of measures relative to causal processes, and the use of well-defined independent measures of stressors, stress processes, and disease. We will discuss these factors in greater detail below. At this point, we wish to emphasize that a longitudinal design may do little to improve one's knowledge of causation and under some circumstances, (e.g. inaccurate timing of measures) may provide *less* accurate data on causal connections than frequently denigrated cross-sectional data (Kessler and Greenberg, 1981; Pelz and Lew, 1970). Thus, the implicit assertion that a longitudinal design gives insight into causation can at best be regarded as a partial truth.

The contribution of biological third factors of genetic or environmental origin to the stress–illness link is one type of confound that cannot easily be isolated in a longitudinal design (Kasl, 1983). These factors may express themselves in both behaviour and disease later in life so as to create the appearance of a connection between stress and illness. Thus, an individual whose autonomic or endocrine system is constitutionally hyperactive (due to genetics, intrauterine exposures, etc.) may be more susceptible to chronic cardiovascular disease or cancer, and may also be more emotionally reactive to social stimuli and generate a higher frequency of life events. The more reactive person may also be more likely to focus on bodily symptoms and seek medical care when under stress (Mechanic and Volkart, 1961). For such individuals, therefore, stressors may induce emotional upset and concern that stimulate health and/or illness behaviours that lead in turn to early discovery of illness. By comparison, their age-matched 'controls' may only detect disease at a later, clinically observable stage (Mechanic, 1974). Both cases would generate the appearance of a link between life events and disease, and there is ample opportunity for the development of such contingencies given the time frame for slowly developing chronic diseases.

A longitudinal design can resolve problems such as those described above when data is available describing the natural history of the specific disease in question and biomedical theory allows us to estimate the time course of the disease, the behavioural stress process (its onset and duration), and the overlap of their temporal windows. To eliminate from the sample those who are ill at the initial time of measurement, it is also necessary that disease be detectable in its pre-clinical stages. If these stringent conditions are met, we can rule out third factors and generate an unbiased estimate of association between stressor and disease (Kessler, 1983).

Before turning to the second major difficulty in stress research with humans, we should emphasize that while the absence of randomization is an important problem, it is in many respects an unavoidable one. Even investigators using long-term prospective designs are unable to insure the initial equivalence of subsequent cases and controls. One potential solution to this difficulty is the development and evaluation of intervention programmes designed to prevent or buffer the effects of stress. In these cases, random assignment to treatment and control conditions may be feasible. However, even here, the implications of findings for an understanding of the stress–illness link may be unclear. In particular the factors or dimensions responsible for the *prevention* of disease may often not be those responsible for its *causation*.

Need for comprehensive theories and methods

In our judgement, stress–illness research can be successful only when investigators make a serious effort to develop a comprehensive, 'causal' model prior to the onset of research. There is general recognition of the need for a model to generate measuring instruments and guide data analysis (e.g. Leventhal and Nerenz, 1983; Pearlin and Schooler, 1978; Pearlin, Lieberman, Menaghan, and Mullen, 1981). What has been less clearly recognized is that it is equally, if not more, important for such a model to specify the complexity of the disease and the stress processes and their interaction, and to specify the vulnerabilities or markers for differentiating sub-populations and individuals. Such models will play a central role in insuring the independent assessment of components of the stress process and disease. They will also include postulates and hypotheses based on the relationships between constructs at the social, psychological and biological levels and specify the time frame for the development and overlap of processes at each level. We shall discuss each of these issues as briefly and specifically as possible.

Correlations versus dependent probability

The absence of a comprehensive theory of the stress process may lead investigators to grossly underestimate the probability of illness given the presence of the stress process. For example, Rabkin and Struening (1976) state that the typical correlation between stressors and disease outcomes is 'embarrassingly' low (they are usually under 0.30). The magnitude of the zero order association between events and disease does not, however, describe the magnitude of the association between the stress process and disease. The correct estimate of the magnitude of association is a statement of the probability of disease given the presence of *all* of the factors theoretically necessary for the stress process to lead to disease. At best, the first or zero order association defines the *presence* of the phenomenon; it tells investigators there is a greater likelihood they will be able to identify and describe the stress–illness process where a zero order relationship exists than where it does not.

This issue is recognized to some degree. Investigators are attempting to assess multiple factors such as the appraisal of the stressor as a threat to self (Pearlin, Lieberman, Menaghan, and Mullan, 1981; Menaghan, 1982), the maintenance or duration of the appraisal, long versus short duration events (Brown and Harris, 1978), continuing hassles versus events (Kanner, Coyne, Schaefer, and Lazarus, 1981) and the presence or absence of mediating factors such as coping resources (Menaghan, 1982; Quayhagen and Quayhagen, 1982) and social supports (Brown and Harris, 1978; Cobb, 1976; Cohen and Hoberman, 1983; Lin, Dean, and Ensel, 1981; Ward, 1985). Investigators now specify and measure these factors and enter them as interaction terms to evaluate the role of moderators in creating vulnerabilities or buffers to life events. They have yet to break with the practice of looking at these interactions as components of the 'overall' or zero order relationship between event and disease. Only when we look at and compare the probability of disease for specific, theoretically structured sequences of factors, will statements of contingencies accurately state the magnitude of relationship between the stress *process* and disease outcome.

We can illustrate our point by drawing upon Pearlin and his associates' sophisticated path analytic models developed to identify the steps by which stressors lead to disease. These authors typically present their data as a process of decomposition, locating the paths that account for relatively meagre zero order relationships between stressor and illness (e.g. Pearlin and Schooler, 1978; Pearlin, Lieberman, Menaghan, and Mullan, 1981). By doing so they inadvertently imply that the stress process can account for no more than 9–15 per cent of the variance in measures of psychological or physical illness. The magnitude of the stressor—disease relationship is *not*, however, the same as the magnitude of the relationship between the stress–emotion process and disease. This latter association requires the participation of the intermediate steps of economic loss, strain experienced from the loss, and loss of self-esteem, and leads to a specific outcome (verbal report of depressive symptoms) for a particular sub-group of the sample. Pearlin et al. (1981) also fail to specify the characteristics of the sub-population that will manifest the stress process. For example, at least a portion of their depressed respondents may be bi-polar depressives or chronic depressives. Life events for these respondents may serve to maintain, intensify, or slow recovery from existent depression (Depue and Monroe, 1986; Gopelrud and Depue, 1985). Thus, the 'true' relationship between the stress process and depression is the probability of depression in the specific subsample responsive to the particular sequence of events defining the stress process.

Stressors, stress, and illness

We have argued that exploration of the stress process and its mechanisms requires a theory that is sufficiently specific and complex to deal with the variety of factors involved in disease, and the social, psychological and biological processes involved in the stress responses of specific subpopulations.

Moreover, this theory must suggest ways of generating independent operations of its variables. Our points have been made at a fairly abstract level and to appreciate their full meaning it is necessary to bring them into contact with central issues in the stress–illness literature. One such issue has been the ongoing effort to define the stressor as distinct from the stress response and illness. It is impossible to test 'causal' hypotheses about the relationship between events and disease outcomes if one cannot generate independent assessments of the stimulus, the process, and disease; such tests are the focus, the *raison d'etre*, of stress–illness research (Kasl, 1983).

Conceptualizing the stressor and the stress process

In our judgement, the issue of independent assessment is insoluble unless approached from a theoretical perspective, that is, from the point of view of a comprehensive, bio-social-psychological theory. While we cannot here provide a systematic presentation of such a theory, the points we will make draw heavily upon such a perspective.

First, one's theoretical perspective determines how and what assessments are made. Both the animal and human data agree on one singularly important fact: exposure to the stressor, whether it be an electrical shock, the loss of a job, or death of a spouse is *not* sufficient to predict disease outcome. Individuals differ in their response to the 'same' stressor. Indeed, the initiation of the stress process by a stimulus depends upon whether the stimulus is, for example, predictable rather than unpredictable, controllable rather than uncontrollable, non-conflictful rather than conflictful. Because a variety of *environmental* variations determine whether the shock stimulus will be linked to the stress process, it is clear that the generation and maintenance of the stress process is a constructive activity of the organism (Neisser, 1967). Specifically, the stressor is *not* simply the stimulus: the response to the stimulus is the key to the generation of the stress process. Thus, *stress* is a product of the representation of the stimulus (how it is perceived and thought about), the responses taken to cope with it (responses to change the situation or to deny or alter its interpretation), and the appraisal of outcomes (successful or unsuccessful). This final appraisal of outcome may be due to temporary or permanent and narrow or global characteristics of one's resources (self and others) and one's environment (Abramson, Seligman, and Teasdale, 1978; Lazarus and Folkman, 1984; Leventhal, 1970; Leventhal and Nerenz, 1983).

Second, efforts to conceptualize the stressor and the variables in the stress process must be designed to develop measures that will be causally linked to one another. In short, we want to measure those aspects of the stressor stimulus that initiate and/or affect the stress process. Stimulus and situational events, habits, images, and thoughts that neither initiate nor change the process are irrelevant to our task.

Third, as stated above, the assessment must not be confounded: we must not use the very same instrument to measure different variables. If our measures share items, their relationships will be confounded. This creates special problems for measures of subjective appraisals of the stimulus. Such measures appear to be the best way of insuring assessments that link to the stress process, but they are also suspect since they are believed to confound outcomes with presumed causes. It is also clear that insufficient attention has been given to the nature of the confounding process. After a brief review of current methods of measurement of stressors, we will explore the various components of the confounding process and discuss the evidence (the little there is) that supports the validity of some of these presumed confounds.

Existent definitions of the stressor

The bulk of empirical work has defined stressors from three distinct frameworks: (a) as *discrete events*, or life change units; (b) as *ongoing role strains*; and (c) as *daily hassles*. Each of these frameworks has been offered as a means of assessing aspects of the environment that initiate or promote the stress process, and each has attempted to provide independent, objective, assessment of variables.

Holmes and Rahe (1967) defined stressors as discrete life change events requiring adaptive effort. Their approach was modelled on psychophysical studies investigating the relationship of stimulus intensity to perception. Thus, groups of judges gave a quantitative score describing the *amount* of behavioural change or effort that would be required to adjust to each event on their Schedule of Recent Events (Holmes and Masuda, 1974; Rahe, 1972). The event was treated as though it were a discrete universal stimulus not embedded in a broader life style. It was assumed that most individuals, in most cultures, would judge events similarly (Holmes and Masuda, 1974), which holds true for the *mean* ratings of the listed events (Fairbank and Hough, 1981).

The role strain approach measures the amount of emotional stress in an individual's life by assessing the strains experienced in ongoing roles. Pearlin (1983) lists six types of strain including task strains such as work overload, both interpersonal and intrapersonal role-induced conflict, role captivity, loss and gain of roles, and role restructuring. The emotional distress induced by a specific event is presumed to be a consequence of the impact of the event upon '... the more structured aspects of social roles.' The idea of role strains emphasizes the importance of interpersonal and self-image factors in the experience of stress and the importance of roles in the maintenance of stress over long periods.

Finally, the third approach, daily hassles, ties the stress process to the myriad of minor nagging and conflictful events that make up our everyday lives (Lazarus and Folkman, 1984; DeLongis et al., 1982). As with role strains, hassles are believed to be the critical stressors intervening between life events and emotional stress, although hassles are thought to produce stress independently.

As we shall note below, these three methods do not exhaust the approaches to stressor assessment: the contextual approach (Brown and Harris, 1978) represents an important fourth approach. Kasl (1983) has also urged consideration of life style assessment, which examines the ongoing texture of daily life in which events are embedded. This approach necessitates the difficult distinction between the contributions of embedded events and daily patterns to the stress process (see discussion in Brown and Harris, 1978). These variations are important and will be commented upon as we deal with the problem of confounds.

Types of confounds

We wish to distinguish two types of confound that beset the stress–illness literature: confounds of content and confounds of process. Confounds of content are widely recognized and have been discussed frequently (see for example the recent interplay between Lazarus, DeLongis, Folkman, and Gruen, 1985, and Dohrenwend and Shrout, 1985). They involve commonality of items between the measures used to assess independent and dependent variables. Confounds of process also involve contamination between the instruments designed to assess independent and dependent variables. In this instance, however, the confounding arises not because of shared content, but because the responses to each item set are biased by the respondent's current psychological or physical state. Since this state is itself a primary dependent variable, the result is a spurious overestimation of the actual relationship between variables.

Confounds of content

Discussions of the confounds between measures of events, mediating processes, and outcomes have focused most commonly on the confound that arises when the measure of events (hassles) have items in common with the measure of illness (psychiatric or physical symptom check lists). Recently, Schroeder and Costa (1984) have identified four types of items that appear in instruments used to assess events (stressors): (a) uncontaminated event reports; (b) subjective event reports; (c) neuroticism-related event reports; and (d) health-related event reports. Each type of item will be correlated with symptom reports for different reasons. First, there may be a 'causal' link between events and symptoms. Second, symptom items on the event report may reflect the same illness assessed by the illness report. Third, the event scale may be related to the illness criteria due to common items that measure neurotic personality dispositions, psychological distress, or response sets.

There is no reason to doubt that factors such as those discussed by Schroeder and Costa may indeed generate a spurious association between an event and a symptom measure and lead to the false conclusion that events cause illness.

While confounds of content apply to all three types of measures (events, strains and hassles) they seem most serious in methods that attempt to describe the many less serious but cumulative factors that make up daily hassles (Dohrenwend, Dohrenwend, Dodson, and Shrout, 1984). One recommended solution to such confounds is the exclusion of shared items (e.g. Schroeder and Costa, 1984). We will discuss the merits of this solution below.

Confounds of process

Confounds of process occur when the experience of illness (its symptomatic and emotional properties) leads to inflated reports of prior events or of mediators between events and illness (Brown, 1974, 1979; Hudgens, 1974; Mechanic, 1974). While this type of bias is most commonly thought to occur in studies using retrospective designs, it is important to note that event reports are *always* retrospective in nature. Thus, prospective studies may also fall prey to process confounds.

At least two distinct components may underlie retrospective bias. These are: (a) bias in the *identification* or retrieval of events; and (b) bias in the *evaluation* of events. Identification bias reflects the tendency to over- or under-report the actual *occurrence* of events. Evaluation bias denotes illness-induced alterations in the *appraisals* or *representations* of events or mediators (e.g. social support, coping behaviours).

It has been argued that the use of subjective evaluations increases the probability of evaluation bias. Such subjective evaluations may be *stimulus*-oriented, focusing on the respondent's perceptions of events, or *response*-oriented, focusing on the respondent's perception of the amount of distress, upset, or similar responses to events. It is generally assumed that response-oriented biases involving emotional appraisals are particularly likely to inflate estimates of the relationship between stress and illness. Indeed, the greater success in predicting illness from negative relative to positive events and from emotionally distressing hassles as compared to neutral hassles is often assumed to be due to failure to separate the measurement of the stressor from the measurement of disease outcome.

Because of the potentially deleterious consequences of response-oriented subjective evaluations in particular, some investigators have relied on more objective assessments of stimulus properties. For example, Cronkite and Moos (1984) obtained reports of depression, symptoms, and alcohol use from both members of 242 couples, treating each of the three behavioural indicators for each spouse as potential sources of stress for the other. While potentially an important advance in assessment, data obtained by observers is still subject to bias. For example, concordance between an observer spouse and a respondent may reflect a commonality of beliefs about the cause of disease that colours the way both parties view events. The observer's report of an event may also reflect shared moods induced by talking about the event or conditioned by vicarious emotional responses to it.

Another approach designed to measure the *objective* representation of a stressor is the contextual approach used by Brown and Harris (1978). These investigators code the uniqueness or meaning of the stressor to the respondent by use of a time-consuming (average six-hour interview) and data intensive procedure. The objective is to obtain enough information about both the event and the objective factors in the respondent's life situation to estimate the impact of that event on that person at that point in time. Their raters are blind both to the respondent's subjective appraisal of the event and to the respondent's classification as depressed or non-depressed. They are, however, extensively informed about the respondent's life situation. This information is used to assess the significance or *magnitude* and expected *duration* of each event. These two factors were deemed most important as initiators of depressive episodes. While Brown and Harris present abundant evidence to rule out alternative hypotheses respecting reporting and forgetting of events, their procedure is time-intensive and obviously very costly.

Current solutions to the problem of confounded measures

Before presenting our own ideas as to how we can best deal with the measurement problems described above, it will pay to examine their plausibility and to look at the possibly more serious problems inherent in some of the solutions suggested in the literature. We will first deal with content confounds and then turn to those of process.

Confounds of content

Schroeder and Costa (1984) and Dohrenwend and Shrout (1985) suggest that we can avoid content confounds by removing shared items from our measures of stressors and illness. Their analysis does, however, point to a serious problem with such a solution: potentially confounding health-related events can be *both consequences and causes* of stress. Thus, an individual's physical illness or depression can be a stressor inducing subsequent psychological and/or physical disturbance. Similarly, reactions such as subjective emotional distress in response to an event can be both a mediator of illness and a stressor (e.g. if the individual conceives of the emotional response as a sign of personal weakness). Indeed, available data suggest such effects play an important role in stress–illness data. For example, Cronkite and Moos (1984) found that depression, physical symptoms, and use of alcohol in index cases were a source of stress for spouses (See also Aneshensel, Frerichs, and Huba, 1984)

As an alternative to the omission of potentially confounding events, Lazarus and his associates suggest that we must accept confounding as a 'theoretically' necessary fact of life (Lazarus, et al., 1985). In our opinion, both sets of 'solutions' should be rejected. It makes no sense to throw away knowledge of health-related stressors (physical and/or mental) and attend only to uncontaminated event reports, and it makes no sense to defend as a causal relationship an association where the predictor and criterion measure reflect the very same factor. What needs to be recognized is that the validity of criticisms of content bias depends as much upon the quality of the measurement of the criterion, the *disease*, as of the measurement of the predictor, the *stressor*. Thus, the problem is most severe in studies using *generic* rather than specific measures of disease. With a generic measure (symptom check-list), one cannot readily distinguish the disease as stressor from the disease as outcome, even in cases where the two diseases differ. This distinction is possible where diagnoses are specific and duration of a disease episode can be determined.

Confounds of process

As noted above, some have argued that the physical and mental status of the respondent may affect both stimulus-oriented evaluations of events and response-oriented evaluations of the emotional distress or upset caused by events. However, studies of the impact of emotional states upon memory suggest that emotional states may impact on the process of recognizing and reporting events, rather than on the appraisal of events (either stimulus-oriented or emotional). Thus, while distress, depression, etc., may increase the likelihood of recall of negative events, these emotions do not appear to affect the evaluation of any given event along a positive–negative dimension (e.g. Teasdale and Fogerty, 1979). Moreover, many studies have failed to find that negative affective states consistently bias recall (for a review, see Leventhal and Tomarken, 1986). Mood-induced bias seems most likely to occur when the emotional state is exceptionally intense and few stimuli are present to cue recall (Bower and Cohen, 1982). Intense emotional outcomes, however, such as depression, appear to depend upon major, not minor, events (Brown and Harris, 1978) and major events are likely to have environmental cues. Bias seems most likely, therefore, for the recall of minor rather than major negative events; Funch and Marshall's (1984) data support this hypothesis. There is an unfortunate dearth of evidence on the degree to which specific, physical conditions bias recall, although experimental techniques could be used to address this question (e.g. Baumann and Leventhal, 1985).

Concerning response-oriented evaluations, extant results suggest less bias than one might have expected in respondents' subjective appraisals of the emotional impact of events. Self-reports of distress by the women in Brown and Harris's (1978) study were highly related to the severity of events as rated by coders; there was agreement with coders for 85 per cent of the events reported by control respondents and 85 per cent of the events reported by the depressives.

As the preceding summary suggests, stimulus- and response-oriented bias induced by negative emotions may not be as potent a factor in life event reports as some have suggested. Indeed, it may be that those biased reports that do occur reflect the under-reporting of negative events by control cases!! Positive states of mind consistently function as potent retrieval cues enhancing memory for positive events (Isen, 1984; Leventhal and Tomarken, 1986).

New directions for dealing with confounds

A well specified theory will offer a variety of solutions to the seemingly intractable problem of confounded measures. A fully specified theory attempts to model the constructive processes that intervene between stressor and disease and to take into account the social, psychological, and biological aspects of the stress process when doing so. As such, it will define mediating mechanisms that can be assessed to test process-based hypotheses, suggest linkages of variables across levels (social to psychological and both to physiological), and specify the temporal windows in which such linkages occur. *The key is to conceptualize and measure those psychological and biological aspects of the stress process that impact on disease processes. Almost certainly this will require distinct conceptual models for different disease outcomes.*

The constructive nature of the stress process makes clear that there will seldom if ever be any simple, direct or univariate link from situational stimuli to physiological processes. The physiological stress responses provoked by job loss are dependent upon the representation and coping responses evoked by the loss (Pearlin, Lieberman, Menaghan, and Mullan, 1981).

One way of dealing with situational variability is to study a single situation, a procedure recommended by Kasl (1983). Thus, if job loss or death of a spouse is reliably associated with disease outcomes, we can study this situation and search for the factors mediating the stress process. By concentrating on a single setting, we can discover the full range of interpretations and coping strategies that occur within its context and develop effective measuring tools for each. We can also develop more detailed knowledge of the types of disease occurring subsequent to stressor onset and focus upon those stress process-disease connections that fit a 'causal' time frame for specific situation-disease combinations. This would require more effective means of disease diagnosis. The animal literature can offer a guide. For example, where situations are interpreted as threatening and susceptible to control by active coping, sympathetic-adrenomedullary reactions may be salient. These may ultimately contribute to cardiovascular disease, especially in individuals of known biological risk. On the other hand, if the situation evokes a sense of hopelessness, pituitary-adrenocortical reactions may dominate and generate diseases in individuals at risk for diseases involving that system (Schneiderman and McCabe, 1985; Steptoe, 1980).

In the present context, the important point is that a research strategy focusing on linkages between specific contexts and disorders would have two beneficial consequences. First, this approach would most likely result in better predictions and greater understanding of the stress–illness process. Second, this strategy would be markedly less susceptible to the interpretive problems created by the process biases noted above. Highly specific linkages between stressors and disease are more likely to emerge as clear 'signals' standing out from the generic 'noise' created by retrospective bias. This is because subjects' common-sense view of the stress process is unlikely to be sufficiently precise to generate biases of a highly focused type.

Bio-psychosocial solutions to the analysis of cause

The power of causal inference can be enhanced by assessing constructs at more than one level: this allows us to connect psychological data to that obtained at the social structural and biological levels (Leventhal, 1983; Schwartz, 1979). Connections between psychological, sociological, and biological constructs will enhance the explanatory power of a model by further increasing the specificity of the connections between environment, psychological mediators, and disease. First, the approach can provide critical clues as to antecedence. For example, if changes occur in reports of subjective strain or loss of control, these psychological variables can possibly be related to a social factor that has a definable onset and duration. If so, this linkage greatly strengthens the hypothesis that the psychological factor reflects an environmentally produced stress process rather than a third factor such as a personality or temperamental trait of the individual.

Psychophysiological data connecting psychological constructs to physiological measures can further strengthen causal analysis. For example, doubt that an event has initiated an illness-producing stress process is substantially reduced if the investigator can show that event onset is reliably followed by psychological change accompanied by specific physiological changes capable of inducing or exacerbating a particular disease process. The likelihood of success with such a psychophysiological strategy is greater if it is guided by detailed knowledge of the physiological aspects of both stress and disease and of the stress–disease interaction. In the absence of the latter, one may locate events that produce physiological change, yet be unconvinced these changes have implications for disease. For example, competitive interactions (Carver and Humphries, 1982) stimulate high levels of catecholamine activity in Type A individuals (Glass et al., 1983), yet it is unclear that competitive events are the source of the physiological changes that lead to coronary disease! Unfortunately, there is insufficient evidence that these changes are sufficiently durable to impact the physiological processes that produce coronary artery disease. (For a possible exception see Krantz and Durel, 1983.) This data is important because so few Type A persons succumb to coronary disease and a number of persons with the disease are Type B: the linkage lacks a high degree of specificity. If both the psychophysiological changes and disease were nearly entirely confined to an identifiable sub-group we could have greater confidence in the causal link of the stress process to disease.

The attitude theory of psychosomatic illness provides an early example of efforts to link psychological events to disease and to do so with a high degree of specificity (Graham, 1972). Specific attitudes were assumed to produce specific changes in physiological patterns that mimicked the physiology of several known illnesses. Attitudes involved two components: (a) a subjective emotion in response to rather vaguely defined events, and (b) a response orientation to the emotional event. Using a double blind procedure for collecting and rating thematic productions, it was found that patients suffering from each of eighteen different diseases were more likely to express the attitude appropriate to their disease than were other patients (Grace and Graham, 1952). For example, a subjective feeling, 'threatened with harm' and a response orientation 'ready for anything', make up the attitude for essential hypertension.

These attitudes were believed to be durable response dispositions that produced the physiological changes appropriate to each disease over long periods of time. In later experimental studies, attitudes were induced hypnotically in normal subjects to see if they produced short-term physiological changes appropriate to the specific disease. Positive results (i.e. appropriate physiological changes) were reported for hypertension (Graham, Kabler, and Graham, 1962), hives, and Raynauds' disease (Graham, Stern, and Winokur, 1958). While there is a substantial jump from short-term to lasting physiological responses, the combination of descriptive and experimental studies established a network of highly specific data points that, if replicated, would greatly enhance the plausibility of the analysis.

Need for a time factor in the model

Accuracy in temporal measurement is one of the most important factors in inferring causation. We have already emphasized the need to establish that stressors antedate disease. Stressors that appear after the onset of disease may appear to be determinants of disease because they provoke the seeking of medical care (Gortmaker, Eckenrode, and Gore, 1982; Roughman and Haggerty, 1973; Mechanic, 1972), intensify symptomatology (Leventhal, in press; Pennebaker, 1982), and/or speed or otherwise promote the rate of development of disease they did not initiate. While accurate assessment of antecedence is important, it is insufficient for the study of stress–illness problems. What must be included in our models are accurate estimates of the *duration* of both the psychological and biological stress processes in relation to the duration of the processes underlying disease.

There are at least three reasons for stressing the importance of time. First, ignorance of the precise causal time course heightens the likelihood that observed relationships are not the product of a causal linkage but are spurious. Second, knowledge of the duration of stress and disease may help us understand variations in the stressor–disease relationship, such as why stress increases vulnerability in some time frames and reduces it in others (Sklar and Anisman, 1981). Many of the physiological processes presumed critical for organismic susceptibility have reasonably well defined and reasonably short time courses that create serious questions about the effects of life events on health. Following the death of a spouse, measures of immune function are suppressed for approximately two to four weeks, but return to normal by six weeks (Bartrop, Luckhurst, Lazarus et al., 1977). This could mean that findings of increased mortality in the following year for the surviving spouse is due to factors other than the initial event alone.

Finally, purely mathematical and statistical considerations dictate that inaccurate specification and estimation of temporal lags can lead to greatly attenuated or even highly misleading estimates of the causal relationships among stressors, their mediators, and illness. Such misspecification would occur, for example, when variable A occurring at time T produces a change in variable B first observable at time T+4, but the researcher has only measured variables A and B at times T and T+2. In this case, the researcher has underestimated the true causal lag.

The results of simulation studies underscore the potentially deleterious consequences of such specification errors (for reviews, see Kessler and Greenberg, 1981, Pelz and Lew, 1970). For example, when two variables have a reciprocal influence characterized by positive feedback (i.e. A has a positive influence on B and vice versa), lagged path coefficients and correlations may strongly underestimate causal relationships unless measurement lags correspond closely to the true causal lag. Even greater difficulties may arise when two variables have a relationship characterized by reciprocal negative feedback (i.e. A has a positive influence on B, while B has a negative influence on A). In this case, inaccurate specification of time lags can result in estimates of parameters with an *incorrect sign*. That is, what are veridically positive coefficients may be estimated as negative and vice versa!

Unfortunately, even when researchers have the luxury of data collected over a wide range of time intervals, it is often not possible to estimate true causal lags. Indeed, the analysis of cross-correlograms showing correlations between variables at various lags may be highly misleading. In cases of one-way causality (A has an effect on B, B has no effect on A), for example, the maximal correlation between two variables may occur at intervals much greater than the true lag. In general, as Kessler and Greenberg (1981) note, cross-correlograms only yield reliable information about causal lags under restricted conditions.

When one considers the rarity with which social science researchers explicitly hypothesize about the duration of causal lags, there is an unfortunately high likelihood that a number of findings in longitudinal investigations of the stress–illness link are biased by the types of misspecifications and inferential errors just enumerated. Readers interested in a more detailed discussion of temporal lag issues, and in some possible solutions to these difficulties, should consult the excellent review by Kessler and Greenberg (1981, chapters eight and nine).

Life style and events; roles and scripts; the problem of timeliness.

In an earlier section we mentioned Kasl's (1983) concern that researchers commonly ignore the integration of events in a patterned life style that may give events specific meanings and that may itself be the source of the stress process. Alterations in the meaning of an event due to its timing in the life span or life sequences (i.e. its 'on-timeness' (Lowenthal and Haven, 1968)) is one example of such integration. We may need, however, a broader social-psychological framework for the analysis of 'nested events'. Most social-psychological models describe the stress process as a sequence of information processing steps that occur during a specific episode or encounter with a stressor. While these processes extend over time, the time interval is typically brief. Thus, these models lack concepts for nesting episodic processes in longer term time frames. The *script* concept (for elaboration, see Abelson, 1976, 1981) may provide a vehicle for such analysis. In elaborating scripts by identifying the temporal sequences or life style units in which an episodic event is nested, we can improve both our analysis of the impact of an event and increase our understanding of how appraisal and coping processes are updated over a series of episodes.

FINAL COMMENTS

Our goal was to present a perspective on the methodological aspects of the stress–illness problem from the social-psychological framework that is characteristic of contemporary health psychology (see Leventhal, 1983; 1986; Leventhal, Zimmerman, and Gutman, 1984).

First, we contrasted animal and human stress research along several dimensions. This comparison highlighted several key problems in human research. In response to these problems, we then suggested several methodological refinements capable of providing more rigorous tests of causal hypotheses concerning the stress–illness link. A major point stressed throughout was the importance of a well developed biopsychosocial model of the stress process. This model should increase the specificity of predictions linking stressors, stress processes, and illness. More specifically, it should define: the attributes of situational representations and coping strategies that generate specific, subjective emotional reactions; the psychophysiological changes contingent upon these appraisals; coping and emotional responses; and the specific disease outcomes expected. The model would also include temporal parameters not only to define the onset of events, appraisals and disease, but also the duration of stressors, mediating processes (social, psychological, and biological), and disease processes.

It may be the rare study that can meet all of our recommended criteria. Thus, our list should be used to define methodological goals for research and not as a set of inflexible prescriptions that rule out further studies. Their intent is to increase the specificity of our predictions and measures. As suggested previously, it will be increasingly implausible to attribute stress–illness outcomes to content or process bias as designs and data move closer to ideal levels of specificity. A critic may have a multitude of good reasons for suspicion of confounds in data showing that negative life events lead to increases in total scores on symptom inventories administered at an arbitrary point in time following the life events assessment. Our critic should have much less suspicion when our data show that a two-week episode of depressed feelings and hopelessness is accompanied by signs of heightened pituitary-adrenocortotrophic activity followed in turn by a specific, medically diagnosed, infectious condition. In summary, increasingly specific assessment of the stress process, individual differences in susceptibility, and disease outcomes should remove existent barriers to testing and 'validating' hypotheses about the stress–illness link.

REFERENCES

Abelson, R. P. (1981) Psychological status of the script concept. *American Psychologist*, **36**, 715–729.

Abelson, R. P. (1976). Script processing in attitude formation and decision making. In J. S. Carroll and J. W. Payne (eds.) *Cognition and Social Behaviour* (pp. 33–45). Hillsdale, N.J., Erlbaum.

Abramson, L. Y., Seligman, M. E. P., and Teasdale, J. D. (1978). Learned helplessness in humans: Critique and reformation. *Journal of Abnormal Psychology*, **87**, 49–74.

Anderson, D. E. (1985). Behavioural stress and experimental hypertension. IN T. M. Field, P. M. McCabe and N. Schneiderman, *Stress and Coping* (pp. 117–33). Hillsdale, N.J., Erlbaum.

Aneshensel, C. S., Frerichs, R. R., and Huba, G. J. (1984). Depression and physical illness: A multiwave, nonrecursive causal model, *Journal of Health and Social Behavior*, **25**, 350–71.

Arnot, W. M. (1954). The changing aetiology of heart disease. *British Medical Journal*, **2**, 887–891.

Bartrop, R. W., Luckhurst, E., Lazarus, L., Kiloh, L. G., and Penny, R. (1977). Depressed lymphocyte function after bereavement, *Lancet*, (Vol. 1), 834–6.

Baumann, L. J., and Leventhal, H. (1985). 'I can tell when my blood pressure is up, can't I?' *Health Psychology*, **4**, 203–18.

Baumann, L. J., Leventhal, H., Zimmerman, R., and Linz, D. (Unpublished manuscript). Effects of false blood pressure feedback on symptom reports.

Bower, G. H., and Cohen, P. R. (1982). Emotional influences in memory and thinking: Data and theory. In M. S. Clark and S. T. Fiske (eds.) *Affect and Social Cognition*, Hillsdale, N.J., Erlbaum, pp. 291–331.

Brown, G. W. (1974). Meaning, measurement, and stress of life events. In B. S. Dohrenwend and B. P. Dohrenwend (eds.) *Stressful Life Events: Their Nature and Effects*, New York, John Wiley & Sons, pp. 217–43.

Brown, G. W. (1979). The social etiology of depression—London studies. In R. A. Depue (ed.), *The Psychobiology of the Depressive Disorders: Implications for the Effects of Stress*, New York, Academic Press, pp. 263–89.

Brown, G. W., and Harris, T. O. (1978). *Social Origins of Depression*. London, Tavistock Press.

Carver, C. S., and Humphries, C. (1982). Social psychology of the Type A coronary-prone behavior pattern. In G. S. Saunders and J. Suls (eds.) *Social Psychology of Health and Illness*, Hillsdale, N.J., Erlbaum, pp. 33–64.

Cassel, J. (1974). An epidemiological perspective of psychosocial factors in disease etiology. *American Journal of Public Health*, **64**, 1040–1043.

Cobb, S. (1976). Social support as a moderator of life stress. *Psychosomatic Medicine*, **38**, 300–14.

Coe, C. L., Rosenberg, L. T., and Levine, S. (in press). Effects of maternal separation on humoral immunity in primates. In N. H. Spector (ed.) *Proceedings of the 1st International Workshop on Neuroimmunomodulation*.

Cohen, S., and Hoberman, H. (1983). Positive events and social supports as buffers of life change stress, *Journal of Applied Social Psychology*, **13**, 99–125.

Cohen, S., and Wills, T. A. (1985). Stress, social support, and the buffering hypothesis, *Psychological Bulletin*, **98**, 310–57.

Conant, J. B. (1947). *On Understanding Science*, New Haven, Yale University Press.

Conway, T. H., Vickers, R. T. Jun., Ward, H. W., Rahe, R. H. (1981). Occupational stress and variation in cigarette, coffee, and alcohol consumption, *Journal of Health and Social Behavior*, **22**, 155–65.

Cronkite, R. C., and Moos, R. H. (1984). The role of predisposing and moderating factors in the stress–illness relationship, *Journal of Health and Social Behavior*, **25**, 372–93.

Delongis, A., Coyne, J. C., Dakof, G., Folkman, S., and Lazarus, R. S. (1982). Relationship of daily hassles, uplifts, and major life events to health status. *Health Psychology*, **1**, 119–36.

Depue, R. A., and Monroe, S. M. (1986). Conceptualization and measurement of human disorder in life stress research: The problem of chronic disturbance, *Psychological Bulletin*, **99**, 36–51.

Dohrenwend, B. S. (1973). Social status and stressful life events, *Journal of Personality and Social Psychology*, **28**, 225–35.

Dohrenwend, B. S., and Dohrenwend, B. P. (eds.) (1974). *Stressful life events: Their nature and effect*. New York: Wiley.

Dohrenwend, B. S., Dohrenwend, B. P., Dodson, M., and Shrout, P. E. (1984). Symptoms, hassles, social supports and life events: The problem of confounded measures. *Journal of Abnormal Psychology*, **93**, 222–230.

Dohrenwend, B. P., and Shrout, P. E. (1985). 'Hassles' in the conceptualization and measurement of life stress variables. *American Psychologist*, **40**, 780–5.

Ekman, P., Levenson, R. W., and Friesen, W. V. (1983). Autonomic nervous system activity distinguishes among emotions. *Science*, **221**, 1208–10.

Engel, B. T. (1985). Stress is a Noun! No, a Verb! No, an Adjective! In T. M. Field, P. M. McCabe, and N. Schneiderman (eds.) *Stress and Coping*, Hillsdale, N.J., Erlbaum. pp. 3–12.

Fairbank, D. T., and Hough, R. L. (1981). Cross-cultural differences in perceptions of life events. In B. S. Dohrenwend and B. P. Dohrenwend (eds.) *Stressful life events and their contexts* (63–84). New York: Prodist.

Fox, B. H. (1978). Premorbid psychological factors as related to cancer incidence. *Journal of Behavioral Medicine*, **1**, 45–133.

Friedman, M., and Rosenman, R. H. (1974). *Type A behavior and your heart*, New York, Alfred A. Knopf.

Funch, D. P., and Marshall, J. (1984). Measuring life stress: Factors affecting fall-off on the reporting of life events. *Journal of Social Behavior*, **25**, 453–64.

Garner, W. R., Hake, H. W., and Eriksen, C. W. (1951). Operationism and the concept of perception, *Psychological Review*, **63**, 149–59.

Glass, D. C., Lake, R., Contrada, R. J., Kehoe, K., and Erlanger, L. R. (1983). Stability of individual differences in physiological responses to stress. *Health Psychology*, **2**, 317–42.

Goldberg, E. L. and Comstock, G. W. (1976). Life events and subsequent illness, *American Journal of Epidemiology*, **104**, 146–58.

Gopelrud, E., and Depue, R. A. (1985). Behavioral response to naturally occurring stressors in cyclothymia and dysthymia. *Journal of Abnormal Psychology*, **94**, 128–139.

Gortmaker, S. L., Eckenrode, J., and Gore, S. (1982). Stress and the utilization of health services: A time series and cross-sectional analysis. *Journal of Health and Social Behavior*, **23**, 25–38.

Grace, W. J. and Graham, D. T. (1952). Relationship of specific attitudes and emotions to certain bodily diseases, *Psychosomatic Medicine*, **14**, 243–51.

Graham, D. T. (1972). Psychosomatic medicine. In N. S. Greenfield and R. A. Sternbach (eds.) *Handbook of psychophysiology*, New York, Holt, Rinehart, and Winston, pp. 839–924.

Graham, D. T., Stern, J. A., and Winokur, G. F. (1958). Experimental investigation of the specificity of attitude hypothesis in psychosomatic disease, *Psychosomatic Medicine*, **20**, 446–57.

Graham, D. T., Kabler, J. D., and Graham, F. K. (1962). Physiological response to the suggestion of attitudes specific for hives and hypertension. *Psychosomatic Medicine*, **24**, 159–69.

Holmes, T. H., and Rahe, R. H. (1967). The social readjustment rating scale, *Journal of Psychosomatic Research*, **11**, 213–18.

Holmes, T. H., and Masuda, M. (1974). Life change and illness susceptibility. In B. S. Dohrenwend and B. P. Dohrenwend (eds.) *Stressful Life Events: Their Nature and Effects*, New York, John Wiley & Sons, pp. 45–72.

House, J. S. (1974). Occupational stress and coronary heart disease: A review and theoretical integration, *Journal of Health and Social Behavior*, **15**, 12–27.

Hudgens, (1974). Personal catastrophe and depression: A consideration of the subject with respect to medically ill adolescents, and a requiem for retrospective life event studies. In B. Dohrenwend and B. P. Dohrenwend (eds.) *Stressful Life Events: Their Nature and Effects*, New York, John Wiley & Sons, pp. 119–34.

Isen, A. M. (1984). Toward understanding the role of affect in cognition. In R. S. Weyer and T. K. Srull (eds.) *Handbook of Social Cognition*, Hillsdale, N.J., Erlbaum, pp. 179–236.

Kanner, A. D., Coyne, J. C., Schaefer, C., and Lazarus, R. S. (1981). Comparison of two models of stress measurement: Daily hassles and uplifts versus major life events, *Journal of Behavioral Medicine*, **4**, 1–39.

Kasl, S. V. (1983). Pursuing the link between stressful life experiences and disease; A time for reappraisal. In C. L. Cooper, (ed.) *Stress Research*, New York, John Wiley.

Kasl, S. V., Cobb, S., and Brooks, G. W. (1968). Changes in serum uric acid and cholesterol levels in men undergoing job loss. *Journal of the American Medical Association*, **206**, 1500–7.

Kessler, R. C. (1983). Methodological issues in the study of psychosocial stress. In H. B. Kaplan (ed.) *Psychosocial stress: Trends and Theory in Research*, New York, Academic Press, pp. 267–342.

Kessler, R. C., and Greenberg, D. F. (1981). *Linear panel analysis: Models of quantitative change*, New York, Academic Press.

Krantz, D. S., and Durel, L. A. (1983). Psychobiological substrates of the type A behavior pattern. *Health Psychology*, **2**, 393–411.

Kuhn, T. (1962). *The structure of scientific revolutions*. Chicago, University of Chicago Press.

LaRocco, J. M., House, J. S., and French, J. R. P. Jun. (1980). Social support, occupational stress, and health, *Journal of Health and Social Behavior*, **21**, 202–218.

Lazarus, R. S. (1966). *Psychological Stress and the Coping Process*. New York, McGraw-Hill.

Lazarus, R. S., and Folkman, S. (1984). *Stress, Appraisal and Coping*. New York, Springer Publishing Co.

Lazarus, R. S., DeLongis, A., Folkman, S., and Gruen, R. (1985). Stress and adaptational outcomes: The problem of confounded measures, *American Psychologist*, **40**, 770–9.

LeShan, L. L. (1959). Psychological states as factors in the development of malignant disease: A critical review. *Journal of the National Cancer Insitute*, **22**, 1–18.

Leventhal, H. (1970). Findings and theory in the study of fear communications. In L. Berkowitz (ed.) *Advances in Experimental Social Psychology, Vol. 5*, New York, Academic Press, pp. 119–86.

Leventhal, H. (1983). Behavioral medicine: Psychology in health care. In D. Mechanic (ed.), *Handbook of Health, Healthcare and Health Professions*, New York, Free Press, pp. 709–43.

Leventhal, H. (in press). Symptom reporting: A focus on process.

Leventhal, H., and Nerenz, D. R. (1983). A model for stress research with some implications for the control of stress disorders. In D. Meichenbaum and M. E. Jaremko (eds.) *Stress reduction and prevention*, New York, Plenum, pp. 5–38.

Leventhal, H., and Tomarken, A. (1986). Emotion: today's problems. *Annual Review of Psychology*, **37**, 565–610.

Leventhal, H., Zimmerman, R., and Gutmann, M. (1984). Compliance: A self-regulatory perspective. In D. Gentry (ed.), *Handbook of behavioral medicine*, (pp. 369–436). New York: Guilford Press.

Levine, S. (1971). Stress and behavior. *Scientific American*, **224**, 26–31.

Lilienfeld, A. M., and Lilienfeld, D. E. (1980). *Foundations of epidemiology. 2nd Edition*, New York, Oxford University Press.

Lin, N., Dean, A., and Ensel, W. M. (1981). Social support scales: A methodological note. *Schizophrenia Bulletin*, **7**, (1), 73–87.

Lipowski, Z. J. (1975). Psychiatry of somatic diseases: Epidemiology, pathogenesis, classification. *Comprehensive Psychiatry*, **16**, 105–124.

Lowenthal, M. F., and Haven, C. (1968). Interaction and adaptation: Intimacy as a critical variable, *American Sociological Review*, **33**, 20–4.

Mason, J. W. (1971). A re-evaluation of the concept of 'non-specificity' in stress theory. *Journal of Psychiatric Research*, **8**, 323–32.
Mason, J. W. (1975a). A historical view of the stress field. *Journal of Human Stress*, **1**, 6–12.
Mason, J. W. (1975b). A historical view of the stress field, II, *Journal of Human Stress*, **1**, 22–35.
Mechanic, D. (1972). Social psychologic factors affecting the presentation of bodily complaints, *New England Journal of Medicine*, **286**, 1132–9.
Mechanic, D. (1974). Discussion of research programs on relations between stressful life events and episodes of physical illness. In B. S. Dohrenwend and B. P. Dohrenwend (eds.) *Stressful life events: Their nature and effects*, New York, John Wiley & Sons, pp. 87–97.
Mechanic, D., Volkart, E. A. (1961). Stress, illness behavior, and the sick role. *American Sociological Review*, **26**, 51–8.
Menaghan, E. (1982). Measuring coping effectiveness: A panel analysis of marital problems and coping efforts. *Journal of Health and Social Behavior*, **23**, 220–34.
Neisser, U. (1967). *Cognitive Psychology*, New York, Appleton-Century-Crofts.
Pearlin, L. I. (1983). Role strains and personal stress. In H. B. Kaplan (ed.) *Psychosocial Stress: Trends in Theory and Research*, New York, Academic Press, pp. 3–32.
Pearlin, L. I., and Schooler, C. (1978). The structure of coping. *Journal of Health and Social Behavior*, **19**, 2–21.
Pearlin, L. I., Menaghan, E. G., Lieberman, M. A., and Mullan, J. T. (1981). The stress process. *Journal of Health and Social Behavior*, **22**, 337–56.
Pelz, D. C., and Lew, R. A. (1970). Heise's causal model applied. In E. F. Borgatta (ed.) *Sociological Methodology*, San Francisco, Jossey-Bass, pp. 28–37.
Pennebaker, J. (1982). *The psychology of physical symptoms*, New York, Springer.
Quayhagen, M. P., and Quayhagen, M. (1982). Coping with conflict: Measurement of age-related patterns. *Research on Aging*, **4**, 364–77.
Rabkin, J. G., and Struening, E. L. (1976). Life events, stress, and illness. *Science*, **194**, 1013–20.
Rahe, R. H. (1972). Subject's recent life changes and their near-future illness reports, *Annals of Clinical Research*, **4**, 250–65.
Rahe, R. H. (1974). The pathway between subject's recent life changes and their near-future illness reports: Representative results and methodological issues. In B. S. Dohrenwend and B. P. Dohrenwend (eds.) *Stressful Life Events: Their Nature and Effects*, New York, John Wiley & Sons, pp. 73–86.
Riley, V. (1981). Psychoneuroendocrine influences on immunocompetence and neoplasia. *Science*, **212**, 1100–1109.
Riley, V., Fitzmaurice, M. A., and Spackman, D. H. (1981). Psychoneuroimmunologic factors in neoplasia: Studies in animals. In R. Ader (ed.) *Psychoneuroimmunology*, New York, Academic Press.
Roughmann, K. J., and Haggerty, R. J. (1973). Daily stress, illness, and use of health services in young families. *Pediatric Research*, **7**, 520–6.
Schnall, P. L., and Kern, R. (1981). Hypertension in American society: An introduction to historical materialist epidemology, In P. Conrad and R. Kern (eds.) *The Sociology of Health and Illness*. New York, St. Martin's Press.
Schneiderman, N., and McCabe, P. M. (1985). Biobehavioral responses to stressors. In T. M. Field, P. M. McCabe, and N. Schneiderman (eds.) *Stress and coping*, Hillsdale, N.J., Erlbaum, pp. 13–61.
Schroeder, D. H., and Costa, P. T., Jun. (1984). Influence of life events on physical illness: Substantive effects or methodological flaws? *Journal of Personality and Social Psychology*, **46**, 853–63.

Schwartz, G. (1979). The brain as a health care system. In G. C. Stone, F. Cohen, and N. E. Adler (eds.) *Health Psychology*, San Francisco, Jossey-Bass, pp. 549–72.
Selye, H. (1973). The evolution of the stress concept, *American Scientist*, **61**, 692–9.
Selye, H. (1975). Confusion and controversy in the stress field. *Journal of Human Stress*, **1**, 37–44.
Selye, H. (1976). *The Stress of Life*. 2nd Edition, New York, McGraw-Hill.
Shekelle, R. B., and Lin, S. C (1978). Public beliefs about causes and prevention of heart attacks. *Journal of the American Medical Association*, **240**, 756–8.
Sklar, L. S. and Anisman, H. (1981). Stress and cancer, *Psychological Bulletin*, **89**, 369–406.
Steptoe, A. (1980). Stress and medical disorders. In S. Rachman (ed.), *Contributions to Medical Psychology*. Oxford, Pergamon Press.
Stout, C., Morrow, J., Brandt, E. N., and Wolf, W. (1964). Unusually low incidence of death from myocardial infarction: Study of an Italian-American community in Pennsylvania. *Journal of the American Medical Association*, **188**, 845–9.
Syme, S. L., and Berkman, L. F. (1976). Social class susceptibility, and sickness. *The American Journal of Epidemiology*, **104**, 1–8.
Teasdale, J. D., and Fogarty, S. J. (1979). Differential effects of induced mood on retrieval of pleasant and unpleasant events from episodic memory. *Journal of Abnormal Psychology*, **88**, 248–257.
Thoits, Peggy A. (1983). Dimensions of life events that influence psychological distress: An evaluation and synthesis of the literature. In H. B. Kaplan (ed.) *Psychosocial Stress: Trends and Theory in Research*, New York, Academic Press, pp. 33–104.
Thomas, C. B., Duszynski, K. R., and Shatfen, J. W. (1979). Family attitudes reported on youth as potential predictors of cancer, *Psychosomatic Medicine*, **41**, 287–302.
Ward, S. (1985). Social support: Reciprocity, the negatives and the person with cancer. Unpublished masters thesis, University of Wisconsin, Madison, WI.
Weiss, J. M. (1971). Effects of coping behavior in different warning signal conditions on stress pathology in rats, *Journal of Comparative and Physiological Psychology*, **77**, 1–13.
Weiss, J. M. (1972). Psychological factors in stress and disease, *Scientific American*, **226**, 104–13.
Weiss, J. M., Glazer, H. I., Pohorecky, L. A., Bailey, W. H., and Schneider, L. H. (1979). Coping behavior and stress-induced behavioral depression: Studies of the role of brain catecholamines. In R. A Depue (ed.) *The Psychobiology of the Depressive Disorders*, New York, Academic Press, pp. 125–60.

Chapter 3

Measurement Bias in Health Psychology Research Designs

Richard J. Contrada

Department of Psychology, Rutgers University, New Brunswick

David S. Krantz

Department of Medical Psychology, Uniformed Services University of the Health Sciences, Bethesda, Maryland

INTRODUCTION

In recent years, the involvement of social and behavioural factors in the aetiology and course of somatic disease has gained widespread attention. Psychological and behavioural variables have been implicated as risk factors for a variety of disorders, including major sources of morbidity and mortality such as cardiovascular disease (Jenkins, 1971, 1976), cancers (Sklar and Anisman, 1981), and diabetes (Fisher, Delamater, Bertelson, and Kirkley, 1982; Surwit, Feinglos, and Scovern, 1983). Our charge in this chapter is to discuss sources of measurement bias encountered in health psychology/behavioural medicine research, with particular emphasis on case-control designs and retrospective studies. Excellent reviews of general methodological issues in epidemiological case-control studies are available elsewhere (Schlesselman, 1982; Kasl, 1985). Therefore, we will borrow freely from these methodological reviews and place a heavy emphasis on conceptual and content issues of particular relevance to behavioural science studies.

Before discussing specific methodological issues, we will consider the types of mechanisms that may link psychosocial and behavioural factors to disease, and the nature of hypothesized relationships between health and behaviour. We will describe conceptual approaches that specify non-causal associations between behaviour and health, as well as those in which behaviour is presumed to play a causal role. Addressing attention to both types of relationships

Preparation of this chapter was supported by NIH grant HL31514 and USUHS grant R07233. The opinions and assertions contained herein are the private ones of the authors and are not to be construed as official views of the DoD or the USUHS.

Research Methods in Stress and Health Psychology. Edited by S. V. Kasl and C. L. Cooper.

establishes a general framework for identifying possible sources of bias in research designs, and for instituting the necessary controls and ancillary measures that will strengthen confidence in the conclusions that can be drawn from the data.

Mechanisms and models linking behaviour and health

If psychosocial factors do, in fact, play a role in the aetiology and course of disease, how might they exert their influence? In this regard, three broad categories of mechanisms linking behaviour to health outcomes have been suggested. First, psychosocial stimuli may have a *direct* effect on physiological systems which sustain health. This mechanism encompasses bodily changes occurring without the intervention of external agents such as smoking or dietary risk factors. Central to this mechanism is the concept of stress, which is often used to explain how environmental events are transduced by the brain into complex neural, hormonal, and metabolic reactions that presumably impair health (Baum, Grunberg, and Singer, 1982; Mason, 1972).

A second means by which behaviour leads to physical illness occurs when individuals engage in habits and life-styles that are damaging to health (e.g. alcohol consumption, poor diet, etc.) (USDHEW, 1979a, 1979b). Cigarette smoking is perhaps the best example of such a behaviour, for it has been implicated unquestionably as a major risk factor for cardiovascular disorders, cancers, and other sources of morbidity and mortality. A third process whereby behaviour can promote poor health involves the individual's perception of symptoms and reactions to being in the role of a sick person. For example, factors contributing to delay in seeking medical attention and to non-compliance with medical treatment certainly jeopardize health-care outcomes, and individual differences in seeking medical care can be an important source of bias in case-control research designs (Kasl and Cobb, 1966; Haynes, Taylor, and Sackett, 1979; Mechanic, 1968).

Psychosocial variables as causal factors in disease

If behavioural variables influence health through any of the above mechanisms, they may be involved in the aetiology of disease before symptoms are present, or be most important for the course and outcome of illness once disease is manifest (cf. Krantz and Glass, 1984). In research adopting the latter perspective, illness is often conceptualized as a stressor, the reactions to which can influence subsequent health changes (Burish and Bradley, 1983; Krantz, 1980). Thus, the outcomes of coping with the stress of illness may alter the course of disease through physiological processes involved in the progression of disease or recovery. Alternatively, coping might affect the course of disease by shaping behavioural reactions to illness, as when individuals choose to ignore important symptoms or fail to comply with medical regimens.

Note that for the examples presented above, non-aetiologic relationships between behaviour and health status can be viewed as potential confounds and threats to internal validity if the working hypothesis under investigation is that behavioural factors play a causal role prior to symptomatology. However, these processes can be and are of considerable interest if non-aetiologic relationships between health and behaviour are under investigation. For example, the study of 'illness behaviour'—the way in which people perceive, interpret, and act upon symptoms—is a thriving area of investigation (e.g. Second International Conference on Illness Behavior, 1985).

Alternatives to a causal role for behavioural factors

An empirical association between a psychosocial variable and health status may, of course, reflect some process other than one in which that variable is causally antecedent to health change. Often, there is good reason to suspect that disease, or processes related to disease, have exerted an influence on the 'risk factor' (cf. Krantz and Glass, 1984). Aspects of the health care system, such as the doctor–patient relationship, or features of the hospital environment and medical treatment can most certainly affect patients' behaviour. Another possibility is that the disease itself may produce behaviourally relevant neurological, endocrine, and metabolic changes. As a result, early stages of the disease may be associated with prodromal symptoms such as fatigue and depression.

It must also be considered that a correlation between a suspected psychosocial risk factor and health status may be brought about by the operation of some third factor, with no direct causal effect in either direction between behaviour and disease. For example, Fox (1978) suggests that many psychosocial variables studied as possible factors in the development of cancers, e.g. socio-economic status, cultural background, and certain personality traits, are associated with risk factors for cancer which may not be of interest to the investigator, such as cigarette smoking and occupational exposure to carcinogens. This type of confounding can produce data giving the false suggestion of an aetiologically significant relationship for the putative risk factor of interest.

In the foregoing example, confounding involved a correlation between the suspected risk factor and a third variable, where that variable is in fact a risk factor for the health outcome under study. By contrast, there are instances where the third variable scenario is entirely a matter of methodological artifact. Here, conceptual and/or measurement overlap between predictor and outcome variables produces a spurious relationship between the two. Thus, it has been suggested that associations between stressful life events and physical illness may be a consequence of the presence in the psychosocial instrument of items which themselves reflect the onset of disease, e.g. 'personal injury or illness', and 'change in eating habits' (Costa and Schroeder, 1984; Hudgens, 1974).

Research designs in health and behaviour research: an overview

Methodologic issues relevant to research designs have been considered in detail from the perspectives of epidemiology (Kleinbaum, Kupper, and Morgenstern, 1982; Schlesselman, 1982), educational psychology (Campbell and Stanley, 1966; Cook and Campbell, 1976, 1979), and developmental psychology (Baltes, 1968; Nesselroade and Reese, 1973). Consequently, our discussion of these issues will be brief, but should provide adequate background for subsequent sections dealing with specific sources of measurement bias. The interested reader is referred to standard texts, such as those cited above, for further detail.

Cross-sectional designs

Cross-sectional research in health psychology/behavioural medicine examines the relationship between health-related outcomes and selected psychosocial variables, as they exist in a defined population at one point in time. One variant of the cross-sectional approach is the case-control study. Here, individuals with the disease are selected from the larger population and compared to a similarly constructed control group consisting of a subset of those individuals without disease.

The fact that all the variables are studied at only one point in time in cross-sectional designs sets the stage for several rather severe impediments to establishing cause–effect relationships (Kasl, 1985). The consequences of these limitations are such that the data may reveal an association (or fail to do so) irrespective of the true nature of the aetiologic process under study. Perhaps the most salient problem is the possibility that psychosocial measurement is biased and does not reflect risk factor status prior to disease onset. More specifically, it is often plausible that the disease, or some disease-related factor has affected the putative risk factor or its assessment.

Other forms of bias in cross-sectional research derive from factors influencing the selection of subjects for study. For example, a sample containing only subjects seeking treatment, or only patients referred for follow-up testing after initial examination, may be biased in complex and unknown ways. Where cases are excluded from study as a result of these or other selection factors (e.g. mortality), the result is an incomplete and non-representative study sample. Matching procedures, used in case-control studies to ensure that subjects with and without disease are otherwise comparable, also introduce the possibility of bias. Failure to match cases and controls adequately with respect to established risk factors for the disease may produce spurious between-group differences (or obscure true differences) for the risk factor of interest.

Prospective designs

In a prospective study, a sample of initially healthy subjects is assessed for known and potential risk factors and then followed with careful monitoring for new disease. By establishing the temporal ordering of suspected cause and effect, the prospective design substantially increases our confidence that the risk factor is of aetiologic significance. This is largely a consequence of a considerable reduction in the possibility that disease-related variables have affected the risk factor or its measurement. In addition, while selection factors cannot be eliminated, it is often possible to evaluate the degree of bias they produce. For example, the effects of attrition may be assessed by comparing subjects lost to follow-up to the rest of the cohort in terms of risk factors and other characteristics assessed at intake.

A major limitation of prospective research is that we cannot distinguish between a causal agent and a marker for causal mechanisms, nor tell how far removed the marker is from the aetiologic process (Kasl, 1985). Indeed, it remains a logical possibility that a common mechanism underlies risk factor and disease, with no causal pathway linking the two. Another shortcoming is that the prospective design is geared toward identifying relatively stable, predisposing factors, or precipitating factors which are produced by stable environmental conditions or personality characteristics. Variables operating through acute effects, occurring only shortly before disease onset, may be missed (Kasl, 1985).

MEASUREMENT BIAS IN CROSS-SECTIONAL RESEARCH

Cross-sectional epidemiologic studies begin with the effect—disease or some other health-related outcome—and work backward to possible causes. As noted earlier, it is this retrospective character of cross-sectional research which sets the stage for the operation of biases that can produce data giving the false impression that the potential risk factor of interest exerted a causal effect upon disease prior to symptom onset. These sources of bias are discussed in the sections that follow.

Disease-related variables affect the suspected risk factor

A wide range of disease-related variables may have effects upon psychosocial risk factors or their measurement, thereby producing associations which may incorrectly be interpreted as reflecting a causal effect of behaviour upon health. It is chiefly for this reason that studies employing retrospective, cross-sectional methodology provide only equivocal support for an aetiologic hypothesis.

Knowledge of disease

There is little doubt that the onset of serious illness constitutes a stressful event of major proportions (Burish and Bradley, 1983). In addition to physical discomfort and fear of death, patients are confronted with uncertainties about employment, family, and quality of life. It is clear, therefore, that negative affect in patients is to be expected, and cannot be taken as a cause of disease, unless it somehow can be shown to have preceded symptomatology (Cohen, 1979).

Consider, in this connection, evidence from retrospective and prospective studies of the relationship between anxiety and distress and myocardial infarction. Reliable associations typically have been obtained in retrospective research (e.g. Thiel, Parker, and Bruce, 1973), but not in prospective studies in which emotionality was assessed in advance of symptomatic coronary disease (e.g. Belgian-French Pooling Project, 1984). Therefore, the conclusion that myocardial infarction produced emotional distress in the retrospective studies appears most compelling.

Knowledge that one is seriously ill also may influence the measurement process, rather than causing real changes in the suspected risk factor itself. For example, the patient may try harder to recall stressful life events, or enhance their significance. Possible explanations for such behaviour include the 'search for meaning', or an attempt to explain the occurrence of disease to oneself (Kasl, 1985), and a desire to please the investigator by confirming his or her hypothesis. The plausibility of this argument is enhanced by evidence indicating that psychological stress is viewed by the public as the primary cause of certain diseases (Marmot, 1982; Shekelle and Lin, 1978).

Motivated distortion in the recall of events preceding acute illness is not ruled out when such reports are collected from friends or family. It is likely that individuals close to the patient are subject to the same attributional processes (Kasl, 1985). Thus, reports of depression in the weeks prior to sudden coronary death, obtained from surviving next of kin (Greene, Goldstein, and Moss, 1972), cannot be assumed to be without bias.

Schmale and Iker (1971) employed a methodology which overcomes some of the problems stemming from patients' knowledge of their illness (see also Greer and Morris, 1978; Horne and Picard, 1979; Wirsching, Stierlin, Hoffman, Weber, and Wirsching, 1982). Women with suspicious pap smear results were interviewed while awaiting biopsy for cervical cancer. Patients were classified as high or low in hopelessness on the basis of their reports of low self-esteem, inability to cope, or self-blame, for the six months prior to the abnormal pap smear. Three-quarters of the women could be correctly classified as having or not having cancer on the basis of the interview data; those with diagnosed cervical cancer showed significantly greater hopelessness.

The Schmale and Iker (1971) study would seem to have minimized the opportunity for retrospective bias, since the women showed no gross evidence of cervical disease at the time of psychological testing. This conclusion presumes that, prior to biopsy, the malignancy had no detectable effects on the psyche. However, the possibility has been raised by Fox (1978) and Kasl (1985) that physicians may be able to predict biopsy results, and unintentionally communicate these expectations to their patients, in which case the design is not as bias-free as might otherwise be thought.

Effects of experience with the health care system

Various experiences encountered as a consequence of undergoing medical examination and treatment can have major effects upon the psychological and behavioural characteristics of patients (Barofsky, 1981; Burish and Bradley, 1983; Weisman, 1979). Among the possible sources of influence are the doctor–patient relationship (Krantz, Glass, Contrada, and Miller, 1981), certain aspects of the hospital environment (Kornfeld, 1972; Krantz, 1980; Plumb and Holland, 1977), and therapeutic treatment (Cohen and Lazarus, 1979; Weisman, 1979). Therefore, experiences with the health care system may be an important confounding factor in research examining psychological correlates of disease (Barofsky, 1981).

The possible operation of bias due to the effects of therapeutic treatment is illustrated in a study concerned with psychological correlates of the progression of cancer (Derogatis, Abeloff, and Melisaratos, 1979). The results indicated that long-term survivors of metastic breast cancer reported greater psychological symptomatology (e.g. anxiety, alienation, and depression) than short-term survivors, whereas initial measures of biological status did not differentiate the two groups. The interpretation advanced by Deragotis et al. (1979) was that these psychological characteristics contributed to survival. However, Barofsky (1981) notes that short-term survivors had a somewhat shorter interval between mastectomy and recurrence, the latter being the point at which they underwent psychological testing. The possibility exists, therefore, that short-term survivors received as much as twice the amount of chemotherapy experienced by long-term survivors, a factor which could account for both psychological and survival differences between the two groups.

Physiologic changes associated with disease

The possible effects of disease upon behaviour have been neglected in aetiologic work in health psychology. There is some evidence, for example, that certain types of cancers, such as leukemia and cancer of the lung, can have direct effects on brain and behaviour, since they often lead to brain metastases (Bunn, Schein, Bankes, and DeVita, 1976; Lister, 1977, Mitchell, 1967; Sklar and Anisman, 1981). Indirect effects of cancers on psychological processes have also been suggested; these may result from metabolic, endocrine, and haematological changes occurring before cancer is clinically evident (Sklar and Anisman, 1981; Mitchell, 1967).

Although the potential importance of cancer having direct and indirect behavioural effects prior to diagnosis is unclear, it cannot be overlooked as a 'somatopsychic' mechanism possibly accounting for correlations between psychosocial variables and neoplastic disease. Thus, in the Schmale and Iker (1971) study described earlier, it is possible that the psychological differences between subjects with and without malignant disease reflected sub-clinical systemic effects of cancer (cf. Sklar and Anisman, 1981). Consider, as another example, a study reporting that advanced cancer patients with mild neurological deficits survived longer and were less distressed than patients without these impairments (Davies, Quinlan, McKegney, and Kimball, 1973). While patients who felt apathetic, or had 'given up', died sooner, the possibility exists that the psychological state, along with earlier death, may have resulted from the disease process.

It is possible that cardiovascular disorders also influence psychological processes (Elias and Streeten, 1980; Miller, Shapiro, King, Ginchereau, and Hosutt, 1984: Shapiro, Miller, King, Ginchereau, and Fitzgibbon, 1982). Research suggests that hypertension is correlated with mild impairments on complex tests of speed and intellectual functioning (e.g. Hertzog, Schaie, and Gribbin, 1978; Spieth, 1964). Similar effects have been observed in patients with increasing levels of coronary atherosclerosis (Matheson, 1979). While there is, at present, little evidence that personality changes can result directly from biological disease processes (Costa, McCrae, Andres, and Tobin, 1980), the findings cited above have led to suggestions that hypertension and other cardiovascular disorders might have such an effect (Shapiro, 1978; Weiner, 1979).

Recent research has generated evidence of interactions between the behavioural effects of cardiovascular disorders and the effects of common medications used to treat the disorders. For example, Miller, Shapiro, and colleagues found in a case-control study that patients diagnosed with mild hypertension showed mild but measureable cognitive and intellectual deficits (Shapiro et al., 1982). However, after patients were medicated to treat high blood pressure, blood pressure was normalized and the deficits disappeared (Miller et al., 1984). In this counter-intuitive example, medications appeared to have had a facilitative effect on cognitive function, perhaps because they acted to remove a portion of the behavioural deficits attributable to disease. However, we should also note that many of the common cardiovascular medications, and no doubt the medications taken for most chronic diseases, can have subtle and occasionally quite pronounced effects on patients' cognitive, emotional, and behavioural state.

The impact of disease also must be taken into account in research on biobehavioural mechanisms presumed to mediate the effects of psychosocial risk factors. For example, recent work has documented differences between coronary patients and matched controls in their hemodynamic reactions to psychological stress (e.g. Schiffer, Hartley, Schulman, and Abelman, 1976; Sime, Buell, and Eliot, 1980). The possibility of heart damage or changes in vascular reactions that are a result of coronary disease tempers the conclusion that enhanced physiologic responsivity was present prior to the development of disease. In addition, in many studies in this area (e.g. Sime et al., 1980) little consideration was made for the physiologic effects of medications.

Non-causal relationships between suspected risk factors and disease

Sources of measurement bias discussed in the preceding section involve the causal influence of physical disease or related variables upon the psychological risk factor of interest, or upon its measurement. A methodological problem which is equally salient in health psychology occurs where the suspected risk factor is correlated with disease despite the absence of a direct, causal effect in either direction. This type of bias may take one of two general forms. In the first form a 'true' risk factor may be correlated with the putative risk factor under study, giving rise to a spurious association between the latter variable and disease. In the second form of bias, the presence of overlap in measurement or in definition of a suspected risk factor and target disease underlies the correlation between behaviour and health. Each of these sources of bias is discussed in turn in the sections that follow.

Confounding with a true risk factor

Formal treatments of design issues in epidemiology devote considerable attention to the problem of ensuring that putative risk factors are not confounded with more established predictors for the disease under study (e.g. Schlesselman, 1982). Indeed, one of the epidemiologic criteria for determining that a new variable is a risk factor is the empirical demonstration that it is predictive of disease after controlling, statistically or otherwise, for the contribution of other known risk factors (Kasl, 1985; Schlesselman, 1982). Since this issue is equally applicable to both psychosocial and biomedical variables, we will not discuss it here at great length. Rather, we shall consider briefly two related points of special relevance to the focus of this chapter.

Established risk factors for somatic disease are often thought of as relatively enduring characteristics which can be expected to remain stable over time. Thus, in prospective epidemiological investigations, the subjects' risk factor status as determined at intake typically is employed in data analysis. Risk factor assessments made on follow-up are less frequently utilized (Kasl, 1985).

Although this approach may be appropriate in many instances, in the case of certain psychosocial risk factors, a more dynamic model may be required. For example, the occurrence of environmental events such as unemployment and bereavement, and related psychological states such as helplessness and depression, may be associated with substantial changes in life-style (Cottington, Matthews, Talbott, and Kuller, 1980; Stroebe, Stroebe, Gergen, and Gergen, 1981). These changes may, in turn, have an impact on established risk factors for the disease under study.

Consider, as an example, the documented life-style changes associated with bereavement, which include increased consumption of cigarettes, alcohol, and drugs (Maddison and Viola, 1968; Parkes and Brown, 1972). Failure to take these factors into account leaves open the possibility that any observed health changes are not directly attributable to alterations in biological functioning associated with psychological stress, but occur as a consequence of attendant changes in life-style. Only through repeated measurement of established risk factors can this potential source of confounding be evaluated.

A related issue concerns the usual statistical model for handling the effects of established risk factors. As noted above, a suspected psychosocial risk factor is considered to have reliably predicted disease only if the relationship is incremental to that involving established (usually biomedical) risk factors. This approach is insensitive to the possibility that social and behavioural variables can be significant yet 'distal' causes of illness, exerting their influence through effects upon more 'proximal' biological variables (cf. Kasl, 1985). Thus, in the example given above, it would be misleading to discount the impact of bereavement simply because its influence on health was mediated by an increase in more traditional risk factors. Many established risk factors for major chronic disorders (e.g. diet, cigarette smoking) have multiple behavioural components. The information to be gained by studying biomedical risk factors in the context of their psychosocial antecedents is of considerable potential value from both aetiologic and preventive points of view.

Confounding between psychosocial risk factors and disease

There are several varieties of confounding which may give the false appearance of an aetiologically significant relationship. These range from outright contamination, where there is overlap in criteria used to assess risk factors and disease status, to cases where there is no apparent redundancy in the measurement of predictor and outcome, but both reflect some latent underlying variable. As with most methodological issues in health psychology, this set of problems is prominent in the literature on stressful life events (Dohrenwend, Dohrenwend, Dodson, and Shrout, 1984; Dohrenwend and Shrout, 1985; Hudgens, 1974; Lazarus, DeLongis, Folkman, and Gruen, 1985;

Schroeder and Costa, 1984). As a consequence, most researchers in this area now delete items that obviously overlap with outcome measures, such as 'major personal injury or illness' and 'hospitalization'.

However, the possibility of more subtle contamination remains. Hudgens (1974) contends that as many as twenty-nine of the forty-three events comprising the Social Readjustment Rating Scale—the most commonly used life events instrument (Holmes and Rahe, 1967)—represent symptoms or consequences of illness. Thus, events such as 'major change in sleeping habits' and 'sexual difficulties', which contribute to scores on symptom checklists or influence physicians' diagnoses, are still included in life events inventories (Schroeder and Costa, 1984). The result may be an association between risk factor and health outcome for which methodological artifact cannot be ruled out as an alternative explanation.

Perhaps a more pervasive problem in health psychology is confounding involving a third variable producing spurious associations between psychosocial factor and disease. A case in point is the growing concern that individual differences in psychopathology may influence scores on life events inventories while, at the same time, producing spurious or exaggerated self-reports of illness (e.g. Dohrenwend et al., 1984). We shall illustrate this form of bias by reviewing recent findings which indicate that the trait of 'neuroticism' may operate to produce a spurious relationship between measures of anxiety, distress, and some clinical manifestations of coronary heart disease.

Neuroticism may be conceived as a broad dimension of personality that encompasses a variety of specific traits, including self-consciousness, vulnerability to stress, and a tendency to experience anxiety, hostility, and depression (Costa and McCrae, 1980). There is ample evidence that psychological instruments tapping one or more of these traits are associated, often in a dose–response manner, with self-report measures of global health as well as scores on symptom check-lists (e.g. Costa and McCrae, 1980; Costa and McRae, 1985). While such data may be taken to indicate that psychological well-being is related to somatic health, an alternative explanation is that psychological maladjustment promotes non-veridical symptom complaints (Costa and McCrae, 1985). This possibility can only be evaluated by comparing the relationship between neuroticism and health using both objective and subjective measures of disease.

Coronary artery disease (CAD) is a condition whose detection may be based on both objective and subjective criteria. *Objective* indicators include EKG evidence of myocardial infarction or ischemia; in contrast, patient complaints of chest pain (angina pectoris) constitute the primary *subjective* symptoms experienced by patients. Recent reviews suggest a prospective association between neuroticism and angina pectoris, but not myocardial infarction (Belgian-French Pooling Project, 1984; Jenkins, 1967, 1971). This finding has been taken to indicate that neuroticism is involved in the development of

CAD, but that its association with the clinical manifestations of this disorder is specific to angina (Jenkins, 1976).

One problem with this conclusion is that between 20 per cent and 30 per cent of patients diagnosed as having angina pectoris solely on the basis of reported chest pain are found to be free of artery disease based on angiographic examination (Kemp, Vokonas, Cohn, and Gorlin, 1973). Moreover, two studies indicate that when evidence of objectively verified CAD is negative, angina is probably not associated with enhanced mortality or morbidity, suggesting that it be a benign condition (Kemp et al., 1973; Banks, Raferty, and Oram, 1971). Thus, a question arises as to whether personality traits such as anxiety are predictive of angina diagnoses which *do* reflect arterial disease.

Costa and associates (Costa, Fleg, McCrae, and Lakatta, 1982) addressed this issue in a longitudinal study of four subject groups: (a) patients with a diagnosis of angina pectoris but no EKG evidence of CAD or myocardial infarction; (b) patients with both angina and EKG signs of CAD; (c) patients with EKG signs of ischemia but no anginal complaints; (d) an age-matched control-group free of both signs and symptoms of CAD. It was found that subjects with high scores on a measures of emotional instability and a somatic complaint check-list were more likely than others to have angina without objective evidence of CAD. However, neither group with verified arterial disease showed elevated scores on personality measures. Even when followed for periods up to twelve years, subjects with angina only and high scores on the neuroticism measure did not have an increased risk for myocardial infarction.

How is it that neurotic individuals come to receive angina diagnoses? Findings summarized above suggest that neuroticism, rather than CAD, underlies the chest pain reports of a subset of angina patients. More direct support for the hypothesis comes from intensive study of chest pain in patients in the two weeks prior to undergoing coronary angiography (Engel, Baile, Costa, Brimlow, and Brinker, 1985; Costa, Zonderman, Engel, Baile, Brimlow, and Brinker, 1985). Neuroticism was strongly related to patients' own pain reports, as well as to physicians' assessment of patients' pain. However, neither neuroticism, nor some forty measures concerning the antecedents, site, and frequency of anginal pain showed a positive association with angiographically-determined arterial stenosis. The sole exception was the report of chest pain brought on by walking. Indeed, there was a tendency toward an *inverse* relationship between neuroticism and arterial occlusion. Other angiography studies have corroborated higher neuroticism-related personality traits in 'false positive' patients referred for cardiac catheterization (Elias, Robbins, Blow, Rice, and Edgecomb, 1982; Shocken, Worden, Harrison, and Spielberger, 1984).

The implication of such findings is that patients come to be referred for CAD diagnostic evaluation either because they have coronary disease or because they present with chest pain complaints deriving from a neurotic personality.

These complaints affect physicians' diagnoses such that patients free of anatomic coronary artery disease are referred for cardiac catheterization. Although these findings may be taken as minimizing the role of personality traits in disease, they also demonstrate how personality characteristics of patients determine the way they are treated and the kinds of health care procedures they receive.

MEASUREMENT BIAS IN PROSPECTIVE RESEARCH

It was noted earlier that the prospective design represents a substantial improvement over cross-sectional methodology by virtue of its ability to establish the temporal ordering of suspected cause and effect. The assessment of risk factor status prior to the development of detectable disease greatly reduces the possibility that disease-related factors have influenced the risk factors or their assessment. Other sources of bias which can be minimized or eliminated by prospective research include factors influencing the interpretation of symptoms and the seeking of medical care, which bias the membership of patient groups in cross-sectional studies where cases are identified after seeking help. In prospective studies, these sources of bias may be avoided by means of periodic, rigorous assessments for new cases of the disease in the entire cohort.

The chief disadvantage of prospective research is that it is often difficult to determine precisely how the risk factor (identified early on) relates to the causal mechanisms underlying the subsequent development of disease in study subjects. When measured, the risk factor may be far removed from the aetiologic process; in addition, the risk factor may or may not represent a link in the causal chain culminating in disease.

Consider, by way of illustration, findings suggesting a prospective association between the propensity for increased stress-induced responses of the cardiovascular system (reactivity) and the later development of essential hypertension (Wood, Sheps, Elveback, and Schirger, 1984). It is possible that the reactivity–hypertension association reflects the operation of an unmeasured central nervous system disruption of autonomic control, which produces *both* the greater cardiovascular reactivity of hypertensive patients to stress and their elevated blood pressure levels (Krantz and Manuck, 1984). Thus, a hyperresponsivity to psychosocial stimuli early in life might be predictive of subsequent hypertension, yet play no direct or causative role in the development of hypertension.

Although prospective designs represent a considerable improvement over cross-sectional approaches, they remain correlational in nature. Aa a consequence, prospective evidence by itself cannot be taken as proof of a cause–effect relationship. Such inferences usually require collateral research (including controlled clinical trials) assessing the effects of risk-factor reduction, and experimental analysis of the causal mechanisms underlying the relationship between risk factor and disease (Schlesselmen, 1982).

Kasl (1985) notes that while the term 'prospective' explicitly means only that healthy subjects are assessed for possible risk factors and then followed for onset of disease, other considerations and assumptions are implied as well. These assumptions concern the precise meaning of subjects being 'initially healthy', the timing of data collection with respect to the course of disease, and the time of maximal impact of the risk factor of interest, and the kinds of risk factors most likely to be detected in prospective studies.

In this connection, Kasl (1985) uses the term 'slice of life' to refer to research designs in which subjects are followed longitudinally, but are not necessarily healthy at the inception of the study. In this type of investigation, there may be no single identified target disease being studied at a stage of development where psychosocial variables are expected to have their maximal impact. Instead, the goal may be to detect non-specific, adverse changes in the subjects' initial health status, whatever initial health may be. To detect such changes, it is necessary to implement statistical controls to correct for the effects of initial health. Unfortunately, as Kasl (1985) points out, these statistical controls eliminate any effects that psychosocial variables may have exerted prior to beginning the study. This may leave little variation in health status for risk factors to predict, given the usually substantial relationship between current health and later health (Hinkle, 1974).

Another problem concerning initial health status has to do with the insidious onset of certain diseases. For example, many cancers undergo a gradual developmental course beginning with precancerous cell changes followed by a 'latency' interval between cancer induction and clinical detection (Fox, 1978). Depending upon the stage of cancer development at which risk factors are assessed, a 'prospective' relationship between a psychosocial variable and cancer diagnosis may or may not reflect an aetiologically significant process. For example, pre-morbid physiological changes may have exerted a causal effect upon behaviour, or a psychosocial variable may have influenced only the clinical expression of existing disease.

In certain cases, suspected psychosocial risk factors may exert pathogenic influences by 'precipitating' clinical events in the presence of subclinical levels of disease. For example, on the basis of current knowledge, it may be argued that Type A behaviour is at least as likely to precipitate clinical events in individuals with existing atherosclerosis as it is to contribute to the atherogenic process itself (Pickering, 1985; Review Panel, 1981). The effects of psychosocial variables exerting an acute, precipitating influence shortly before disease onset may be missed in prospective studies focusing on risk factor assessments made only at the inception of a prospective study. This problem may be avoided when the precipitating variable is associated with relatively stable dispositional and environmental factors. Examples of such stable factors are the Type A behaviour pattern, and occupational settings giving rise to periodic deadline pressures (cf. Kasl, 1985).

Kasl (1985) also suggests a number of strategies for modifying prospective designs to increase their sensitivity to 'precipitating' risk factors. One is to reassess the psychosocial variable retrospectively, at the time of follow-up contact for the identification of cases who have developed disease. As Kasl notes, this strategy has the disadvantage of introducing all the methodological problems inherent in retrospective data. As an alternative, risk factor status may be reassessed at multiple points prior to final follow-up, in order to increase the probability of identifying precipitating events prior to disease onset. Still another strategy is to take advantage of natural experiments, or situations where subjects are selected for study because they are about to undergo a psychosocial event expected to influence health, such as unemployment, bereavement, or migration. Each of these strategies carries with it its own advantages and disadvantages, and these have been discussed in detail elsewhere (Kasl, 1985; 1983; Kasl, Gore, and Cobb, 1975).

OTHER SOURCES OF BIAS

There are sources of bias in health psychology/behavioural medicine research that are not specific to any particular research design. Three of these possible sources of error are discussed briefly in the sections that follow.

Sampling bias

The validity of both retrospective and prospective epidemiologic studies depends on the procedures used to select subjects for study and to classify them with respect to the presence/absence of disease, and the presence/absence of suspected risk factors (Schlesselman, 1982). Sampling procedures are biased to the extent that they influence the proportion of subjects falling into risk factor/disease categories in a way that is independent of the aetiologic process being studied. A spurious association between risk factor and disease may result if that risk factor increases the likelihood of undergoing diagnosis, the thoroughness of diagnosis, or the probability of referral for further examination (Schlesselman, 1982).

Matthews and Haynes (1986) have raised the possibility that a sampling bias of this sort may account for reported inconsistencies in the relationship between Type A behaviour and severity of coronary artery disease in studies of patients undergoing cardiac catheterization. This argument suggests that physicians may consider chest pain complaints of their Type A patients more seriously than similar complaints made by Type B patients because the physicians recognize Type A behaviour as a risk factor for coronary heart disease. As a result, samples of patients referred for examination may be biased in the direction of being overrepresentative of Type A individuals with little or no arterial disease. It can be seen that this type of interaction between patients' behaviour and physician referral would have the effect of biasing against the detection of an association between Type A behaviour and severity of atherosclerosis.

The selection factors which shape the composition of patient groups referred for cardiac catheterization also illustrate another form of bias that may occur wherever samples of convenience are employed. As noted by Pickering (1985), individuals undergoing coronary angiography are heavily biased toward a preponderance of patients with coronary artery disease. This is because prior non-invasive testing is frequently reliable in detecting the *presence* of disease, with the purpose of subsequent referral for angiography being to determine the *severity* of disease. In effect, this referral process restricts the range of the dependent variable (coronary disease) in studies correlating possible risk factors with angiographic findings. It is a truism that a restriction in the range of a variable works against detecting significant correlates of that variable. As Pickering (1985) notes, selection bias of the sort described here may be partially responsible for the fact that cigarette smoking and hypertension, two risk factors for coronary disease firmly established in prospective research, have shown weak and inconsistent relationships to degree of coronary artery disease in cross-sectional angiographic studies.

Reliability and validity of psychosocial measures

In any area of research, failure to confirm the hypothesis under study implies one of two possibilities: either the hypothesis is false, or it has not been subjected to an adequate test in a given research design. Therefore, for epidemiologic research in health psychology, as in other areas, a minimum requirement for adequate hypothesis testing is the use of reliable and valid measures of the psychosocial variables and of the target disease. It follows that failure to employ adequately validated psychosocial measures (or diagnostic procedures) may contribute to weak and inconsistent findings.

Consider a study by Greer, Morris, and Pettingale (1979), who investigated the psychological characteristics of women with breast cancer. Data derived from their clinical interviews indicated that women displaying a 'fighting spirit' and willingness to combat their disease showed more favourable outcomes on five-year follow up than women exhibiting stoic acceptance of disease and helplessness. However, in seeming contradiction, questionnaire measures of dispositional tendencies toward hostility and anger suppression collected in the same study failed to predict cancer prognosis. In the absence of information concerning reliability and validity, one can only speculate as to whether the inconsistencies in these data are real, or that the interview versus the questionnaires are measuring distinct psychological characteristics with different implications for the clinical outcomes of breast cancer.

The problem of heterogeneous disorders

Many disease categories used as end points in health psychology actually comprise two or more distinct disorders, or different developmental stages of a single disorder. It is imperative that these distinctions be taken into account, since various forms of a disease may be associated with different aetiologies, mortality rates, and so on (cf. Weiner, 1977). We have seen, for example, that with respect to clinical manifestations of coronary disease, angina pectoris, and myocardial infarction cannot be considered as equivalent and therefore interchangeable markers for coronary artery disease. Similarly, cancers differ in many respects, including site and histological type. In some cases, the incidence of one cancer site/type is inversely related to that of another (Fox, 1978). As a consequence, the combining of patient groups with heterogeneous cancers may introduce a systematic bias against detecting an association with a suspected risk factor.

SUMMARY AND CONCLUDING COMMENTS

In this chapter we have identified major sources of measurement bias in research concerning the influence of psychosocial and behavioural variables on physical illness. To establish a general framework for this discussion, three ways of conceptualizing the relationship between health and behaviour were described. These approaches encompass both causal and non-causal effects of behaviour on health.

Obviously, defining what is or is not a possible source of bias depends on which of the above models best matches the investigator's working hypothesis. For example, if traits such as anxiety and depression lead to increased symptom reporting and case-finding, this association may be a source of bias if the hypothesis being tested is that these emotions play a role in the aetiology of disease. However, if the investigator is interested in psychosocial factors that lead to increased physician utilization, associations between traits an illness behaviour are of considerable interest. By contrast, correlations between psychosocial variables and disease may be brought about entirely as a result of methodological artifact, such as confounding with a true risk factor, or overlap in the measurement of predictor and outcome.

It was also noted that cross-sectional studies are the most susceptible to alternative explanations concerning direction of causality, since psychosocial and health-status data are collected at the same point in time. In prospective studies, the possibility that disease affects risk factors and their assessment is greatly reduced. Although this increases the confidence that can be placed in causal inferences, we noted that a prospective relationship does not establish causality. To confirm the causal status of a risk factor, additional research focusing upon aetiologic mechanisms is required.

In cross-sectional studies, the collection of both psychosocial and disease data at one point in time sets the stage for ambiguities of interpretation. However, the situation is greatly exacerbated by the sole reliance on subjective and retrospective self-report measures of psychosocial or biobehavioural variables. The practice of using only subjective measures increases the plausibility of alternative explanations that subjects have biased their reports of risk factor status prior to illness. This is true because many subjectively assessed variables, such as self-reported coping behaviours and emotional distress, can be altered or affected by social, psychological, and biological components of the experience of illness and treatment (Barofsky, 1981; Burish and Bradley, 1983; Krantz and Glass, 1984).

REFERENCES

Baltes, P. B. (1968). Longitudinal and cross-sectional sequences in the study of age and generation effects, *Human Dev.*, **11**, 145–71.

Banks, D. C., Raferty, E. B., and Oram, S. (1971). Clinical significance of the coronary arteriogram, *Br. Heart J.*, **33**, 863–70.

Barofsky, I. (1981). Issues and approaches to the psychosocial assessment of the cancer patient, in C. K. Prokop and L. A. Bradley (eds) *Medical Psychology: Contributions to Behavioral Medicine,* pp. 57–64.

Baum, A., Grunberg, N. E., and Singer, J. E. (1982). The use of psychological and neuroendocrine measurements in the study of stress, *Health Psychol.*, **1**, 217–36.

Belgian-French Pooling Project. (1984). Assessment of Type A behaviour by the Bortner scale and ischaemic heart disease, *Eur. Heart J.*, **5**, 440–6.

Bunn, P. A., Schein, P. S., Bankes, P. M., and DeVita, V. T. (1976). Central nervous system complications in patients with diffuse histiocytic and undifferentiated lymphoma: Leukemia revisited, *Blood*, **47**, 3–10.

Burish, T. G., and Bradley, L. A. (eds.) (1983). *Coping with Chronic Disease: Research and Applications*, Academic Press, New York.

Campbell, D. T., and Stanley, J. C. (1966). *Experimental and Quasi-Experimental Designs for Research*, Rand McNally, Company, Chicago.

Cohen, F. (1979). Personality, stress, and the development of physical illness, in (G. C. Stone, F. Cohen, and N. E. Adler (eds.) *Health Psychology*, Jossey-Bass, San Francisco. pp. 77–111.

Cohen, F., and Lazarus, R. S. (1979). Coping with the stresses of illness. In G. C. Stone, F. Cohen, and N. E. Adler (eds.) *Health Psychology*, pp. 217–54.

Cook, T. D., and Campbell, D. T. (1976). The design and conduct of quasi-experiments and true experiments in field settings. In M. D. Dunnette (ed.) *Handbook of Industrial and Organizational Psychology*, Rand McNally, Chicago, pp. 223–26.

Cook, T. D., and Campbell, D. T. (1979). *Quasi-Experimentation: Design and Analysis for Field Settings*, Rand McNally, Chicago.

Costa, P. T., and McCrae, R. R., Andres, R. and Tobin, J. D. (1980). Hypertension, somatic complaints, and personality, in M. F. Elias and D. P. H. Streeten (eds.) *Hypertension and Cognitive Processes*, pp. 95–110.

Costa, P. T. and McCrae, R. R. (1980). Somatic complaints in males as a function of age and neuroticism: A longitudinal analysis, *J. Behav. Med.*, **3**, 245–57.

Costa, P. T., Fleg, J. L., McCrae, R. R., and Lakatta, E. G. (1982). Neuroticism, coronary artery disease and chest pain complaints: Cross-sectional and longitudinal studies, *Exper. Aging Res.*, **8(1)**, 37–44.

Costa, P. T., and Schroeder, D. H. (1984). Influence of life event stress on physical illness, *J. Pers. Soc. Psychol.*, **46**, 853–63.

Costa, P. T., and McCrae, R. R. (1985). Hypochondriasis, neuroticism, and aging: When are somatic complaints unfounded?', *Am. Psychol.*, **40**, 19–28.

Costa, P. T., Zonderman, A. B., Engel, B. T., Baile, W. F., Brimlow, D. L., and Brinker, J. A. (1985). The relation of chest pain symptoms to angiographic findings of coronary artery stenosis and neuroticism, *Psychosom. Med.*, **47**, 285–93.

Cottington, E. M., Matthews, K. A., Talbott, E., and Kuller, L. H. (1980). Environmental events preceding sudden death in women, *Psychosom. Med.*, **42**, 567–74.

Davies, R. K., Quinlan, D. M., McKegney, F. P., and Kimball, C. P. (1973). Organic factors and psychological adjustment in advanced cancer patients, *Psychosom. Med.*, **1**, 159–76.

Derogatis, C. R., Abeloff, M. D., and Melisaratos, N. (1979). Psychological coping mechanisms and survival time in metastatic breast cancer, *J. Am. Med. Assoc.*, **242**, 1504–8.

Dohrenwend, B. S., Dohrenwend, B. P., Dodson, M., and Shrout, P. E. (1984). Symptoms, hassels, social supports, and life events: Problem of confounded measures, *J. Abnorm. Psychol.*, **93**, 222–30.

Dohrenwend, B. P., and Shrout, P. E. (1985). 'Hassles' in the conceptualization of life stress variable, *Am. Psychol.*, **40**, 780–5.

Elias, M. F., and Streeten, D. H. P., (eds.) (1980). *Hypertension and Cognitive Processes*, Beech Hill, Mount Desert, Maine.

Elias, M. F., Robbins, M. A., Blow, F. C., Rice, A. P., and Edgecomb, J. L. (1982). Symptom reporting, anxiety, and depression in arteriographically classified middle-aged chest pain patients, *Exper. Aging Res.*, **8**., 45–51.

Engel, B. T., Baile, W. F., Costa, P. T., Brimlow, D. L., and Brinker, J. A. (1985). A behavioural analysis of chest pain patients suspected of having coronary artery disease, *Psychosom. Med.*, **47**, 274–85.

Fisher, E. B., Delamater, A. M., Bertelson, A. D., and Kirkley, B. G. (1982). Psychological factors in diabetes and its treatment, *J. Consult. Clin. Psychol.*, **50**, 993–1003.

Fox, B. H. (1978). Premorbid psychological factors as related to cancer incidence, *J. Behav. Med.*, **1**, 45–133.

Greene, W. A., Goldstein, S., and Moss, A. J. (1972). Psychosocial aspects of sudden death, *Arch. Int. Med.*, **129**, 725–731.

Greer, S., and Morris, T. (1978). The study of psychosocial factors in breast cancer: Problems of method, *Soc. Sci. Med.*, **12A**, 129–34.

Greer, S., Morris, T., and Pettingale, K. W. (1979). Psychological response to breast cancer: Effects on outcome, *Lancet*, **13**, 785–7.

Haynes, R., Taylor, D. W., and Sackett, D. L. (1979). *Compliance in Health Care*, Johns Hopkins University Press, Baltimore.

Hertzog, C., Schaie, K. W., and Gribbin, K. (1978). Cardiovascular diseases and changes in intellectual functioning from middle age to old age, *J. Gerontol.*, **33**, 872–83.

Hinkle, L. E. (1974). The effects of exposure to cultural change, social change, and changes in interpersonal relationships on health. In B. S. Dohrenwend and B. P. Dohrenwend (eds.) *Stressful Life Events: Their Nature and Effects*, Wiley, New York, pp. 9–44.

Holmes, T. H., and Rahe, R. H. (1967). The social readjustment rating scale, *J. Psychosom. Res.*, **11**, 213–8.

Horne, R. L., and Picard, R. S. (1979). Psychosocial risk factors for lung cancer, *Psychosom. Med.*, **42**, 11–24.

Hudgens, R. W. (1974). Personal catastrophe and depression: A consideration of the subject with respect to medically ill adolescents, and a requiem for retrospective life-event studies. In B. S. Dohrenwend and B. P. Dohrenwend (eds.) *Stressful Life Events: Their Nature and Effects* Wiley, New York, pp. 119–34.

Jenkins, C. D. (1967). Recent evidence supporting psychologic and social risk factors for coronary disease, *New. Eng. J. Med.*, 294, 987–94, 1033–8.

Jenkins, C. D. (1971). Psychologic and social precursors of coronary disease, *New Eng. J. Med.*, 284, 244–55, 307–17.

Kasl, S. V. (1985). Environmental exposure and disease: An epidemiological perspective on some methodological issues in Health Psychology and Behavioral Medicine. In J. E. Singer and A. Baum (eds.) *Advances in Environmental Psychology, Vol. 5: Methods and Environmental Psychology*, Erlbaum, Hillsdale, New Jersey, pp. 119–46.

Kasl, S. V., and Cobb, S. (1966). Health behavior, illness behavior, and sick role behavior. *Arch. Environ. Health*, **12**, 246–66, 531–41.

Kasl, S. V., Gore, S., and Cobb, S. (1975). The experience of losing a job: Reported changes in health, symptoms, and illness behavior, *Psychosom. Med.*, **37**, 106–22.

Kemp, H. G., Vokonas, P. S., Cohn, P. F., and Gorlin, R. (1973). The anginal syndrome associated with normal coronary arteriograms: Reports of a six-year experience, *Am. J. Med.*, **54**, 735–42.

Kleinbaum, D. G., Kupper, L. L., and Morgenstern, H. (1982). *Epidemiologic Research: Principles and Quantitative Methods*, Lifetime Learning Publications, Belmont.

Kornfeld, D. S. (1969). The hospital environment: Its impact on the patient, *Adv. Psychosom. Med.*, **8**, 252–70.

Krantz, D. S. (1980). Cognitive processes and recovery from heart attack: A review and theoretical analysis, *J. Human Stress*, **6(3)**, 27–38.

Krantz, D. S., Glass, D. C., Contrada, R. J., and Miller, N. E. (1981). Behavior and health, in *Five Year Outlook of Science and Technology: 1981*, National Science Foundation, Washington, DC. (Source materials, Vol. 2), pp. 561–88.

Krantz, D. S., and Glass, D. C. (1984). Personality, behavior patterns, and physical illness: Conceptual and methodological issues. In W. D. Gentry (ed.) *Handbook of Behavioral Medicine*, The Guilford Press, New York, pp. 38–86.

Krantz, D. S., and Manuck, S. B. (1984). Acute psychophysiologic reactivity and risk of cardiovascular disease: A review and methodological critique, *Psychol. Bull.*, **96**, 435–64.

Lazarus, R. S., DeLongis, A., Folkman, S., and Gruen, R. (1985). Stress and adaptational outcomes: The problem of confounded measures, *Am. Psychol.*, **40**, 770–9.

Lister, T. A. (1977). Early central nervous system involvement in adults with acute non-myelogenous leukemia, *Br. J. Cancer*, **35**, 479–83.

Maddison, D., and Viola, A. (1968). The health of widows in the year following bereavement, *J. Psychosom. Res.*, **12**, 297–306.

Marmot, M. G. (1982). Hypothesis-testing and the study of psychosocial factors, *Adv. Cardiol.*, **29**, 3–9.

Mason, J. W. (1972). Organization of psychoendocrine mechanisms: A review and reconsideration of research. In N. S. Greenfield and R. A. Sternbach (eds.) *Handbook of Psychophysiology* Holt, Rinehart, and Winston, New York, pp. 3–91.

Matheson, L. H. (1979). *Cardiovascular Disease, the Coronary Prone Behavior Pattern, and Central Nervous System Function*. Unpublished doctoral dissertation, University of Southern California.

Matthews, K. A., and Haynes, G. G. (1986). Type A behavior and coronary risk: Update and critical evaluation, *Am. J. Epidemiol*, **123**, 923–60.

Mechanic, D. *Medical Sociology*, Free Press, New York.

Miller, R. E., Shapiro, A. P., King, H. E., Ginchereau, E. H., and Hosutt, J. A. (1984). Effect of antihypertensive treatment on the behavioral consequences of elevated blood pressure, *Hypertension*, **6**, 202–8.

Mitchel, W. M. (1967). Etiologic factors producing neuropsychiatric symptoms in patients with malignant disease, *Int. J. Neuropsychiat.*, **3**, 464–8.

Nesselroade, J. R., and Reese, H. W., (eds.) (1973). *Life-Span Developmental Psychology*, Academic Press, New York.

Parkes, C. M., and Brown, R. J. (1972). Health after bereavement: A controlled study of young Boston widows and widowers, *Psychosom. Med.*, **34**, 449–61.

Pickering, T. G. (1985). Should studies of patients undergoing coronary angiography be used to evaluate the role of behavioral risk factors for coronary heart disease?, *J. Behav. Med.*, **8**, 203–13.

Plumb, M. M., and Holland, J. (1977). Comparative studies of psychological function in patients with advanced cancer: 1. Self-reported depressive symptoms, *Psychosom. Med.*, **39**, 264–76.

Review Panel. (1981). Coronary-prone behavior and coronary heart disease: A critical review, *Circulation*, **63**, 1199–215.

Schroeder, D. H., and Costa, P. T. (1984). Influence of life event stress on physical illness: Substantive effects or methodological flaws?, *J. Pers. Soc. Psychol.*, **46**, 853–63.

Shapiro, A. P. (1978). Behavioral and environmental aspects of hypertension, *J. Human Stress*, **4**, 9–17.

Shapiro, A. P., Miller, R. E., King, H. E., Ginchereau, E. H., Fitzgibbon, K. (1982). Behavioral consequences of mild hypertension, *Hypertension*, **4**, 355–60.

Shekelle, R. B., and Lin, S. C. (1978). Public beliefs about causes and prevention of heart attacks, *J. Am. Med. Assoc.*, **240**, 756–8.

Schlesselman, J. J. (1982). *Case-Control Studies: Design, Conduct, Analysis*, Oxford University Press, London.

Second International Conference on Illness Behavior: Issues in Measurement, Evaluation, and Treatment (1985). Toronto, Ontario, Canada, August 14–16, 1985.

Schmale, A. H., and Iker, H. P. (1971). Hopelessness as a predictor of cervical cancer, *Soc. Sci. Med.*, **5**, 95–100.

Schiffer, F., Hartley, L. H., Schuman, C. L., and Abelmann, W. H. (1976). The quiz electrocardiogram: A new diagnostic and research technique for evaluating the relation between emotional stress and ischemic heart disease, *Am. J. Cardiol.*, **37**, 41–7.

Schoken, D. D., Worden, T. J., Harrison, E. E., and Spielberger, C. D. (1984). Anxiety differences in patients with angina pectoris, nonanginal chest pain, and coronary artery disease. Paper presented at the 57th Scientific Sessions, American Heart Association, Miami Beach, Florida.

Sime, W. E., Buell, J. C., and Eliot, R. S. (1980). Cardiovascular responses to emotional stress (quiz interview) in post-infarct cardiac patients and matched control subjects, *J. Human Stress*, **6(3)**, 39–46.

Sklar, L. S., and Anisman, H. (1981). Stress and cancer, *Psychol. Bull.*, **89**, 369–406.

Spieth, W. (1964). Cardiovascular health status, age and psychological performance, *J. Gerontol.*, **19**, 277–84.

Stroebe, M. S., Stroebe, W., Gergen, K. J., and Gergen, M. (1981). The broken heart: Reality or myth?, *Omega, J. Death Dying*, **12**, 87–105.
Surwit, R. S., Feinglos, M. N., and Scovern, A. W. (1983). Diabetes and behavior, *Am. Psychol.*, **38**, 255–62.
Theil, H. G., Parker, D., and Brice, T. A. (1973). Stress factors and the risk of myocardial infarction, *J. Psychosom. Res.*, **17**, 43–57.
United States Department of Health, Education, and Welfare. (1979a). *Healthy People: A Report of the Surgeon General on Health Promotion and Disease Prevention*, Government Printing Office, DHEW Publ. (PHS) 79–55071, Washington, DC.
United States Department of Health, Education, and Welfare. (1979b). *Smoking and Health: A Report of the Surgeon General*, Government Printing Office, DHEW Publ. (PHS) 79–50066, Washington, DC.
Weisman, A. D. (1979). *Coping with Cancer*, McGraw-Hill, New York.
Weiner, H. (1977). *Psychobiology and Human Disease*, Elsevier, New York.
Weiner, H. (1979). *Psychobiology of Essential Hypertension*, Elsevier, New York.
Wirsching, M., Stierlin, H., Hoffman, F., Weber, G., and Wirsching, B. (1982). Psychological identification of breast cancer patients before biopsy, *J. Psychosom. Res.*, **26**, 1–10.
Wood, D. L., Sheps, S. G., Elveback, L. R., and Schirger, A. (1984). Cold pressor test as a predictor of hypertension, *Hypertension*, **6**, 301–6.

Chapter 4

Methodological Designs for the Evaluation of Occupational Stress Interventions

Terry A. Beehr and Kirk O'Hara

Department of Psychology, Central Michigan University

It is commonly accepted that stress and strain are major problems in modern life, and there are many professional recommendations for coping with them. Precise understanding of these concepts and unequivocal evidence for the effectiveness of recommended stress treatments is more rare, however. Reviews (e.g. Beehr and Newman, 1978; Cooper and Marshall, 1976; Kasl, 1984; Schuler, 1980) of general stress and job stress in particular have noted that the concept of stress is used inconsistently in the literature. Ivancevich and Matteson (1980) have gone so far as to compare stress to sin, since both terms are emotionally charged but different people think they mean different things.

While a definitive conceptualization of stress will not be offered here (see for example Schuler, 1980), the following key terms require brief definition: stressor, strain, stress. Stressor refers to an environmental characteristic or event thought to produce an adverse reaction in the person (either psychological or physiological). This is consistent with Selye's (1974) definition and is used here primarily because few people misinterpret stressor to mean the person's reaction. Stressors of primary interest in this chapter are psychosocial characteristics of employees' work environments.

Strain refers specifically to the adverse reactions of the individuals to the environmental event or stressor. These individuals are usually employees in the present chapter. The term stress itself is used here only to refer to the general domain of research and practice involving stressors and strain (Beehr, 1984). Consistent with this, a recent trend in the literature away from attempts to define stress precisely has been observed, combined with more effort invested in strengthening the research methods (Kasl, 1984). This chapter reviews designs used in stress-reduction programmes commonly reported in the literature, with an emphasis on examples from

C. Merle Johnson provided helpful comments on a draft of this chapter.

Research Methods in Stress and Health Psychology. Edited by S. V. Kasl and C. L. Cooper.

occupational settings. In reviewing the literature, it became apparent that stress-treatment programmes can logically target stressors, strains, *or* both, but the overwhelming tendency has been to try to reduce strains directly.

Although research investigating the effects of occupational stress on productivity began in the early 1950s (Hoiberg, 1982), worksite programmes to improve employee health and to reduce the effects of stressors began much later. Nevertheless, a significant trend toward greater corporate involvement in promoting employee health through a variety of programmes has been noted recently (e.g. Fielding, 1984; Murphy, 1984). Such programmes have often been justified as cost-savers. Governmental studies estimate a $17 billion annual decrease in US industry productivity due to stress-induced mental dysfunction, with another $75–90 billion lost due to stress-induced poor health (Rosen, 1984). The President's Council on Physical Fitness puts the figure at $25 billion lost in productivity and $132 million lost workdays annually due to premature deaths alone—presumably related to stress (Fielding, 1984). Many such figures have been presented in various publications, and the numbers are often in the tens of billions of dollars yearly, but putting price tags on occupational stress is fraught with difficulities. It is hard enough to determine how much time was lost from the workplace and how many dollars of productivity were lost due to specific illnesses or deaths of employees, but attributing those illnesses or deaths to stress (job stress or otherwise) is little more than that—an exercise in attribution. While one can assert the importance of job stress by invoking dollar figures, there is usually little more than assertion behind the figures. For whatever reason, however, people working in the field of job stress, and increasingly company managements, do appear to believe that some aspects of stress are widespread, important, and worth trying to reduce. The development of work-based stress reduction programmes are thought to benefit both employers and employees, but this is of course true only if they are effective.

Although there are a variety of stress-management programmes available, it is not always clear which are actually effective in reducing stress. Demonstration of effectiveness requires not only that levels of stressors or strains are reduced but that such effects can reasonably be attributed to the programme. This is not necessarily the same as observing that stress was reduced after the programme was implemented. Factors other than effective treatment programmes can result in reduced levels of strain and hence masquerade as programme or treatment effects. Before methodological problems are discussed, however, it is necessary to understand ethical issues involved in stress-management research as they serve to define the acceptable research limits in assessing treatment effectiveness.

ETHICAL CONCERNS

Investigators interested in evaluating stress-reduction programmes have certain ethical restrains to consider. For example, except within relatively mild ranges, it is not acceptable to expose the participants intentionally to different levels of stressors in order to assess programme effects (Beehr, 1984). For the study of high levels of stress, therefore, it is more ethical to find stress where it occurs naturally than to create it. Most people would probably agree, however, that the exposure of people to treatments that are expected to reduce stress is a more acceptable manipulation. Even so, the basic experimental design often used in research can pose an ethical dilemma for the investigator. Some commonly recommended research designs in investigating stress-management programmes are variations of the traditional experimental-control group design. The paradigm is for one group to receive the treatment while the control group does not. Although this allows for comparison between changes in the level of strain between the experimental and control group, the investigator must ask whether withholding treatment from a group of potentially stressed participants is ethical. This is particularly salient when the participants have specifically volunteered for the study in search of relief from stress (Beehr, 1984).

The counter-argument, however, is that the investigator is not knowingly withholding effective treatment from the control group until it has been demonstrated that the treatment is indeed effective. At that point, the experimenter is obliged to provide such treatment to the control group, and most articles reviewed here have done this. In fact, that practice can make a nice blend of ethics and methodological rigour, since evaluating the treatment given to the control group is a way of replicating the results found with the experimental group. The argument goes on to state that temporarily withholding treatment from a group is in fact more humanitarian as it allows for more certain identification of effective programmes that can be applied to all stress sufferers. Furthermore, in organizational stress as well as stress in general, at least moderately large numbers of people often appear to be experiencing stress simultaneously—so many that treatment resources are not capable of dealing with everyone at once anyway. As is typical with ethical dilemmas, the issues are not simple.

A final ethical issue addresses a fundamental problem inherent in almost all reported stress-management studies in occupational settings. With very few exceptions, the stress-management programmes described attempt to teach the employee how to cope with the stressors present in the work environment. This is essentially an inoculation approach (Ganster, Mayes, Sime, and Tharp, 1982), which does not address the issue of changing the work environment to make it inherently less stressful. While employers are likely to make physically dangerous machinery more accident-proof, they and professionals working on employee health in the workplace have rarely attempted to change the presumed causes (stressors) of poor employee health (strain) in the job stress process. Instead, the favoured approach has been to train employees to withstand the dangers of stress better. Teaching employees to cope with stress treats the effect while ignoring the cause. Because of this, it is a less desirable and perhaps less ethical strategy than improving the work environment. There has been only rare mention of this issue (e.g. Ganster, et al., 1982; Jackson, 1983; Karasek, 1979; Love and Beehr, 1981) in the literature.

TYPICAL PROBLEMS RELATED TO VALIDITY

The essence of identifying effective stress-reduction programmes lies in developing methodological designs that allow one to rule out competing causes or artifacts that may otherwise account for the observed effect. Once a stress-management method has been demonstrated to have a reliable effect, the investigator typically addresses the issue of whether that effect can be generalized to other subjects and situations. Broadly, the first issue is referred to as internal validity and the second as external validity. Although the notion of internal and external validity was first introduced by Campbell and Stanley (1963), Cook and Campbell (1979) have written one of the current definitive resource books for experimental and quasi-experimental design and analysis for field research. This chapter uses their language and the reader is encouraged to read their book if general background information and detailed clarification is needed. For another approach to research methodology in general and programme evaluation in particular, readers are referred to Cronbach (1982).

While the establishment of what constitutes truth is probably best left to philosophers, Cook and Campbell (1979) defined validity as 'the best available approximation to the truth or falsity of proposition, including propositions about cause' (p. 37). Four types of validity are related to experiments in field settings, and each has a set of common 'threats' or problems. These four are: statistical conclusion validity, internal validity, construct validity, and external validity. The following section discusses internal and external validity in stress-management evaluation in more detail than the other two, because statistical conclusion validity is discussed in another chapter and construct validity is less relevant to the applied focus of this chapter.

The use of inferential statistics

When one conducts an experiment, there is an initial attempt to determine whether changes in the outcome (i.e. the dependent variable) covary with changes in the treatment (i.e. the independent variable). The demonstration of this covariation is the first step towards inferring causation. Inferential statistics are the preferred method of demonstrating such covariation (e.g. Hays, 1981), and their use often depends on moderately large sample sizes. Some studies have not treated many people and consequently have not used inferential statistics. Some of these will be described later in the chapter as examples because their designs (other than their use of statistics) illustrate classical types: they are nearly always weaker, however, for their failure to use inferential statistics. These statistics allow the evaluator to be certain, within known levels of confidence, that the results of the stress intervention actually covary with the treatment. Not using inferential statistics leads to the necessity of relying on more subjective judgements (which are more susceptible to bias) regarding whether effects covary with the treatments.

Because conclusions about covariation are generally made on the basis of statistical evidence, Cook and Campbell (1979) refer to this as statistical conclusion validity. In designing experiments to evaluate stress treatments, the researcher should be reasonably certain that the study is sensitive enough to measure this covariation; this concerns sample size and statistical power (Cohen, 1970). Since this chapter is concerned more with methodological design than with statistics, readers with a need for further, more detailed knowledge of statistical usage in stress treatment evaluations are referred to the chapter by Kessler and to traditional statistical books (e.g. Ferguson, 1981; Hays, 1981).

Internal Validity

If it has been demonstrated statistically that the independent and dependent variables in a stress management programme covary, the second type of validity, i.e. internal validity, still needs to be established. As has often been stated, correlation (covariation) does not demonstrate causation. Potential causal factors other than the stress-treatment programme might account for the observed covariation. Internal validity goes to the heart of demonstrating effective stress-management interventions and is a major reason for needing strong research designs in evaluating stress treatments. Scientific investigation is merely a more formal, systematic method of observation, in which one attempts to control extraneous variables. Some extraneous variables are threats to internal validity, and some designs control these threats better than others. Cook and Campbell (1979) have developed a list of threats to internal validity, and these are presented in Table 1. While the list in the table gives a good overall impression of the types of threats to internal validity, it is not an exhaustive list that should be used as the only 'check-list' in designing job stress treatment evaluations. Researchers need to examine each situation separately, asking themselves what could be a problem with a study's design.

Historical events which occur between the time of the pretest (before any stress treatment) and the posttest can affect these scores and hence masquerade as a treatment effect. This is especially true if only members of the control or experimental group experience the event, as often occurs in field research. An example is a company deciding to reorganize and eliminate certain departments. This action, or even rumours of it, are potential causes of

Table 1: Some Threats to Internal Validity

History	Effect is due to events that occur between the pretest and posttest that are not part of the research. Example: Employing organization decides to cut a selected 10% of its workforce because of a sluggish economy.
Maturation	Effect is due to the participants growing older, wiser, more tired etc. Example: Employees learn 'on their own' how to deal with stress.
Selection	Effect is due to differences between the individuals who compose the experimental groups. Example: Only volunteers are treated in a company's stress programme, and the volunteers are more motivated to improve than the non-volunteers.
Testing	Effect is due to participants' familiarity with the measurement itself, usually because measurements are taken more than once. Example: Employees remember how they answered the anxiety scale before the treatment, and this memory influences their answers after treatment.
Instrumentation	Effect is due to changes in the measuring instrument or the way people use it. Example: After the treatment, participants believe a high number on the depression scale describes a situation that they previously thought a lower number described.
Statistical regression	Effect is due to the fact that extreme scores tend to regress toward the average (mean) on repeated measures. It usually occurs if people with extreme scores are chosen for treatments and if the scores have low reliability. Example: Employees tested once for blood pressure are assigned to a treatment group only if they have high blood pressure.
Mortality	Effect is due to the kinds of people who drop out of the treatment programme. Example: Employees who do not experience immediate relief from stress drop out of a programme, and others do not.
Resentful demoralization of people receiving less desirable treatments	Effect is due to respondents in one group becoming resentful or demoralized. Example: Employees not receiving a stress-treatment programme (while others are) become resentful and score lower on a self-report measure of job burnout than they would otherwise.
Compensatory rivalry or competition by people receiving less desirable treatments	Effect is due to respondents in one group becoming (socially) competitive with other experimental groups.

Table 1: Some Threats to Internal Validity *Contd*

	Example: A department not receiving the stress treatment tries to 'score better' on a criterion such as days of sick leave than the treatment group does.
Diffusion or imitation of treatments	Effect is due to respondents in one group communicating to respondents in another and thereby distributing the treatment. Example: Employees in one department participate in a stress reduction programme, and they 'teach' employees in another (control group) department how to reduce their stress.
Compensatory equalization of treatment	Effect is due to administrators or others 'correcting' the perceived inequalities between experimental groups. Example: Employees in one department were receiving the benefit of a stress programme. In the name of fairness, high-level managers ordered similar programme for the other departments (control groups).

changes in the level of psychological and even physiological strains. If stress programmes are in operation while such historical events occur, they may mistakenly be attributed causation for the changes in strains.

Maturation or changes within the respondents solely as a function of the passage of time (e.g. employees who are gradually adjusting after being transferred to a new geographical location) can also threaten internal validity of stress programme assessment, since it may account for changes in stress-related variables absent of any treatment effect.

When random asignment to groups is not used, unequal *selection* of different types of people into one group as opposed to another can create spurious treatment effects. Employees' personal characteristics that are likely to be related to some strains include, for example, hardiness (Kobasa, 1979) and Type A behaviour (Friedman & Rosenman, 1974). This threat can also interact with others (e.g. history, maturation, instrumentation), resulting in differential rates of change for treated and non-treated groups.

Merely being exposed to the *pretest*, e.g. a questionnaire assessing anxiety, can change the responses of the subjects the next time the questionnaire is administered. They may remember how they answered it before and let this affect their answers the second time. Similarly, the measuring *instrument* itself may change, as when human observers (e.g. supervisors or spouses asked to report on a participant's stress-related behaviours) become more experienced and change their 'standards' between the pretest and posttest measures. In this instance, the change in scores is a function of the change in the observer and not a treatment effect. Instrumentation effects can also be due to equipment malfunctions or other mechanical problems if mechanical equipment is used (e.g. in biofeedback treatments).

When treatment is applied to only those individuals who fall at the extremes of a continuum, for example, only highly anxious individuals, the change in posttest scores may be confounded by *statistical regression* (towards the mean). Statistical regression is a phenomenon in which extremely high or extremely low scores regress toward the average on a second measurement, often due to the unreliability of the measuring instrument. Statistical regression occurs because some of the extremely high scores are high primarily because most of the measurement error in them is positively biased. Since a second measurement is less likely to contain as much positive bias in the measurement error, extremely high scores will regress somewhat toward the mean. Obviously the reader is advised to take caution in interpreting the results of any stress-management study that treats only the high or low scorers on a pretest. This is a strong temptation in stress treatment programmes, since those people with extreme scores appear to be most in need of some type of treatment.

Fortunately, all the above threats to internal validity are reduced when random assignment to groups is employed. By definition, unequal selection is eliminated as all members have an equal chance of being placed in any of the groups. By extension, regression toward the mean is also eliminated as it is unlikely that all high scorers or low scorers on the pretest will be placed in the same group. Similarly, differing maturational trends between groups should be the same, as random assignment tends to create (roughly) equivalent groups. Since all groups should experience the same testing conditions, research instrument, and global history occurrences (i.e. events occurring to all groups), these threats should also not cause differential effects between participants receiving and not receiving stress treatment.

A word of caution is in order, however; for random assignment to be beneficial there must be a relatively large number of participants available for each group. The exact number required is impossible to specify, as it depends on the particular situation. An important determining factor in this regard is the influence of individual differences on the phenomenon of concern. That is, the more there is variability between individuals on the dependent measure, the more subjects are required in order to diminish the influence of individual differences. Perhaps stated more succinctly, randomly assigning four individuals to two groups is unlikely to control many of the threats to internal validity. This is an important issue in stress-management research where it is known that individuals vary greatly in their general (i.e. typical) stress levels and in their reactions to stressors (Bandeira, Bouchard, and Granger, 1982). Moreover, many stress studies have relatively few subjects in each group, for whatever reason. It may be that the dominance of stress treatment strategies that target the individual tends to lead to the use of small numbers of participants, since these strategies have historically focused on individual (one person at a time) treatments, e.g. individual sessions with psychiatrists or psychologists, usually aimed at directly reducing strains. If stress is a large-scale problem in organizations, however, these types of treatments are probably not as cost-effective as treatments that would change the psychological environment of large parts of the organization, affecting many people with a single intervention by changing the stressors that are common to all of them. Thus, organizational stress has built-in reasons for treating large numbers of people, and this meshes well with methodological reasons for large numbers.

In spite of the fact that, when properly used, random assignment controls many threats to internal validity, there are some threats it does not eliminate. For example, even in randomly created groups if the *mortality* or drop out rate is high in one group compared to another between the pretest and posttest, there is no assurance that the groups are equivalent when the critical posttest is made. An example would be people dropping out of a stress-treatment group because they had too much work to do, leaving in the group only those with light workloads and therefore presumably lower job stress.

Further, there are certain group reactions that are made more likely if participants are all members of a single, interdependent organization. These reactions can threaten the internal validity of the study. Members of the control group may perceive themselves to be receiving a less desirable treatment or less attention than the experimental group. This can lead to *resentment and/or demoralization* and produce a significant difference between the two groups at posttest even if the treatment actually had no effect. Or the converse may occur, where the control group becomes *competitive* with the treatment group and attempts to 'out-perform' the experimental group. In this situation a significant difference may not be found even if the treatment was effective. In a related vein, members of the control group may *imitate* the treatment group members by seeking their own treatment outside the research-setting to obtain the perceived advantages of the treatment. This is particularly a problem for stress management interventions where the *Zeitgeist* is towards reducing levels of stress. Finally, administrators within the field setting may perceive inequitable treatment between the experimental and control group and attempt to *compensate* by providing the same or substitute treatments. This tends to break down the planned contrast between the two groups and weakens the design. In very large organizations or in organizations in which people do not often interact with each other, however, some of these problems can be avoided if it is possible that the treatment and no-treatment groups can be unaware of each other's situation.

Internal validity and statistical conclusion validity are related to each other to the extent that both are concerned with whether there is a demonstrable relationship between the treatments and the stress variables. Experimentation in and of itself would not be very interesting, however, unless the observed effects can be generalized. This ability to generalize effects also has two validity components. Construct validity involves the ability to generalize the independent and dependent variables to higher-order constructs, whereas external validity entails the extent to which the results can be generalized to and across populations of persons, settings, and times.

Construct validity

In experimental work the researcher must operationalize definitions of the concepts of interest in order to manipulate and/or measure them. For example, the experiment may operationalize the stressor, role overload, as the number of assignments to be completed in a specified period of time or may operationalize strain as the level of certain catecholamines (i.e. epinephrine or norepinephrine) in urine samples. This specificity of definitions is necessary in the design and conduct of experiments. If a significant result is obtained, however, the researcher often desires to make a case that the operationalized variables actually represent higher-order constructs such as stressors and stains. If the case is successfully made, the results contribute to the theoretical knowledge of the subject matter, and construct validity is demonstrated. In the above example, a significant finding that the levels of epinephrine and norepinephrine in the urine positively covary with the number of job assignments would be of little theoretical interest unless the researcher could convincingly argue that the number of assignments represents the stressor construct and the level of catecholamines represents the strain construct. Establishing construct validity is often of only minor interest to many developers of stress-treatment programmes. Instead, the assessment of the effectiveness of a single specific programme is often considered useful knowledge in itself. Since stress programmes are developed explicitly or implicitly from theory, however, it is often wise at least to know the extent to which the treatment may have adequately tested the theory. If an unsuccessful programme did not test the theory adequately, for example, one would realize that the theory could still be useful in developing other stress-management programmes—programmes that would also need evaluation.

Since this chapter is more concerned with evaluations of specific applications than with theory testing, construct validity is not of direct, major importance here. Briefly, however, Cook and Campbell (1979) advise that threats to construct validity include using only one measure of the effect construct (i.e. the dependent variable) or one method of manipulating the treatment construct (i.e. independent variable). Other threats include evaluation apprehension about being evaluated by an experimenter and mixing treatments so that the effects of any individual treatment cannot be assessed.

External validity

Not only are the variables in stress-treatment programmes usually intended to be generalizable to higher-order constructs, but it is nearly always desirable if the effects can be generalized to other people at other places and at other times. The ability to do this is the embodiment of external validity (Cook and Campbell, 1979). As with internal validity, external validity is especially important in the evaluation of stress-management programmes. Without it one does not know whether similar programmes would be equally effective if implemented again. Issues of generalizability involve whether or not the treatment interacted with either the specific subjects, settings, or times (Table 2).

Table 2: Some Threats to External Validity

Interaction of selection and treatment	Generalizability of treatment is limited to certain types (or classes) of respondents. Example: A stress-treatment programme requiring a lot of homework is found to be effective with volunteer participants, but it may not be effective with non-volunteers.
Interaction of setting and treatment	Generalizability of treatment is limited to certain organizational or environmental settings. Example: A stress-treatment programme using counselling techniques is found to be effective with employees of mental health clinics, but it may not be effective with assembly-line workers.
Interaction of history and treatment	Generalizability of treatment is limited to certain periods of time, e.g. special days. Example: A stress-treatment programme aimed at helping laid-off employees cope with the stress of unemployment through improving their job-seeking skills is found to be effective during periods of low national or regional unemployment rates, but it may not be effective during periods of widespread high unemployment.

If there is a *subjects-by-treatment* interaction, a treatment may work well with one set of participants and not at all with another set. Therefore, any one evaluation of the treatment will provide misleading results. There might be treatments, for example, that work well with hard-driving coronary prone Type A employees and not with Type B (See Powell's chapter on Type A and associated constructs).

If there is a statistical interaction between the *treatment and the setting* (e.g. the type of job or industry in which an employees' stress management programme is implemented), there is a particular relevant attribute in the setting that determines whether the treatment has an effect or not. For example, some stress treatments might be effective for employees whose jobs require them to work closely with other people, but the same treatments might not be effective for employees whose jobs do not involve working with others. If the relevant attribute (e.g. required interaction on the job) can be identified, appropriate and inappropriate uses of the treatment can be specified.

If there is a *history-by-treatment* interaction, a treatment is effective at some times and not at others. This could happen, for example, if a company's stress treatment programme worked well in normal times but not during periods of peak work activities such as tax deadline time for accounting agencies or peak tourist seasons in travel agencies. Again, the problem is that results of evaluations done at any one time might not generalize to other times.

Meta-analysis of the empirical research on job stress has recently led Jackson and Schuler (1985) to conclude that there probably are moderators of the stressor-strain relationships in the workplace. It seems likely also that there are moderators or variables that interact with stress treatments to affect the treatment outcomes. Although Cook and Campbell (1979) offer three models to enhance external validity, they conclude that in the final analysis both external validity and construct validity are a matter of replication of the experiment, especially replication at many times and with a variety of situations and people.

COMMON STRESS MANAGEMENT EVALUATION PROBLEMS AND ATTEMPTED SOLUTIONS

Cook and Campbell (1979) have provided a valuable service by conceptualizing validity and listing common threats to it in field settings. There are also, however, a host of methodological concerns and issues that tend to be more specific to stress-management evaluation designs, and this section focuses on these particular problems. Proper evaluation of the stress-management research designs typically employed requires a firm grasp of these difficulties.

Non-Specific Effects

Perhaps the most pervasive problem regarding the evaluation of stress-management programmes involves the development of appropriate control groups. In the ideal case, a control group is exposed to all aspects of the treatment regimen except that which is hypothesized to be the active ingredient. All variables not held constant across the groups compete with the stress management programme as a viable explanation for the treatment effects (Hatch, 1982). If some of these extraneous variables are not held constant it is impossible to identify the specific mechanism that accounts for the effect. In addition to halting the advancement of the stress-management theory, it is not known whether future implementations of the treatment are likely to be effective. This is seen clearly in the use of biofeedback, where practical application has far outpaced theoretical advancement (Kimmel, 1981). In fact, it is entirely possible that much of what goes into the typical biofeedback stress-management packages (e.g. the apparatus and elaborate instrumentation) is superfluous to their effectiveness. For example, Yates (1979) claims that normal subjects who are asked to try to decrease muscle actitivy, heart rate, etc. succeed as well as normal subjects who are provided with feedback. Empirical evidence comes from Holroyd and his co-workers (1984). They had biofeedback subjects view bogus video displays designed to convince them they were either achieving large (high success) or small (moderate success) reductions in EMG activity. Regardless of actual changes in EMG activity, subjects in the high-success condition showed substantially greater improvement on the dependent variable (headaches). Apparently the effectiveness of their EMG biofeedback training was mediated by cognitive changes and not primarily by reductions in EMG activity. Unless appropriate control group procedures rule out the impact of non-specific effects, (a) the theoretical mechanism for change cannot be identified; (b) research may follow unproductive avenues; and (c) stress sufferers may experience needlessly cumbersome and expensive stress treatments.

The nature of adequate control groups is not always simple. Several types of control groups have been used in evaluating biofeedback, for example (Hatch, 1982). If it is desirable to control potential placebo effects, waiting-list control groups are not usually ideal, since they allow a control only between total treatment and no treatment at all; they do not attempt to disentangle treatment effects from non-specific (e.g. placebo) effects. Non-specific factors are agents not specific to any treatment paradigm that nevertheless affect the dependent variable measures. For example, treatment credibility, expectations for therapeutic gains, and even sitting in a comfortable chair with the intent to relax can all be considered non-specific factors in stress-management research (Murphy, 1984).

The effect of non-specific factors in stress reduction interventions was recently discussed in a review of occupational stress-management programmes (Murphy, 1984). Of nine studies that employed control groups, six reported significant benefits for *both* the experimental and control groups on some outcome measures. Moreover, direct empirical evidence of expectancy effects exists. Shaw and Blanchard (1983) varied the instructional set for two experimental groups, one receiving high expectations instructions and the other more neutral expectations, and they compared both to a waiting list control. Not only did the high expectancy group rate themselves as more able to cope with stress but they also showed significantly greater reductions in systolic blood pressure reactivity to laboratory stress tests. In another study (Onoda, 1983), eight subjects were taught to increase their fingertip temperature and eight other subjects to decrease fingertip temperature (warmer hand temperature is regarded as a sign of relaxation as it indicates freer blood circulation). After eight practice sessions there was a significant difference in temperature change between the two groups, but no significant changes in reported subjective relaxation. A clear pattern between changes in hand temperature and subjective relaxation was not established, and the use of hand warming to enhance relaxation was largely due to placebo effects. The effect of high expectancies in work-based stress reduction programmes is especially great, as many workers have a great deal of interest in stress-management programmes and positive attitudes are generated when organizations develop them for their employees (Murphy, 1984).

A particular method has been developed in drug evaluations to deal with expectancy effects, i.e. double-blind designs. In a double-blind experiment neither the therapist (treater) nor the subject (patient) is aware of whether the treatment received contains the active treatment ingredient or an inert placebo. The design works reasonably well in the control of non-specific effects of experimental drugs, and although it has been applied by some biofeedback researchers (e.g. Guglielmi, Roberts and Patterson, 1982), others argue that it is an inappropriate technique for the control of placebo in stress-management studies (Steiner & Dince, 1981; Surwit & Keefe, 1983). These authors argue that the design tends to isolate the therapist from the subject and thus eliminates the use of clinical judgement, an important component in most stress reduction programmes. Disentangling specific treatment effects from non-specific placebo is a major challenge facing stress reduction researchers. Frank (1982), and Miller and Dworkin (1977) suggest not attempting to eliminate or circumvent expectancy effects but to design research to study it in its own right.

If placebo effects are not controlled in stress management evaluations, serious evaluation problems result. Fortunately, however, many if not most possible stress strategies do not require the use of clinical judgements. The idea that most of them do is probably related to the preoccupation with a narrow range of individual-centred (i.e. person as the target) stress treatments mentioned earlier. There are many other potential treatments that require less clinical judgement, especially those that would attempt to reduce the causes of stress in the environment rather than attack the symptoms or strains. For the few types of treatment that are thought to require clinical judgements, an effect of not using control groups that include some attention and/or expectations may lead to continued use of unnecessary treatments and to continued use of belief in incorrect theories. Double-blind experiments and other methods for assessing placebo effects need not eliminate clinical judgements in all experimental groups, only in some control groups. If the judgement is considered one of the active ingredients of the stress treatment, then it should also be assessed for its effectiveness. Groups could even be compared which had varying degrees of clinical judgements, e.g. such judgements used during varying percentages of the treatment time or varying levels of skill in the judgements (e.g. expert clinician, para-professional, untrained college student, etc.).

There are several types of control groups with promise for assessing and controlling potential non-specific effects. One typical control group is the attention placebo group. In contrast to a waiting list control, they are generally brought into the experimental setting and exposed to a variety of events and procedures similar to the experimental group. The type of attention the control group receives varies according to the nature of the treatment the experimental group receives. It should match the attention and expectations to the experimental treatment but not the presumed active ingredient. For psychotherapy groups, attention placebo groups are often involved in discussion groups with experts to simulate the therapist attention. This often fails to match the treatment credibility and expectations to improve, however, and hence is not entirely comparable to the treatment group. In biofeedback treatments, pseudo–feedback groups are sometimes used. This type of control group generally receives the same instructional set and treatment rationale as the contingent feedback group, but as the name indicates the feedback stimulus is not contingent upon the participants' actual response.

Another typically employed procedure in biofeedback stress treatments is the yoked design. In this format the subjects are run in pairs where the experimental subject receives the contingent feedback, and the control subject is yoked to him or her. Thus the control subject receives the same amount and temporal distribution of feedback but in a non-contingent manner. There is, however, reason to suspect that subjects can discriminate between contingent and non-contingent feedback for at least some biological responses. For example, in frontal EMG training it takes little ingenuity to wrinkle one's forehead and see if the machine responds accordingly. Detecting false feedback could easily have a demoralizing effect on the control group causing reduced expectations and subsequently not controlling the effect of expectations on strains. This would tend toward concluding that the treatment is successful even if it really is only due to expectations.

Finally, altered contingency groups have been suggested as a way of meeting some of the problems of pseudo-feedback groups (Katkin and Goldband, 1979). In this design the contingencies of the feedback are altered to observe the effects on behaviour. For example, the feedback stimulus may be delayed. In this way the feedback contingency is not eliminated but merely altered in some manner. This may allow the subject the opportunity to experience a sense of control between changes in muscle tension and the feedback stimulus, but it is not clear whether this control procedure induces the expectancy effects of unaltered contingent feedback and hence is probably not a total solution to the problem. The examples offered above focus on clinically oriented treatments since their problems are the most often reported in the literature. Other types of stress-mangement programmes may have less trouble with this (but they could have their own unique problems).

Obviously, there are several types of useful control groups, and the choice has important implications for interpretation of results. The use of more than one type of control group is an obvious solution.

Individual differences

Non-specific effects are not the only methodological problem faced by stress management researchers. Another issue concerns the effects of individual differences in the object of study (e.g. levels of strain). In the traditional between-group experimental design, individual differences are treated as random error. Hence random assignment to groups is used, which in the ideal case will evenly distribute the individual differences thus counterbalancing their influence. As indicated previously, the random assignment principle works best with relatively large numbers of subjects. It has been noted that many biofeedback stress reduction experiments employ less than twelve subjects per group (Bandeira, et al., 1982). Obviously, the logical solution is to increase group size.

Subjects who have higher pre-training baseline levels on measures of strains will typically achieve greater decreases at posttest simply because there is greater room for improvement. Two solutions are available for handling unavoidable individual differences. One is analysis of covariance, which statistically equates the pretest measure for all groups, reducing error variance and increasing statistical power. Another is within-subjects experimental designs, in which the group of subjects serve as their own controls, eliminating the problem of individual differences between groups. Bandeira et al. (1982) report that the literature suggests rather large heterogeneity between individuals regarding autonomic nervous system activity (potential strains) but considerable intra-subject consistency, which argues in favour of within-subject designs. There are, however, weaknesses of these designs, e.g. the difficulty of detecting the type of placebo effects previously discussed.

While within-subject designs have some advantages over the more traditional between-group procedure, the optimal arrangement would be for both designs to be used in stress reduction research so that the inadequacies of one approach could be corrected by the other.

Reactivity of measures

Another important issue is the reactivity of the measures themselves. For example, when electronic recording instruments are used (e.g. EMG training), time may be required for participants to adapt to the measuring instruments. Sallis and Lichstein (1979) reported a study in which subjects required approximately eleven minutes to obtain a stable EMG recording level. That is, after sensory electrode placement, EMG readings decreased for eleven minutes before the physiological adaptation (i.e. measure) stabilized. Obviously experiments employing this type of training should allow time for adaptation to occur, but in their review of twenty-five articles, Sallis and Lichstein report that 44 per cent clearly permitted no time for stabilization. If within-subjects designs were used, significant results could be due to the adaptation response rather than to the treatment. Control groups in which participants were also attached to the machine could eliminate this problem.

Inherent differences among types of treatments

Finally, regarding control groups, the basic model employed by virtually all between-groups stress reduction studies that target the person rather than the environment may have problems. Many person-targeted stress reduction programmes focusing on alleviating strains directly regardless of whether responses (strains) are cognitive or physiological, involve learning a task (Lang and Twentyman, 1974). These stress-management programmes almost always allow a fixed number of sessions for training and then compare the experimental and control groups. This can be troublesome primarily when comparing the effectiveness of two different stress reduction programmes, since learning one technique may be more difficult and require a longer time than learning another. Steiner and Dince (1981), regarding biofeedback, suggest a more appropriate model would be training to a criterion before assessing for treatment effects. For example, if temperature training was used to reduce the frequency of migraine headaches, the subjects might be required to increase their hand temperature to 90 °F or above before expecting a reduction in migraine headaches. The trouble with this model is that it would be necessary to specify a criterion that is different from the dependent measure. Otherwise the researcher might always conclude that (a) the treatment was successful or (b) it would be successful if only more time were allowed. In some other types of treatments, a related technique is simply a variation of the tradition of manipulation checks, e.g. one could test to see whether the work load had been altered in treatments targeted at changing that job stressor.

GENERAL DESIGNS FOR ASSESSING EFFECTIVENESS OF STRESS TREATMENTS

With the identification of common methodological concerns relating to stress management studies complete, it is appropriate to review example designs used to evaluate stress treatments cited in the literature. This section reviews a sample of stress-management studies selected to highlight methodological problems and how some of them have been overcome. Again, Cook and

Campbell's (1979) language and conceptual scheme for identifying different designs is used.

Generally uninterpretable designs

Many trade and professional journals describe how workers can deal with the stresses that are present on the job. There are, for example, many articles in the nursing journals describing procedures for recognizing and dealing with nursing burnout (e.g. Wandelt, Pierce, and Widdowson, 1981; Zindler-Wernet, & Bailey, 1980). Since these articles and the projects upon which they are based do not purport to be scientifically rigorous, it is not surprising that such descriptions often report designs that are not interpretable. These results do not represent good evidence for or against the stress-treatment programme.

In one study with such a design, for example, a questionnaire (entitled 'Health, Stress and Your Lifestyle') was administered as a pretest and posttest to a group of top managers in a processing plant who went through a two-day stress management workshop (Adams, 1981). The questionnaire contained twenty-nine items measuring such areas as current health risks, levels of stress and strain, nutritional habits, etc., on a seven-point scale. The pre- and post-test measures were separated by a six-month interval, and a two-point difference was used as an indication of 'significant' improvement or decline. Eleven of eighteen patients made significant overall improvements in their lifestyle and one made a significant decline. Similar evidence and analysis was reported for nineteen workers in a research and development facility.

Perhaps the biggest design weakness in this and similar studies resides in the fact that no control groups were developed to provide a comparison. Consequently most threats to internal validity cannot be ruled out in the *one-group pretest-posttest design*, and the results are generally uninterpretable in the sense that strong conclusions cannot be made (Cook and Campbell, 1979). A multitude of (historical) events, for example, could have occurred during the six-month interim to produce the effect. Since inferential statistics were not used, we cannot be sure that the changes covaried with the treatment. Moreover, the managers who participated in the programme may have been particularly concerned about their level of strain, and it is impossible to know whether or not the results can be generalized to other managers since a selection bias may have been operating (although the fact that the study reports results in two different facilities allows for some inference of generalizability). While still other specific difficulties are inherent in this design, the overall point is that the observed effects cannot be attributed to the stress-management programme with any degree of certainty. Hence, one cannot establish that the time, money, and effort invested in the specific programme were worthwhile (especially in light of the large placebo effect known to operate in stress reduction interventions).

Even without conducting true experiments some designs can yield results that are more interpretable than others. A few of these are described below.

Non-equivalent control group designs

The most often used, generally interpretable design is the *untreated control group design with pretest and posttest* (Cook and Campbell, 1979). Except that it may not be possible to randomize participants between groups, this is the familiar experimental-control group design with stressor and/or strain measures taken before and after the stress treatment is administered. Because of its frequent use, an example of it is followed by four examples of variations of it.

Recently advocated by Hendrix, Ovalle, and Troxler (1985) for evaluating wellness programmes in work settings, the *untreated control group design with pretest and posttest* is illustrated by a stress management programme for school psychologists (Forman, 1981). In this example eight school psychologists in one school district served as the experimental group while eight school psychologists from another district composed the control group. Hence random assignment to groups was not employed, making this a quasi-experiment. The eight participants attended six two-hour training sessions held on a weekly basis. The training programme was based on Meichenbaum's (1977) stress inoculation model. Anxiety (strain) measures from both groups were obtained via the State-Trait Anxiety Index (STAI; Spielberger, Gorsuch, and Luchene, 1970), and work satisfaction measures were obtained from the Job Descriptive Index (JDI; Smith, Kendall, and Hulin, 1969). Both measures were administered one week prior to training and again during the last week of training. There was a significant decrease in self-reported state and trait anxiety for the experimental group but not for the control group. An effect was found, but it is instructive to examine the study for methodological flaws.

First, since intact groups were used selection and the interaction of selection with other threats to internal validity (e.g. maturation, history, instrumentation) may have been operating. Selection was especially a threat if the groups could have plausibly been different on attributes that interact with the treatment. To some extent it can be argued that the groups were different, since there was a substantial difference between them on the pretest measure of trait anxiety. A difference, although not as large, also existed on the state anxiety pretest. In this situation a more appropriate statistical analysis would have been an analysis of covariance (multivariate and univariate analysis of variance were actually employed). Analysis of covariance would have equated the two groups, at pretest, at least on the attribute measured by the dependent variable. It would also have been preferable to employ measures of the dependent variable from sources other than self-report, especially in light of the fact that the posttest measures were gathered during the last week of training, which could have biased the experimental group's perceptions of their anxiety-reducing abilities. As always, long-term follow-up measures would have aided in the assessment of the permanence of the effects.

As a general principle, *inclusion of more than one type of control group* is a variation that strengthens an experiment as it allows for more comparisons to be made and therefore enhances researchers' ability to assess treatment effects. In a stress-management evaluation a completely satisfactory single control group is usually not possible, so it is especially helpful to have more than one type of control group. Thirty middle-level business managers were placed into one of three groups in one study (Allen and Blanchard, 1980). One control group participated only in the assessment procedures and served primarily as a waiting-list control. The second control group was intended to be an attention-placebo control group, and the subjects participated in individual and group discussions. In this control group time off the job and time spent with the trainer were controlled but expectancy and treatment credibility effects may not have been. The experimental group received six once-per-week sessions of EMG biofeedback coupled with an assortment of other stress reduction techniques including instructions in progressive relaxation and stress inoculation training (Meichenbaum, 1977). A number of dependent variables were employed. These include self-report measures (four), job performance measures (including absenteeism), and physiological assessment (EMG and fingertip temperature). Overall the results showed little consistent effects of the treatment and did not support the use of biofeedback to decrease distress or to improve the job performance of managers. Moreover, the article cites evidence that the typical stress-reduction programme in business is relatively brief (i.e. one or possibly two consecutive days) and speculates whether the reward systems of most organizations may not override the effects of most worksite stress management programmes. This might again argue for the use of organization- rather than person-targeted stress treatments, since the former attempts to use and/or change the organization instead of ignoring its potentially powerful influence on employees. Finally, in light of the non-significant results, a power analysis (Cohen, 1970) would have been helpful in determining if the experiment itself was likely to be powerful enough to detect an effect.

Of course if the basic experimental-control group design can be expanded to include additional control groups, it can also be expanded to include *more than one experimental group*, each implementing a separate independent variable (treatment). In some cases, this variant is barely distinguishable from the previously discussed design, since the difference between control groups receiving special treatment and experimental groups receiving some treatment may be indistinguishable. The main difference is that all experimental groups in the present design are expected to be more effective than any control group in the previous design. In this design the effectiveness of various treatments can be compared and interaction effects between the treatments can even be assessed if the independent variables are combined in one or more experimental groups.

One stress-treatment programme (Yorde and Witmer, 1980) compared EMG biofeedback with a lecture-discussion treatment that presented cognitive coping and relaxation skills. Thirty-eight subjects drawn from the general population of a small university community were matched on the basis of age and sex (no minority races participated to match on the basis of race) and were randomly assigned to one of five experimental groups: (a) lecture only group (N=7); (b) lecture plus contingent biofeedback group (N=9); (c) lecture plus non-contingent biofeedback group (N=7); (d) contingent biofeedback group (N=8); and (e) non-contingent biofeedback group (N=7). The majority (58 per cent) of these volunteer participants were employed, making the selected sample potentially relevant to the topic of occupational stress. The lecture-discussion treatment consisted of four one-and-one-half-hour sessions providing information about stressors and strain and presenting a variety of coping suggestions including autogenic training, progressive relaxation and breathing exercises. The biofeedback training was limited to four one-half hour training sessions (frontal EMG training was used). Subjects in the non-contingent feedback conditions were yoked to receive feedback that the subjects in the contingent feedback condition received. Two dependent measures were used, both self-report indices of anxiety level. The State-Trait Anxiety Index and the Subjective Stress Scale (Kerle and Bialek, 1958) were administered one week prior to treatment and one week after treatment. Anxiety scores for participation in the lecture-discussion format declined and there was no evidence that frontal EMG biofeedback contributed to the reduction of stress.

Such results imply that expensive biofeedback equipment is unnecessary in stress management and that reductions in levels of strain can be accomplished by relatively low-cost discussion and lectures. As always though, it is important to consider methodological weaknesses before firmly accepting such conclusions. An obvious difficulty is that the biofeedback training time was quite short. It is conceivable that weekly thirty-minute training sessions spaced over one month simply did not allow the subjects enough time to learn the relaxation response. Perhaps the most disturbing weakness involves the fact that only self-report measures of anxiety were used as dependent measures. Although some justification for this was provided by citing evidence that the Subjective Stress Scale has been correlated with physiological measures (Appley and Trumbull, 1967), self-report indices are generally more subject to confounding than are physiologic measures. This is especially worrying when one realizes that the groups participating in the lecture treatments decreased their scores on the Trait-Anxiety subscale of the STAI. It is overly optimistic to believe that a valid measure of a trait can be changed by a total of six hours of lecture and discussion.

A third variation of the quasi-experimental, non-equivalent control group design is the *cohort design* (Cook and Campbell, 1979). 'Cohort' in this usage denotes a group of respondents who follow each other through formal or informal institutions. Such cohorts are useful for experimental purposes because some cohorts receive a particular treatment while preceding or following cohorts do not. It is often reasonable to assume that a cohort differs in only minor ways from its contiguous cohort, therefore assuming only minor selection effects. Although the degree of achieved comparability of cohort designs does not reach that of designs using random assignment, this 'quasi-comparability' can often be useful. An example of this design used four cohorts of forty subjects each, with subjects randomly assigned to one of ten groups (Hiebert and Fitzsimmons, 1981). At any one time there were forty subjects in the study, i.e. four subjects per group. Although participants were partially solicited through public media, the majority (69 per cent) were college students—making the study only partially relevant to work-related stress. When one group of subjects (cohort) finished their respective treatment programme there was a one-week break, after which forty more subjects began treatment. Three anxiety treatment procedures were investigated: frontal EMG biofeedback training, cognitive self-monitoring, and systematic desensitization. These treatments were used individually and in combination with each other. In addition, a waiting list group and a high expectation discussion group were used as controls. Checks of treatment credibility and expectations of effectiveness resulted in no significant effects, suggesting that non-specific effects were reasonably well controlled. Two dependent variables were used: the 40-item IPAT Self-Analysis Form (an anxiety scale; Cattell, 1957), and a five-minute frontal EMG. EMG treatment subjects received six fifty-minute treatment sessions. The dependent measures were taken at three different times. The first measure served as a conventional pretest, the second measure was taken at the beginning of session three, and the third measure was taken during the sixth session and constituted a posttest. Subjects experienced anxiety reductions regardless of the treatment conditions, but treatment groups receiving EMG feedback achieved more consistent reductions on both dependent measures. Combining desensitization or cognitive monitoring with EMG did not appear to enhance the treatment effect of EMG alone. A one-month follow-up of a random sample of the original subjects revealed a significant relationship between the initial impression of treatment effectiveness and the maintenance of the treatment effect.

By and large this is a reasonably well controlled study, especially given the fact that random assignment to groups was employed and a check of treatment credibility indicated that non-specific placebo effects were controlled. Some methodological flaws still leave room for improvement, however. For example, one of the dependent measures consisted of a five-minute frontal EMG baseline. It is reported that the subjects were only given thirty seconds to settle themselves before recording began. Consequently, it appears as though this measure was confounded by the adaptation response (Sallis and Lichstein, 1979) and it is no wonder that subjects in all treatment conditions showed decreases on this measure. A second major flaw of the study is that it does not assess the efficacy of the three stress-management procedures very well, as it adheres to the model of allowing only a fixed number of treatment sessions before assessing for effects. It is entirely possible that either systematic desensitization or cognitive monitoring (or both) are just as effective as EMG training but require more than six sessions to be effective. Training to a specific criterion might have been a better test of the three methods—if some criterion other than the dependent variables was available.

Although Cook and Campbell (1979) discuss other between-group designs, a final useful variant of the non-equivalent control group design commonly found in the stress literature (although not in the occupational stress literature) is the *reversed-treatement (non-equivalent) control group design with pretest and posttest*. In this design the control group receives the conceptually opposite treatment from the treatment of the experimental group. Obviously this would be expected to reverse the pattern of findings in the experimental group. An example of this design is from the study (not job-related) that trained subjects to either increase or decrease their hand temperature (Onoda, 1983). Sixteen subjects were randomly assigned to either of two conditions. The dependent variable was subjects' feelings of relaxation as measured by the Subjective Rating Sheet. The Subjective Rating Sheet requires the subject to rate the degree of subjective relaxation in a range from 1 to 100. Both groups received eight one-half hour practice sessions. Posttest measures demonstrated a significant difference in temperature change, but no significant main effects in subjective relaxation.

Interrupted time series designs

Thus far all the designs discussed have been some version of the traditional between-group design in which certain groups receive treatment of interest while others do not. Usually measures are only taken at two points in time, i.e. before the treatment and after it. There is a different type of design available for research purposes, however, the primary characteristic of which is that measures are taken at several points in time. They are therefore labelled time-series designs (Cook and Campbell, 1979). These designs may incorporate the between-group approach, resulting in especially strong designs (e.g. Cook & Campbell's time-series with switching replications, 1979). Several authors in the (non-job-related) stress management literature have argued for increased use of time-series designs (i.e. Bandeira, et al., 1982; Barlow, Blanchard, Hayes and Epstein, 1977) although thus far it appears that they are rarely employed. The distinct advantage of the time-series designs is that by taking measures at several points in time a functional relationship can be established between the independent and dependent variables. In contrast, between-group designs that take only a single pretest and a single posttest can only assess changes in level. That is, they ask the question 'did the mean level of a dependent variable change significantly as compared to the mean level for the control group?' While time-series designs can assess changes in level (often called intercept changes since time-series measures can be plotted on a graph), they can also assess for slope changes (often referred to as trend or drift). With intercept and slope values determined for an independent and dependent variable, a functional relationship can be established (often a linear relationship). Said another way, with multiple measures, time can serve as the independent variable and the dependent variable can be regressed on it. Then the researcher can use regression procedures and visual graphs to assess abrupt changes in level or changes in the slope of the relationship. Also, since posttest measures are taken at several points in time, it is possible to determine whether an effect is continuous or tends to decay over time, an obvious advantage for stress research where maintenance of treatment effects is important.

As will be seen shortly, experimental conditions and procedures are possible in a time-series framework to control for many threats to validity. With proper experimental controls and the opportunity to assess the functional relationship between the dependent and independent variable, time-series designs represent a potentially powerful procedure for researchers in all field settings.

Although Cook and Campbell (1979) describe six time-series designs, only three of them appear to be used with any degree of frequency—and none are used frequently in occupational stress research. In part this is undoubtedly due to the fact that at least two of the infrequently used designs can be strengthened by additional procedures that are often relatively easily implemented (thereby becoming a different design). The *interrupted time-series with switching replications* is among the most powerful of the quasi-experimental designs. It involves multiple measures taken on two groups. The treatment is introduced at different times, however, so that each group is able to serve as a control group while the other is receiving the treatment. By introducing the treatment in a staggered fashion a kind of replication is achieved, and it is possible to limit most threats to internal validity.

A study by von Baeyer and Krause (1983–4) illustrates a time-series design with switching replications applied to stress management. Fourteen nurses working on a burn unit were given three hours of individual training in cognitive-behavioural stress-management skills. The nurses were randomly divided into two groups with the second group beginning their individualized training one week after the first group completed theirs. Two self-report scales were used as the dependent measures of strain: The State-Trait Anxiety Index administered weekly during the study (five administrations) and then once more two weeks later, and the Daily Record Sheet (DRS), a scale specially constructed for this study, administered daily for the first thirty-four days of the study. In addition, a retrospective evaluation questionnaire was administered two days after the final STAI administration to assess impressions of benefits of the treatment and the extent of practice (a manipulation check). Because the treatment was introduced at different times for the two groups, two comparisons were possible. The first comparison was made at the point at which the first group had completed the training and the second group had not yet begun. Because the groups were created by random assignment, the experiment at that point resembled the traditional experimental-control group design. A one-way analysis of covariance using pretest scores as the covariate indicated a significant difference between the two groups on all three dependent measures at that time.

The second legitimate comparison of designs of this type involves changes in the dependent variable over time. That is, one would expect lower posttest scores as compared to pretest scores, for both groups. In von Baeyer and Krause (1983–4) this comparison resulted in an effect of training for the first group but no apparent effect for the second group. Further analysis suggested the treatment was more effective for nurses who had relatively little experience in general nursing, while more experienced nurses apparently benefited little from the training. Nurses in the second group had an average of five years experience while those in the first group averaged less than two years (despite the random assignment). The retrospective evaluation questionnaire indicated a moderately positive evaluation of the programme but that the modal subject did not practise relaxation after the treatment was completed. This example highlights one of the advantages of the time-series design with switching replications when random assignment is used. That is, two comparisons are possible, i.e. comparisons within each group over time and comparisons between groups when one group has completed treatment and the other has not yet begun.

On the other hand, in many organizational settings, introducing treatment in a staggered manner allows subjects in the first group to discuss the treatment with members in other groups which can alter expectations. With all nurses in the same burn unit, this is made more likely, but in large organizations it is more possible to treat two groups that have little contact with each other.

Ganster, Mayes, Sime, and Tharp (1982): A strong design example

The designs discussed above represent models that can be followed in field work, but it is also possible to combine these designs, sometimes in ways that increase their ability to rule out threats to validity. In fact, the time-series design with switching replications can be considered such a combination (e.g. of time-series, untreated control group with pretest and posttest with a replication). This combination is what makes it such a powerful design.

Ganster, et al. (1982) report one of the best examples of a stress-management field experiment in a work setting. It was a true experiment combined with switching replications (not time-series, however) of the treatment using the control group. In addition, a four-month follow-up measurement of the first group allowed a test for moderately long-term effects. Seventy-nine public agency employees were randomly assigned to the treatment or control group, constituting larger groups than most studies. The authors took some care in diminishing the possible effects of demoralization of being placed in a less favourable treatment condition (i.e. control group) by explaining to all participants that demand for the treatment exceeded the supply. Hence a lottery was conducted to determine who would receive the treatment first. The authors perceived that the subjects accepted this as fair and reasonable. Additionally the construct validity of the effect was enhanced by taking measures on three classes of strain responses, i.e. psychological, physiological, and somatic complaints. Psychological strain was measured by the STAI supplemented by a six-item measure of depression and a three-item measure of irritation. Somatic complaints were measured by a seventeen-item scale that was averaged to yield a total somatic complaint score. Physiological strain was measured by levels of epinephrine and norepinephrine in urine samples. All subjects completed the measures on the same day of the week (if something happened only on that particular day of the week, i.e. extra coffee breaks, this would be a confound) at each of the three measurement waves of the study.

The independent (treatment) variable was an integrated approach to coping with stress that was based primarily on the work of Meichenbaum (1975) and Ellis (1962). The treatment utilized a cognitive restructuring approach that was supplemented by progressive relaxation training and biofeedback, the combination of which should constitute a powerful treatment. No attempt was made, however, to keep the treatment approaches separate in order to identify which ingredient(s) accounted for most of the treatment effect, and potential expectation and placebo effects were not controlled. Treatment consisted of sixteen hours of training by an experienced clinical psychologist over eight weeks, a more extensive treatment than many appearing in the literature.

Because the design consisted of a true experiment supplemented by switching replications and a long-term (four-month) follow-up posttest, the results were analyzed in several stages. Analysis of the true experiment indicated that the treatment subjects exhibited significantly lower level of epinephrine and depression than control subjects. Further, these effects did not regress to pretest levels during the four-month follow-up. The treatment effects were not replicated, however, when the treatment was extended to the control group. The authors' recommendations are also instructive in that they are a good example of logical interpretation of the results of a strong design. They did not recommend widespread adoption of such stress-management programmes. There are several reasons for not endorsing work-based stress-management programmes based on this study, despite the fact that some significant effects were found. First, there was the failure to replicate the effect when the control group was treated. Second, despite statistical significance, the effect size of the treatment was not particularly dramatic. For epinephrine, the dependent variable affected most strongly, only seven per cent of the variance was accounted for by the programme. Third, the treatment package lasted much longer and was conducted by people who were more expert in their fields than many of the commercial stress-management programmes available from many consulting firms and used by many organizations. Therefore if *it* had little effect, the others are also unlikely to be successful.

SUMMARY, COMMENTS, AND A FINAL EXAMPLE

This chapter provided examples and evaluations of several types of research designs for investigating the effects of stress treatments, with an emphasis on stress in work settings. Since the references cited are neither exhaustive nor randomly chosen from all published evaluations of occupational stress treatments, readers should not conclude that the studies described here are representative of those found in the literature generally. In reality, those included here tended to be somewhat 'better', i.e. stronger in design than the average study encountered reading the literature. A few comments are therefore in order regarding the state of the art of evaluation of work-related stress-treatment programmes.

Types of strain investigated

Perhaps because stress has become a very popular topic among psychologists, many studies rely primarily or exclusively on psychological strains as dependent variables. It is obviously important to assess the impact of stress-management programmes on behaviours and physiologic reactions as well as on psychological reactions (Newman and Beehr, 1979), and this chapter purposely reported some studies doing that; practice and science in the field would be advanced more quickly if more studies would include a variety of dependent variables, however.

Placebo effects

The discussion of placebo or non-specific effects illustrated the difficulty of developing ideal control groups. In many studies that tested for placebo effects, they were found. Therefore, it is possible that many gains shown by participants in stress-management programmes are not due to specific treatments but are placebo effects. This highlights the need for strong designs in assessing treatment effects and questions the validity of the claims for many specific programmes.

Long-term benefits of stress treatments

Few studies encountered in reviewing the literature assessed the impact of the treatment much beyond the length of the treatment. In order for a programme to be worthwhile, it usually needs to have an impact beyond the time of contact with the employees experiencing stress. Otherwise, the effective cost-benefit ratio is very poor. Related to this, many of the treatments reviewed were supposed to become self-administered and to continue in the long term. Relaxation, for example, is traditionally assumed to work only if the individual continues to practise it after the training sessions are terminated (e.g. Budzynski, Stoyva, Adler, and Mullaney, 1973). Recent studies of biofeedback and progressive relaxation techniques have suggested that such long-term continued practice of the treatment may not be necessary to sustain gains, however (e.g. Andrasik, Blanchard, and Neff, 1984; Carrington, Collings, Benson, Robinson, Wood, Lehrer, Woolfolk, and Cole, 1980; Libo and Arnold, 1983). Those who make long-term decreases in self-administration of a stress programme act similarly to patients who do not follow physicians' orders regarding following diets or taking medicines. There may be treatments that would work quite well if only they were administered 'correctly', and the people who are experiencing stress are often partly responsible for applying their own long-term treatment in any cost-effective programme. It is too easy to attribute such failure to apply treatments to participants' laziness, forgetfulness, or apathy; just as likely, however, some treatments may be difficult to apply, embarrassing or painful to experience, of low social acceptability in the participant's culture or subculture, or require changing strongly engrained habits. This is an area in need of study and one that is often disregarded in assessing the efficacy of stress treatments. Some studies reviewed here included manipulation checks in at least the short run to see whether the participants were adhering to their treatment programmes, and this is a necessary step in assessing programmes that require participants to administer part of their own programme. This may be less of a problem if organizationally-targeted treatments were applied (Newman and Beehr, 1979), since individuals would be less responsible for administering their own treatments. The parallel problem in organizationally-targeted programmes would be acceptability by those managers responsible for changing the organization or the stressful parts of it. At any rate, such programmes have seldom been tried to date.

Stressors as targets of change

In organizationally-targeted stress programmes, the causes or the job stressors are attacked rather than attempting to inoculate employees to withstand the existing stressors. Ganster et al. (1982) argued that the predominant person-centred approach, inoculation, even has ethical problems since the causes of the problems are not even considered for change. Instead, the attempt is to strengthen and patch up people so that they can continue to work in an inherently unhealthy workplace.

Regardless of the ethics of the person-as-target approach, it is logical that a stronger, more serious approach would attempt to treat the causes instead of only the effects of stress. Ganster, et al. (1982) argued that person-targeted occupational stress treatments are doomed to failure because of their relative weakness compared with other forces in the workplace. They cited a study (Timico and Gentili, 1976) in which the manipulation of pay systems (i.e. piecework versus salary) had a much larger effect on levels of catecholamines than the treatment programme used in their own study. This represents a dim view of the likelihood of success for person-targeted approaches to stress in the work setting; it is certainly true, however, that some stressors will not be susceptible to change with any reasonable chance of success. For example, the adverse weather conditions faced by farmers are nearly unalterable. In such cases, the inoculation approach is the only hope for success in treating work-related stress. If organizations are interested in the health of their employees, however, there are undoubtedly many more organizationally targeted possibilities than have been attempted.

Another consequence of the overwhelming use of person-targeted treatments in virtually all published reports of stress treatments in the workplace is that there is no evidence that the treatment is treating stress at all. Certain individual responses have apparently been accepted as stress (strains) by definition, and any attempt to treat them is labelled stress treatment. Typical of these personal reactions thought to be stress related are depression, anxiety, catecholamine secretions, cholesterol in the blood stream, and almost any risk factor in coronary heart disease. When programmes are designed to treat these and similar dependent variables, the problems are apparently labelled stress treatments and the label is accepted by employees and journal editors alike. The point is that they are not stress treatments unless there is some stressor known to have caused or at least been related to these responses, and the literature on stress-management programmes is virtually devoid of any such evidence. While it is certainly laudable to treat these problems, from a scientific and theoretical viewpoint these are not strictly stress treatments. For example, since diet is thought to be related to cholesterol in the blood stream, it is just as logical to assume that a participant's cholesterol level is due to his or her diet as to occupational stress (or any other type of stress). Similarly, since heredity is believed to be a major causal factor in coronary heart disease, it is just as logical to assume that a participant's coronary heart disease is due to his or her inherited factors as to job stress. Therefore, labelling such treatments as stress management or stress treatments in the absence of evidence gathered using the sample of participants themselves is nothing more than an unsubstantiated guess.

For those who are actually interested in stress, its treatments, and evaluation of its treatments, therefore, it is recommended that stressors be assessed as well as strains and that at least an association be established between the two in future work. Thus, in the workplace, such theoretically stressful organizational characteristics as role ambiguity, role overload, role conflict etc. should be measured in order to establish their relationship (if not causal role) with strains. Also stress treatments aimed at changing these presumed job stressors would be a welcome addition to the many programmes attempting to treat solely the 'strains'. Evaluating treatment-programmes without doing this amounts to a task of evaluating the general effectiveness of nearly all psychological and behavioural medicine treatments and many other medical treatments. While this would be a worthy and monumental task, it is not the same as evaluating occupational stress or other stress-treatment programmes.

Jackson (1983)—An organization-targeted treatment example

An experiment by Jackson (1983) provides an example of treatments targeting the organization and aimed at changing stressors directly instead of changing potential strains directly. The project used the Solomon four-group design (Campbell and Stanley, 1963) with an additional long-term (six-months) posttest. This design includes two experimental groups, one receiving a pretest and one not, and two control groups, one receiving a pretest and one not. It is a variation of the traditional experiment, with most threats to internal validity controlled.

In an outpatient facility of a university hospital, experimental groups of nurses' and white collar employees' working practices were changed by requiring unit heads to hold twice-per-month staff meetings. This intervention or treatment was conceived as a step toward participative management style, which some writers (e.g. Beehr, 1985; French and Caplan, 1973; Morris, Steers and Kock, 1979) have argued would lead to reduced stressors, particularly role stressors. Unit heads were trained in a two-day workshop in conducting meetings and especially in the use of the Nominal Group Technique (Delbecq, Van de Ven, and Gustafson, 1975), and they were provided with a list of potential meeting topics that was developed from structured interviews and a pilot survey of the facility's employees. Pretests were used to assess the effectiveness of the randomization procedure, and manipulation checks were undertaken to see whether the experimental groups had actually met twice per month and the other groups not. The primary dependent variables of interest for present purposes were the presumed job stressors, perceived role conflict and role ambuiguity, and these were indeed affected by the treatment. In addition, path analysis was used to assess the likelihood that these stressors could cause some other variables, including psychological strain. Demonstrating associations between stressors and strains is an important step in a complete approach to evaluating occupational stress treatments. The main point for present purposes, however, is that the final issue discussed in this chapter, the recommendation that organization treatments focus on changing stressors instead of only strains, is practical. This has been advocated by Newman and Beehr (1979), Ganster, et al. (1982), Jackson (1983), and Jayaratne and Chess (1984), among others, but it has rarely been attempted. The Jackson (1983) study illustrates this recommended approach.

REFERENCES

Adams, J. D. (1981). Health, stress and the manager's lifestyle, *Group and Organizational Studies*. **6**, 291–301.

Allen, J. K., and Blanchard, E. B. (1980). Biofeedback-based stress management training with a population of business managers, *Biofeedback and Self-Regulation*, **5**, 427–38.

Andrasik, F., Blanchard, E. B., and Neff, D. F. (1984). Biofeedback and relaxation training for chronic headache: A controlled comparison of booster treatments, and regular contacts for long-term maintenance. *Journal of Consulting and Clinical Psychology*, **52**, 609–15.

Appley, M., and Trumbull, R. (1967). *Psychological Stress*, New York, Appleton-Century-Crofts.

Bandeira, M., Bouchard, M. A., and Granger, L. (1982). Voluntary control of autonomic responses: A case for a dialogue between individual and group experimental methodologies. *Biofeedback and Self-Regulation*, **7**, 317–30.

Barlow, D. H., Blanchard, E. B., Hayes, S. C., and Epstein, L. H. (1977). Single-case designs and clinical biofeedback experimentation. *Biofeedback and Self-Regulation*, **2**, 221–39.

Beehr, T. A. (1984). Stress research: Approaches and issues. In A. S. Sethi and R. S. Schuler (eds.) *Handbook of Organizational Stress Coping Strategies*, Cambridge, MA., Ballinger.

Beehr, T. A. (1985). Organizational stress and employee effectiveness: A job characteristics approach. In T. A. Beehr and R. S. Bhagat (eds.) *Human Stress and Cognition in Organizations: An Integrated Perspective*, New York, Wiley & Sons.

Beehr, T. A., and Newman, J. E. (1978). Job stress, employee health, and organizational effectiveness. *Personnel Psychology*, **31**, 665–98.

Budzynski, T., Stoyva, J., Adler, C., and Mullaney, D. (1973). EMG biofeedback and tension headache: A controlled outcome study, *Psychosomatic Medicine*, **35**, 484–96.

Campbell, D. T., and Stanley, J. C. (1963). Experimental and quasi-experimental designs for research on teaching. In N. L. Gage (ed.) *Handbook of Research on Teaching*, Chicago, Rand McNally.

Carrington, P., Collings, G. H. Jr., Benson, H., Robinson, H., Wood, L. W., Leher, P. M., Woolfolk, R. L., and Cole, J. W. (1980). The use of meditation-relaxation techniques for the management of stress in a working population, *Journal of Occupational Medicine*, **22**, 221–31.

Cattell, R. B. (1957). *Self-Analysis Form*. Champaign, IL, IPAT.

Cohen, J. (1970). *Statistical Power Analysis for the Behavioural Sciences*, New York, Academic Press.

Cook, T. D., and Campbell, D. T. (1979). *Quasi-Experimentation: Design and Analysis Issues for Field Settings*, Chicago, Rand McNally.

Cooper, C. L., and Marshall, J. (1976). Occupational sources of stress: A review of the literature relating to coronary heart disease and mental ill health, *Journal of Occupational Psychology*, **49**, 11–28.

Cronbach, L. (1982). *Designing Evaluations of Educational and Social Programs*, San Francisco, Jossey-Bass.

Delbecq, A. L., Van de Ven, A. H., and Gustafson, D. H. (1975). *Group Techniques for Program Planning: A Guide to Nominal Group and Delphi Group Processes*. Glenview, IL, Scott, Foresman.

Ellis, A. (1962). *Reason and Emotion in Psychotherapy*, New York, Lyle Stuart.

Fergusen, G. A. (1981). *Statistical Analysis in Psychology and Education*, New York, McGraw-Hill.

Fielding, J. E. (1984). Health promotion and disease prevention at the worksite, *Annual Review of Public Health*, **5**, 237–65.

Forman, S. G. (1981). Stress-management training: Evaluation of effects of school psychological services, *Journal of School Psychology*, **19**, 233–41.

Frank, J. D. (1982). Biofeedback and the placebo effect. *Biofeedback and Self-Regulation*, **7**, 449–60.

French, J. R. P., jun., and Caplan, R. D. (1973). Organizational stress and individual strain. In A. J. Marrow (ed.) *The Failure of Success*, New York, AMACOM.

Friedman, M., and Rosenman, R. H. (1974). *Type A behavior and your heart*, New York, Alfred A. Knopf.

Ganster, D. C., Mayes, B. T., Sime, W. E., and Tharp, G. D. (1982). Managing organizational stress: A field experiment. *Journal of Applied Psychology*, **67**, 533–42.

Guglielmi, R. S., Roberts, A. H., and Patterson, R. (1982). Skin temperature biofeedback of Raynaud's disease: A double-blind study. *Biofeedback and Self-Regulation*, **7**, 99–120.

Hatch, J. P. (1982). Controlled group designs in biofeedback research: Ask, 'What does the control group control for?' *Biofeedback and Self-Regulation*, **7**, 377–401.

Hays, W. L. (1981). *Statistics for the Social Sciences* (3rd ed.). New York, Holt, Rinehart, and Winston.

Hendrix, W. H., Ovalle, N. K. Jun., and Troxler, R. G. (1985). Behavioral and physiological consequences of stress and its antecedent factors. *Journal of Applied Psychology*, **70**, 188–201.

Hiebert, B. A., and Fitzsimmons, G. (1981). A comparison of EMG feedback and alternative anxiety treatment programs. *Biofeedback and Self-Regulation*, **6**, 501–16.

Hoiberg, A. (1982). Occupational stress and illness incidence. *Journal of Occupational Medicine*, **24**, 445–51.

Holroyd, K. A., Penzien, D. B., Hursey, K. G., Tobin, D. L., Rogers, L., Holm, J. E., Marcille, P. J., Hall, J. R., and Chila, A. G. (1984). Change mechanism in EMG biofeedback training: Cognitive changes underlying improvements in tension headaches. *Journal of Consulting and Clinical Psychology*, **52**, 1039–53.

Ivancevich, J. M., and Matteson, M. T. (1980). *Stress and Work: A Managerial Perspective*, Glenview IL, Scott, Foresman.

Jackson, S. E. (1983). Participation in decision making as a strategy for reducing job-related strain. *Journal of Applied Psychology*, **68**, 3–19.

Jackson, S. E., and Schuler, R. S. (1985). A meta-analysis and conceptual critique of research on role ambiguity and role conflict in work setting, *Organizational Behavior and Human Decision Processes*, **36**, 16–78.

Karasek, R. A. Jun. (1979). Job demands, job design latitude, and mental strain: Implications for job redesign. *Administrative Science Quarterly*, **24**, 285–308.

Kasl, S. V. (1984), Stress and health, *Annual Review of Public Health*, **5**, 319–41.

Katkin, E. S., and Goldband, S. (1979). The placebo effect and biofeedback. In R. J. Gatchel and K. P. Price (eds.) *Clinical Applications of Biofeedback: Appraisal and Status*, New York, Pergamon Press.

Kerle, R. H., and Bialek, H. M. (1958). The construction validation, and application of a subjective stress scale (Staff Memorandum, Fighter IV, Study 23). Presidio of Monterey, CA: Human Resource Research Office (NTIS No. AD-489 875).

Kimmel, H. D. (1981). The relevance of experimental studies to clinical applications of biofeedback. *Biofeedback and Self-Regulation*, **6**, 263–71.

Kobasa, S. C. (1979). Stressful life events, personality, and health: An inquiry into hardiness, *Journal of Personality and Social Psychology*, **37**, 1–11.

Lang, P. J., and Twentyman, C. T. (1974). Learning to control heart rate, Binary vs. analogue feedback, *Psychophysiology*, **11**, 616–29.

Libo, L. M., and Arnold, G. E. (1983). Relaxation practice after biofeedback therapy: A long-term follow-up study of utilization and effectiveness, *Biofeedback and Self-Regulation*, **8**, 217–27.

Love, K. G., and Beehr, T. A. (1981). Social stressors on the job: Recommendations for a broader perspective, *Group and Organizational Studies*, **6**, 190–200.

Meichenbaum, D. H. (1975). A self-instructional approach to stress management: A proposal for stress inoculation training. In C. D. Spielberger and J. G. Sarason (eds.) *Stress and Anxiety* (Vol. 1), New York, Halsted Press.

Meichenbaum, D. H. (1977). *Cognitive Behavior Modification*. New York, Plenum Press.

Miller, N. E., and Dworkin, B. R. (1977). Critical issues in therapeutic applications of biofeedback. In G. E. Schwartz and J. Betty (eds.) *Biofeedback: Theory and Research*, New York, Academic Press.

Morris, J. H., Steers, R. M., and Koch, J. L. (1979). Influence of organizational structure on role conflict and ambiguity for three occupational groups, *Academy of Management Journal*, **22**, 58–71.

Murphy, L. R. (1984). Occupational stress management: A review and appraisal, *Journal of Occupational Psychology*, **57**, 1–15.

Newman, J. E., and Beehr, T. A. (1979). Personal and organizational strategies for handling job stress: A review of research and opinion. *Personnel Psychology*, **32**, 1–43.

Onoda, L. (1983). Handwarming and relaxation in temperature feedback: Positive placebo effects. *Biofeedback and Self-Regulation*, **8**, 109–14.

Rosen, R. H. (1984, August). The picture of health in the workplace, *Training and Development Journal*, **38**, 24–30.

Sallis, J. F., and Lichstein, K. L. (1979). The frontal electromyographic adaptation response: A potential source of confounding, *Biofeedback and Self-Regulation*, **4**, 337–9.

Schuler, R. S. (1980). Definition and conceptualization of stress in organizations, *Organizational Behavior and Human Performance*, **25**, 184–215.

Selye, H. (1974). *Stress Without Distress*, Philadelphia, J. B. Lippincott.

Shaw, E. R., and Blanchard, E. B. (1983). The effects of instructional set on the outcome of a stress management program, *Biofeedback and Self-Regulation*, **8**, 555–65.

Smith, P. C., Kendall, L. M., and Hulin, C. L. (1969). *The Measurement of Satisfaction in Work and Retirement*, Chicago, Rand McNally.

Spielberger, C., Gorsuch, R., and Lushene, R. (1970). *State-Trait Anxiety Inventory Manual*. Palo Alto, Consulting Psychologist Press.

Steiner, S. S., and Dince, W. M. (1981). Biofeedback efficacy studies: A critique of critiques, *Biofeedback and Self-Regulation*, **6**, 275–88.

Surwit, R. S., and Keefe, J. F. (1983). The blind leading the blind: Problems with the 'double blind' design in clinical biofeedback research. *Biofeedback and Self-Regulation*, **8**, 1–2.

Timio, M., and Gentili, S. (1976). Andrenosympathetic overactivity under conditions of work stress, *British Journal of Preventive Social Medicine*, **30**, 262–5.

von Baeyer, C., and Krause, L. (1983–4). Effectiveness of stress management training for nurses working in a burn treatment unit. *International Journal of Psychiatry in Medicine*, **13**, 113–26.

Wandelt, M. A., Pierce, P. M., and Widdowson, R. R. (1981). Why nurses leave nursing and what can be done about it, *American Journal of Nursing*, **81**, 72–7.

Yates, A. J. (1979). The physiopathology and treatment of functional disease: Including anxiety states and depression and the role of biofeedback training (G. B. Whatmore and D. R. Kohli authors; review essay). *Biofeedback and Self-Regulation*, **4**, 189–92.

Yorde, B. S., and Witmer, J. M. (1980). An educational format for teaching stress management to groups with a wide range of stress symptoms. *Biofeedback and Self-Regulation*, **5**, 75–90.

Zindler-Wernet, P., and Bailey, J. T. (1980). Coping with stress through an 'on-site' running program for Stanford ICU-nurses, *Journal of Nursing Education*, **19**, 34–7.

Chapter 5

The Interplay of Research Design Strategies and Data Analysis Procedures in Evaluating the Effects of Stress on Health

Ronald C. Kessler

Department of Sociology and Institute for Social Research
The University of Michigan, Michigan

The most fundamental question asked by stress researchers is whether stress causes ill health. Yet, despite an enormous amount of research over several decades, we still have only limited information about this fundamental question. The slow pace of our progress is due largely to the fact that experimental investigations of major stress effects cannot be carried out on humans for ethical reasons. The effects of major stresses like job loss and widowhood have consequently been studied primarily with naturalistic methods, and these methods provide evidence about causation which is inherently equivocal.

Three sorts of experimental literatures have nonetheless developed to provide indirect information about the effects of major stresses. One of these involves the physiological effects of stress on animals (Turkkam et al., 1982). A good deal has been learned from these investigations about the links between a stressful situation and short-term physiological responses. The second sort of experimental evidence comes from laboratory studies in which humans are exposed to mild forms of stress (Selye, 1982). We have learned a considerable amount about the effects of psychological mediating variables from this paradigm, but it is not clear whether studies of such mild stresses generalize to more serious stress situations (Silver and Wortman, 1980). Finally, a series of field experiments has been conducted among people who experienced some serious stress like job loss of widowhood (Price et al., 1980). These experiments manipulate some of the presumed intervening or moderating variables in the stress–health relationship to study the preventive effects of interventions. While not designed in such a way that the effects of stress can be evaluated directly, these studies document the range within which an association between stress and health can be modified.

Despite their importance, all of these experimental paradigms are limited in

Research Methods in Stress and Health Psychology. Edited by S. V. Kasl and C. L. Cooper.

the evidence they provide about the effects of stress. Even the intervention experiments, which provide the most direct evidence of this sort, are based on extensive non-experimental research aimed at selecting the most likely candidates among the many different resources and vulnerabilities which could be targets of intervention. Other non-experimental research is also needed to trace out intervening links between stress and health. When reliable evidence about pathways is available, research is needed on the factors which help short-circuit the relationship between stress and health and on the factors which increase resistance to the effects of stress.

All of these research agendas raise questions about causal associations which have to be studied non-experimentally. As our understanding increases, the causal links investigated become more complex, but the basic problems of carrying out causal inquiries with non-experimental data remain the same. The poverty of our methods for making causal imputations retards our progress here. Uncertainty about causal links is an inherent part of non-experimental investigation. Nonetheless, it is important to make whatever efforts one can to discount rival hypotheses about the influence of stress. This is not done in conventional practice. This failing can only work against efforts to isolate potent stress effects.

In this chapter, I discuss the main approaches available for making reliable causal imputations with non-experimental data. It is my hope that this discussion will serve as a guide to stress researchers who work with non-experimental data and who are concerned about the validity of their causal interpretations. Several data analysis and design strategies are discussed which have not been presented before to stress researchers. Each of these has promise for reducing the range of ambiguity about causal links. In addition, I discuss limitations of several design and analysis strategies which are commonly used by stress researchers.

The problems of documenting whether a particular stress causes a particular health outcome differ considerably depending on whether the stress under consideration is a specific event or an ongoing situation. Therefore, I treat life events and chronic stresses separately.

DOCUMENTING THE HEALTH-DAMAGING EFFECTS OF LIFE EVENTS

Measurement bias

There are two basic types of life event studies. One focuses on a single event, like job loss or widowhood. Studies of this type often obtain data at multiple points in time in order to study the process of adjustment. Yet they are usually retrospective in the sense that they draw the sample of respondents after the event has occurred. They sometimes include a control group of respondents who did not experience the event.

The other type of life event study obtains information on a wide variety of events in a general population survey. Respondents are usually presented with a check-list of events and asked to report which of these occurred to them over some recent interval of time. Studies of this type vary in the time interval and in the length of the life event inventory investigated. Some of these surveys are longitudinal, in which case they can assess the occurrence of events after some baseline health assessment.

Accuracy of event measurement is problematic in each of these approaches. In the focused assessment of a particular event, it is usually necessary to sample from an incomplete sampling frame. For example, if rape victims who experience the most intense emotional reactions are least likely to contact the police, a researcher using police records to obtain a sample of rape victims will probably underestimate the emotional impact of this event (Burgess and Holmstrom, 1979).

A different type of measurement problem arises in surveys which assess many events at once. In this design, the respondent is asked to report restrospectively any event that occurred over an interval of time. The problem is that respondents may incorrectly recall events which occurred at an earlier time but which they report as having occurred in the time interval under investigation (the problem of 'telescoping'), or they may forget to report events that actually occurred in the time-interval under investigation. If people who are most distressed by an event are also most likely to telescope and/or to recall, then the observed association between self-reported exposure and distress will be larger than the true association. There is evidence that this sort of systematic bias exists in retrospective life event reports (Clark and Teasdale, 1982; Nelson and Craighead, 1977).

If a researcher seriously wants to evaluate the health damaging effect of a life event, every attempt must be made to assure that these measurement biases are removed from his data. Samples of people who experienced a particular event should be selected from a representative sampling frame, even if this requires expensive screening. Retrospective reports about exposure to events on a check-list should be dated carefully to minimize telescoping and respondents should be asked about exposure in ways that trigger recall (Biderman and Moore, 1980; Jabine et al., 1984).

The case of random exposure

Once measurement problems are resolved, the most simple case to consider is one in which exposure to a life event occurs for reasons which are random with respect to the health outcome under investigation. This situation occurs by design in experiments and sometimes happens in nature, as when a tornado touches down and destroys one particular block of homes but none on adjoining blocks. In a situation of this sort, it is conventional to interpret an association between event exposure and the health outcome as evidence that the event had a health-damaging impact.

This association can be described as:

$$H_i = b_0 + b_1 LE_i + e_i, \tag{1}$$

where H_i is the health outcome for person i, LE_i is a dichotomous variable describing that person's exposure to the life event, and e_i is his prediction error. The coefficients b_0 and b_1 are parameters which can be estimated from the observed values of LE and H across a sample of people who are sampled in such a way that there is variance in LE_i.

When exposure to LE is randomly assigned and LE is measured accurately, the association between LE_i and e_i will be random and the parameters of the model can be estimated without bias. In particular, $\hat{b}_1$ is an unbiased estimate of the life event effect. This is true no matter what the distributions of the variables, so long as the sample was drawn using probability methods. If a further assumption is made about the distribution of e_i in the population from which the sample is drawn, confidence intervals can be placed around the parameter estimate for b_1.

The practical problem here is that very few life events occur that are entirely random with respect to the outcomes of interest. Even seemingly random events like the death of a loved one occur more often to lower-class than middle-class people and to the old more often than to the young. These structural determinants are associated with a wide variety of health outcomes, which means that an attempt to estimate the health damaging effects of such events on the assumption that they occurred randomly would yield biased estimates of life event effects.

In some cases, though, it is possible to regain inferential power by constructing a matched comparison group.

Matching

There are many cases where the assumption of random event exposure is plausible *within some range* of comparison. Indeed, this is true in most cases if the researcher is willing to consider a sufficiently narrow range of comparison.

Most uses of matching are fairly mechanical—like making sure that the age, sex, and other demographic distributions of cases and controls are comparable. The real power of matching, though, comes in finding a subpopulation within which it can plausibly be assumed that exposure to the event under investigation was truly random. In an investigation of job loss, for example, it is not enough to determine that respondents were part of a plant closing that occurred for reasons which were random with respect to their behaviours. If the health damaging effects of this event are to be assessed accurately, it is also necessary to select a comparison group of stably employed people who are as similar as possible to the job losers in all respects related to the health outcomes.[1] A general population sample of stably employed people will not do here, because plant closings occur more often in some industries than others. This means that the social class backgrounds and occupational health risks to which job losers have been exposed will differ from those of 'typical' workers in the general population. Failure to select an appropriate comparison group will consequently introduce bias into the estimate of b_1 based on Eq.(1).

The limiting condition in finding a comparison group is that the range within which exposure to the event can be considered random is often quite narrow. For example, even though we would not normally think that a drunk driver's involvement in an automobile accident was a random event, it would be legitimate to think of it as random within a matched sample of drunk drivers who were on the road the same time of night and differed in accident involvement for reasons which were random with respect to their own behaviours (like hazardous driving conditions which varied from one road to another).

Some researchers might not find the population within which an event can be considered a random occurrence an interesting one to study. Yet it is important to recognize that no matter what data analysis strategy or research design one uses to study the effects of life events, each event has a well defined range of the population over which exposure was random. This range is not always apparent to the researcher, but it exists, it varies from one event to another, and it plays a part in shaping estimates of life event effects even when the researcher fails to take it into consideration. The researcher should develop sufficient knowledge about the events he studies to define this range of valid inference and understand the implications of matching for making estimates of event effects.

This kind of careful analysis and understanding of the appropriate matched comparison group is seldom made in stress research. The far more common strategy is to use control variables in a multivariate analysis to approximate matching. This approach can yield valid inferences of causal impact if certain restrictive conditions are met by the data. It is my impression, though, that neither the nature of these restrictions nor their low likelihood of being fulfilled empirically are appreciated by most stress researchers. The next few subsections review variants on this multivariate control approach and make explicit the conditions under which they can be used to make valid causal inferences.

The regression–discontinuity approach

Although only rarely used to make causal inferences, it is useful to consider a special case of the multivariate control approach before turning to the more general case. The regression–discontinuity approach is possible when exposure to the life event is known and *completely* determinate. For example, the impact of retirement might be evaluated with this approach by focusing on industries where retirement is totally determined by age. The impact of job loss could be studied in precisely the same way in plants where seniority completely determines who is laid off.

The regression–discontinuity approach creates a synthetic comparison group with adjusted levels of the outcome variable by studying the relationship between the selection variable—age or seniority in the above examples—and the outcome among respondents who were not exposed to the event. This relationship is imputed to the sample of respondents who experienced the event to provide an expected value of the outcome in the absence of the event. The expected value is compared to the observed value to estimate the impact of the event (Trochim, 1984).

This adjustment procedure is typically carried out in a revised version of Eq.(1) as follows:

$$H_i = b_0 + b_1 LE_i + b_2 S_i + b_3 S_i^2 + e_i \qquad (2)$$

where S is the selection factor which determines exposure to LE.[2] For an elegant example of this approach, see Berk and Rauma (1983).

The multivariate control approach

The multivariate control approach uses the logic of multivariate analysis to estimate the causal impact of a life event in cases where exposure to the event is assumed to be non-random with respect to H. A typical model might be:

$$H_i = b_0 + b_1 LE_i + b_2 C_{1i} + \ldots + b_{n+1} C_{ni} + e_i, \qquad (3)$$

where C_1 through C_n are determinants of H which are correlated with LE. If this model is correct in expressing the causal links to H, then $\hat{b}_1$ yields an unbiased estimate of the life event effect.

The practical problem in using this approach is that we seldom understand the determinants of H sufficiently well to include all relevant control variables in the prediction equation. Sometimes unmeasured causes can be very subtle. For example, in studying the emotional impact of being in an industrial accident, we should take into consideration that people who select themselves into dangerous jobs are temperamentally quite different from people who choose low-risk jobs. Personality determinants of job selection have been documented (Kohn and Schooler, 1982). Yet it is a nearly hopeless task, given our primitive understanding, to think that we could measure all such relevant variables in a multivariate control analysis.[3]

No statement whatever can be made about the direction or magnitude of bias introduced into the estimate of b_1 by the omission of a relevant control variable unless the researcher has more understanding about the omitted variables than one usually has. This is one of the main results in the literature on specification error (Duncan, 1975, 101–12). It means, among other things, that there is no reason to believe that an estimate of b_1 obtained in a model with incomplete controls will be any more accurate than an estimate obtained in a model which omits control variables entirely.

The longitudinal analysis approach

A popular corrective to this problem is to measure the outcome variable prior to the time when the event occurred. In this approach, the assumption is made that by controlling the earlier value of H one can successfully adjust for initial differences between subjects who subsequently were exposed to the event and those who were not, thus yielding an unbiased estimate of b_1.

This assumption is seldom based on a clear consideration of the ways in which bias is produced. As we will see below, the use of H_{t-1} as a control variable will correct for missing variable bias only in a restrictive set of situations. Three cases will be considered: (a) where H_{t-1} is the only omitted variable from the prediction equation that both affects H_t and is associated with LE; (b) where some predictors other than H_{t-1} are omitted from the prediction equation and H_{t-1} itself is not a significant predictor of H_t; and (c) where both H_{t-1} and other omitted variables are important predictors of H_t.

(a) The first case to consider is one in which the outcome variable affects exposure to the event. For example, alcohol problems can lead to job loss and this fact can pose problems for a researcher who is interested in evaluating the impact of job loss on drinking habits. If we attempted to estimate the impact of this event using Eq.(3) without controlling for prior drinking behaviour, we would obtain a biased estimate.

This problem can be overcome if we obtain longitudinal information (or accurate retrospective information) and control for earlier levels of drinking. However if we are mistaken in the time lag we pick between measures of H in the longitudinal analysis, we can introduce bias into the prediction equation even when we have data collected prior to the occurrence of LE. To see how this might happen, assume that H affects LE with a time lag of one unit. A situation of this sort might exist, for example, if we obtained data once a year over several years and found out that a worker's emotional functioning (H) predicted whether he would be fired (LE) over the next year. We also assume that LE affects H without a lag, which in this case would mean that job loss would affect emotional functioning immediately (within the year).

If we accurately obtained data of this sort over two waves of a panel we could estimate all the coefficients in this model without bias. In particular, we could estimate the equation:

$$H_3 = b_0 + b_1 LE_3 + b_2 H_2, \tag{4}$$

The subscripts for individuals have been dropped from this equation for ease of presentation. This means that the term e_i, included in earlier equations, has also been dropped. The subscripts associated with the variables now refer to time, with H_3 representing the expectation of the H score in the aggregate at time 3, and the other variables having similar interpretations.

Let us now consider the case where we incorrectly assumed that the causal lag was two years rather than one, so that we measured H_1 rather than H_2. In this situation, we would estimate the equation:

$$H_3 = b_0^* + b_1^* LE_3 + b_2^* H_1, \tag{5}$$

and interpret the estimate of b_1^* as if it were the same as b_1 in Eq.(4). Calculations of the reduced-form equations show that b_1^* yields a biased estimate of b_1. This bias is equal to:

$$b_2 b_{H_2LE_3}(1- R^2_{H_1H_2}). \tag{6}$$

which is the fraction of the missing variable bias due to H_1 not being a perfect proxy for H_2. Typically this bias will act to inflate the estimate of b_1 in Eq.(5) because both b_2 and $b_{H_2LE_3}$ will be positive.

This bias will not be severe when the health outcome is highly stable over time because H_1 will be a good proxy for H_2 (Kessler and Greenberg, 1981). In situations where H is unstable, though, the bias can be enormous. For example, imagine a situation where a worker's emotional functioning deteriorated rapidly in an acute episode of major depressive disorder and his supervisor fired him. A prediction equation which assessed baseline levels of emotional functioning several years earlier would totally miss this process of selection into unemployment and would overestimate wildly the impact of unemployment on emotional functioning.

This problem of time misspecification is almost never considered by stress researchers. Yet in those few cases where time lags are examined—largely in time-series investigations focused on the relationship between unemployment and health—estimates of stress effects have been extremely sensitive to both the choice of time period and the time lag structure (Gravelle, et al., 1981).

(b) The next case to consider is one in which the outcome variable is affected by some unmeasured common causes of H and LE, but where the lagged value of H does not directly affect the outcome. This situation applies most readily to an acute health problem which has no meaningful internal consistency over time.

In this case, the true structural equation would be as in Eq.(3), and the researcher would attempt to correct for the inability to measure C_1 through C_n by using H_{t-1} as a control in Eq.(4). This approach would yield a biased estimate of the life event effect for the same reason sketeched out in case (a) above; namely, that H_{t-1} is almost certainly an inadequate proxy variable for all of the relevant variables which were omitted from the prediction equation.

This limitation is seldom grasped by researchers who work with two-wave panel data. The intuitive form of the argument against this approach is that while measurement of H_{t-1} adjusts for baseline differences in *levels* of H it does not adjust for baseline differences in *trajectories* of H.[4]

There is no way to correct for this bias completely. However, it is possible to estimate the magnitude of the bias by bounding the estimate of b_1. This approach makes use of the fact that when H_{t-1} does not appear in the structural equation it is possible to use first differences to eliminate all unmeasured C variables which are constant over time. In a similar fashion, by making certain restrictive assumptions about the ways in which the unmeasured C variables change it is possible to estimate upper and lower limits on the true value of b_1. In some cases, these two bounds will be close to each other, in which case the researcher will have evidence that omitted control variables did not importantly distort the estimate of b_1. The technique used to generate these bounded estimates is discussed in Kessler (1983) and will not be repeated here.

(c) The situations considered so far are those in which H_{t-1} is either the only omitted variable or other C variables but not H_{t-1} appear in the true structural equation. In each of these two cases it is possible to use H_{t-1} to improve the estimate of b_1. The third case we will consider is one in which H_{t-1} and other C variables are all important predictors of H_t in the true structural equation. In this third situation, the use of H_{t-1} as a control variable will not lead to an improved estimate of b_1 if some of the other important C variables are omitted from the equation. This is a special case of the general conclusion stated above (see the section: Multivariate control approach), that incomplete control for omitted variables will not produce estimates of b_1 which are better than those obtained in a model which omits control variables entirely. In this third case—which I judge to be much more common than the two cases considered earlier—use of longitudinal data yields no improvement whatever in the researcher's ability of evaluate the impact of stress on health.

Overview

Our review has shown that there are serious problems with most approaches used to assess the impact of life events. The only exception is the case where we can assume that exposure to the event was random. This assumption is plausible in a far wider variety of situations than most researchers realize, especially when we recognize that any assumption of this sort requires the researcher to specify an appropriate matched comparison group.

The use of matching is not possible, though, in research which uses a life event inventory to study the effects of events. Selection factors are too complex to generate meaningful comparison groups for an analysis based on a single measure of life event exposure constructed from a list containing many different events. For all such research, then, other less rigorous approaches are required if we want to make some provisional assessment of life event effects.

Yet these other methods are all limited in serious ways. The regression–discontinuity design offers a powerful solution but the requirements for its use are strict. Furthermore, violation of these assumptions has a profound effect on the estimation of b_1.

Outside this fairly powerful strategy we have either non-experimental standardization through multivariate regression procedures or the somewhat more flexible approach made possible with panel data. The latter is more general in that no special insight is required into the confounding influences but it requires that specification of the time lag is exact or that the outcome variable is highly stable or that some restrictive assumption can be made about the behaviour of the unmeasured variables. We seldom have sufficient understanding of the processes under investigation to meet these requirements. This is an important and widely overlooked fact among researchers who call for the collection of longitudinal data to help resolve uncertainties about causal order.

DOCUMENTING THE HEALTH-DAMAGING EFFECTS OF CHRONIC STRESS

It is common to find that people who report chronic emotional distress also report that they are experiencing problems in one or more of their central life roles—difficulties at work, a troubled marriage or ongoing financial problems. The researcher would like to assess the extent to which chronic stresses like these are causes of the distress.

A major problem in making this assessment is that both the emotional disability and the chronic stress typically have been going on for such a long time that an unambiguous decision as to which one came first is difficult to make. Respondents have a hard time retrospectively reconstructing the temporal order. There is usually no particular event that marks the beginning of the stress period, nor any clear way to date the time when the distress first began.

The task of making a causal imputation is even more difficult because one can seldom assume that stress exposure occurred for reasons which were random with respect to the respondent's emotional functioning. In fact, there can be selection *into* exposure (e.g. mate selection as a precursor of a troubled marriage) and *out* of exposure (e.g. differential likelihood of seeking a divorce) once the stress has occurred.

The technical problems that arise in attempting to develop explicit mathematical models of these selection processes are overwhelming.

As we shall see below, these complexities make it much more difficult to make reliable assessments of chronic stress effects than life event effects. Nonetheless, there are some opportunities for making inferences about the effects of chronic stress which are feasible. These require somewhat different research designs and analysis strategies than we have reviewed so far.

Measurement bias

A central problem that arises in studies of chronic stress involves the use of self-report stress measures. These are widely used because chronic stress is difficult to measure objectively. The problem in using such measures is that we are never sure what we are measuring, because influences other than the actual stress situation can play a part in shaping perceptions. In particular, a relationship between self-reported exposure to a stressful situation and emotional functioning might reflect the influence of emotional functioning on perception as much as the influence of the situation on functioning.

There is an analysis strategy available to help separate reciprocal influences like these. This approach has not been used in any study of chronic stress effects which I know about. It is ideally suited to the case where subjective appraisal of the stress situation mediates the relationship between the situation and the health outcome. This is the case suggested by Lazarus' influential model of the stress process (Lazarus and Folkman, 1984). An unbiased estimate of the influence of appraisal on the outcome requires the researcher to adjust for the reverse influence of the outcome on self-reported stress (Dohrenwend et al., 1984; see also Dohrenwend and Shrout, 1985; Lazarus et al., 1985).

This kind of adjustment can be made when there is an indicator of the objective stress situation available which is independent of the respondent's perception. This indicator need not be as complete a measure as if this were the only stress measure used in the prediction equation, but it has to be sufficiently strong to have a meaningful association with the outcome variable. This kind of situation is often encountered in studies of occupational stress, when an objective measure of the job environment is available from independent ratings. Even an indirect indicator would do here, like a measure based on Dictionary of Occupational Titles job condition ratings (Roos and Treiman, 1980).

The critical assumption required to make the necessary adjustment for measurement bias is that the objective stress condition affects health only through the intervening mechanism of subjective stress appraisal. This assumption is particularly plausible when the health outcome is some measure of emotional functioning. In this case, we can assume that the partial regression of H on the objective stress measure (S) is zero once the subjective measure of stress appraisal (A) is controlled. This means that we can express the effect of A on H at the individual level as:

$$H_i = b_0 + b_1 A_i + e_i. \tag{7}$$

The reciprocal effect of H on A can be expressed as:

$$A_i = d_0 + d_1 H_i + d_2 S_i + f_i. \tag{8}$$

Control variables could be introduced into either of these two equations without loss of generality in the results to be derived below.

The important feature of these two equations is that A appears as a predictor of H and H appears as a predictor of A. In general, coupled equations like these cannot be solved without bias. In particular, conventional single-equation estimation procedures cannot be used to derive an unbiased estimate of b_1 from Eq.(7) because A_i and e_i cannot be assumed to be uncorrelated. (There is an association between e_i and A_i because e_i helps determine H_i and H_i helps determine A_i.)

However, in the special case considered here—where we are willing to assume that S affects A but does not affect H—it is possible to obtain an unbiased estimate of b_1 by the method of *instrumental variables*. This method was developed by econometricians and has a long history of use in econometrics, where problems of reciprocal influence are common occurrences (Fisher, 1965).

An instrumental variable is a variable which is assumed to affect one and only one of two variables in a reciprocally related pair. The instrumental variable can 'stand in' for the variable it is assumed to cause in a reduced-form equation, thereby identifying the influence of the variable for which it is standing in even though the latter is not included in the equation.

It is relatively simple to demonstrate how this is done in the present example. We begin by obtaining the reduced-form equations in which the effects of A on H and H on A are removed from the structural equations. This is done by substituting the expression for A_i on the right side of Eq.(8) into Eq.(7) and by substituting the expression for H_i on the right side of Eq.(7) into Eq.(8). After rearranging terms, these manipulations yield the following expressions:

$$H_i = \frac{b_0 + b_1 d_0}{1 - b_1 d_1} + \frac{b_1 d_2}{1 - b_1 d_1} S + \frac{e_i + b_1 f_i}{1 - b_1 d_1} \tag{9a}$$

$$= b_0^* + b_1^* S + e_i^* \tag{9b}$$

$$A_i = \frac{d_0 + d_1 b_0}{1 - b_1 d_1} + \frac{d_2}{1 - b_1 d_1} S + \frac{f_i + d_1 e_i}{1 - b_1 d_1} \tag{10a}$$

$$= d_0^* + d_1^* S + f_i^* \tag{10b}$$

The causal influence of S on H—b_1 in Eq.(7)—is estimated by the ratio b_1^*/d_1^* in the reduced-form equations. The latter can be estimated by conventional single-equation regression procedures. The effect of H of S—d_1 in Eq.(8)—is not identified. Indeed, none of the coefficients in Eq.(7) or Eq.(8) other than b_1 is identified.

In cases where multiple intervening variables are assumed to exist—for example, when we believe that several different perceived job stresses affect emotional adjustment to the occupational setting—an extension of this approach is possible in which multiple reciprocal relationships are estimated simultaneously, using the same logic as above. All that one needs is at least one instrumental variable for each of the subjective stress measures.

This approach can also be used to estimate the influence of H on A if an instrumental variable for the H equation is available. The single-equation estimation procedure described here, which is known as indirect least squares, can only be used when there is a single instrumental variable in an equation. A more precise estimate of b_1 is possible when there are two or more instrumental variables. A discussion of estimation procedures for this more general case can be found in any standard text on simultaneous equation models (Duncan, 1975, 91–100).

Matching

The above discussion assumed that selection into chronic stress exposure was random with respect to the outcome variable. We have already noted that this is unlikely to be the case in most applications. So some design adjustment is needed if a valid estimate of b_1 is to be made, even with the sophisticated instrumental variable approach we have yet outlined.

As in the case of life event analysis, the most appealing way to make such an adjustment is by matching cases and controls. This can most easily be done for chronic stresses which are essentially random within some well-defined subsample of the population and which are relatively *inescapable* once they have occurred. A good example is the matched comparison of parents whose children have a chronic health problem with those whose children are healthy. The impact of the child's health problem on the parents can be evaluated directly by using Eq.(1).

It is important to focus on chronic stress situations that are relatively inescapable because selection *out* of exposure to the stress can lead to bias in the estimate of stress effects even when initial exposure is random. For example, it might be that the supervisory style of one's foreman is a random situation which has implications for the job stresses to which blue collar workers are exposed. Nonetheless, if job turnover rates are higher in work groups with demanding foremen, it is possible that an estimate of b_1 will be biased even though initial exposure to different levels of demand was random.

Under some circumstances, it is possible to use an analysis approach which corrects for selection bias in situations where initial exposure was random but continued exposure is related to the health outcome under investigation. This approach is due to Heckman (1979). The fundamental insight in this approach is that selective attrition from a chronic stress situation leads to bias in the estimation of stress effects identical to the bias introduced by the omission of an important predictor variable from the structural equation. The adjustment procedure to correct for this bias creates a synthetic variable which measures each respondent's probability of attrition from the stress situation and then uses a transformation of this variable in the prediction equation to control for the bias introduced by attrition.

I will not explain this approach technically. The mathematical derivation is complex and cannot easily be summarized without assuming more statistical background on the part of readers than is reasonable. A detailed technical description can be found in Heckman (1979). Instead, I will provide an intuitive introduction for readers who might want to know if they should invest the time and energy needed to master the technical details of the approach.

The basic strategy is to estimate a pair of equations. The first estimates the probability of attrition from the sample while the second is a substantive equation which estimates the influence of stress on the health outcome. Results from the first equation are used to create a control variable for the second equation.

In the first equation, the researcher compares people who have remained in the stress situation to those who have left it. The estimation of this equation might require some ingenuity on the part of the investigator in tracking down people who have quit undesirable jobs or left unfulfilling marriages or in some other way selected themselves out of stressful situations. A probit equation should be used here to use information about the individual and the situation to predict whether he remained in the situation or left.

This equation yields a predicted probability of attrition for each person studied. These probabilities, in turn, can be used to calculate a *hazard rate* (*HR*) of attrition for respondents who actually remained in the situation under study. The hazard rate is a non-linear function of the attrition probability which can be used as a control variable in the substantive equation to remove selection bias. Under the assumption that *initial* exposure to the stress was random, an unbiased estimate of the stress effect can be obtained by solving an equation with the expectation:

$$H = b_0 + b_1S + b_2HR. \qquad (11)$$

In a situation where one is evaluating the effect of appraised stress and some adjustment is required for measurement bias, an instrumental variable approach can be combined with this hazard rate correction procedure by including *HR* as a predictor in each of the instrumental variable reduced-form equations.

The main difficulty in implementing the hazard rate correction procedure is that information about people who have left stressful situations is usually unavailable. Typical studies of chronic stress obtain information from workers who remain on the job but not from those who quit, from people who remain in their marriages but not from those who divorced, and so on. In the absence of some information about the people who selected themselves out of situations which they might have considered stressful, and about the characteristics of these situations, it is not possible to use the analysis scheme described here.

Three feasible approaches are possible for solving this problem. The first is to draw a sample of attriters at the same time one draws the sample of respondents who are currently in the stress situation. A sample of people who have been divorced could be selected at the same time one draws a sample of people in their first marriages. Interviews with the attrition sample can be much shorter than with respondents in the sample of substantive interest because our concern is only with obtaining information from attriters which can be used to estimate an attrition probit equation. Furthermore, attriters can be sampled at a different rate than the substantive sample. We might design a study, for example, in which 1000 married people are targeted for interviews about the stresses of marriage while a sample of only 100 divorced people are targeted for interviews about the determinants of their divorces. When differential probabilities of selection are used in this way, weighting to population probabilities can be used to adjust probit estimates of attrition probabilities or a logistic approximation to the probit equation can be estimated from the unweighted data (Hanushek and Jackson, 1977, 187–205).

This first strategy is infeasible when the sampling frame is a small fraction of the general population because extensive screening would be required to obtain a sample of attriters. (The exception is when there is a comprehensive list of attriters, as there may be of people who quit their jobs in a certain company.) A second approach is to collect panel data and observe attrition over time. Data obtained at baseline could be used in this design to predict subsequent attrition within subgroups of the panel defined by their tenure in the situation at baseline. These sub-group probit equations could then be used to generate a set of predicted probabilities of *cumulative* attrition in a discrete time approach. The hazard rate adjustment could then be applied to substantive analysis of the panel sample.

In some special cases a third strategy is possible which is more easy to implement than the first two. This uses information about attrition rates in an analysis based on a two-part sampling scheme of situations and individuals. For example, we might want to study the impact of job stress by assessing the health of fifty employees in each of 100 different job settings. Aggregate information about the settings would be used to generate information about job stress and the 100 settings would be selected in such a way that selection into one particular setting compared to the others could be assumed to be random. In a design of this sort, we could make an adjustment for attrition bias merely by obtaining information on attrition rates in each of the settings. No attempt need be made to interview any of the people who quit their jobs in these settings. Information on attrition rates could be used to estimate a *group-level* probit equation, where the sample size is set at n = 100 settings and the observed probits are used as outcomes (Hanushek and Jackson, 1977, p. 189). The hazard rates calculated from this equation could then be applied to the substantive equation where the health damaging effects of the job stresses are examined among the $n = 5000$ individual respondents. This adjustment would automatically remove the bias introduced by the fact that attrition rates are likely to be higher in those settings which are most stressful and by the fact that workers who experience the greatest health impairments from the stressful situations are most likely to leave their jobs.

The multivariate control approach

In situations where exposure is clearly not random, the conventional approach is to introduce control variables which the researcher hopes will adjust for specification bias. As we already discussed (see the first section on Matching, above), the problem of incomplete control makes this approach hopelessly inadequate in most applications.[5]

The inadequacy of the naive multivariate control approach is demonstrated clearly by considering recent work on the relationship between job demands and worker health. (For a review, see Kahn, 1981.)[6] A common research design used here is to conduct a general population survey of employed men in which each respondent is asked to describe the conditions of his work. A multivariate approach is then used to assess relationships among a variety of different work stresses and the health of these respondents.

These analyses typically introduce controls for selection factors which are preconditions for certain jobs—like education. Yet even if we grant that controls of this sort might be adequate, it is still doubtful whether the results of such analyses would yield valid information about the health damaging effects of job conditions.

The problem with this approach can be understood intuitively if we begin with a consideration of the experimental analogue. Control variables are used in multivariate analysis to adjust for non-random exposure to job stresses so that the relationship between these stresses and health outcomes can be interpreted *as if* jobs had been randomly assigned. But think for a moment about this ideal. Imagine what would happen if we actually carried out an experiment in which we randomly assigned respondents within each education category to the full array of jobs which exist in the general population. People with a grade school education would be proportionally assigned to jobs which require complex technical skills while those with technical training would be proportionally assigned to jobs which require heavy physical labour and little decision latitude. The mismatch of people and jobs would be immense and the result would almost certainly be that aggregate rates of stress-related illness would be much higher in the experimental sample than in the normal population.

This hypothetical experiment would fail to provide useful information about the influence of job stress on worker health because it would lack external validity. It would assign people with diverse backgrounds across a range of job conditions that is considerably greater than the actual distribution in the general population.

Yet researchers who work with general population samples that include such a diverse array of people engage in an enterprise which has the same validity problems as this experiment. Such an exercise cannot provide valid information about the effects of job stress on worker health.

It is important to note that an analysis of this sort can provide useful *descriptive* information about the types of job settings which are associated with high rates of particular health problems. No control variables are needed for such an analysis. Once high risk jobs are isolated, more focused efforts can be used to develop matched comparisons which would justify causal inferences about the effects of particular job settings.

The longitudinal analysis approach

We already discussed (see the section: Longitudinal analysis approach, above) that longitudinal analysis has limitations which are much more serious than many researchers realize. The limitations are particularly clear in the analysis of chronic stress effects, for stresses of this type are slow to change. In those few cases where change does occur, furthermore, it tends to occur in an uneven way which is often associated with some life event. This makes it difficult to determine whether it was the event or the change in chronic conditions which caused any associated change in health (Converse et al., 1983).

A good example of the complexities involved here can be found in the analysis of machine-paced repetitive work. It has been observed consistently that blue collar workers whose jobs are paced by machines (as they are on an assembly-line) have poorer mental health than blue collar workers who control the pace of their work (Kasl, 1978). The substantive question is whether this association can be taken as evidence that this particular job condition causes poor mental health. Other plausible interpretations are that (a) workers who are in poor mental health are less capable of obtaining a more desirable job and that (b) workers who hold machine-paced jobs are less likely to advance to a more desirable job if they are in poor mental health.

The issue I want to consider is whether longitudinal data could help us adjudicate among these contending interpretations. This could happen if change between waves of data collection could be used to provide insight into the causal dynamics of the association between the control of work pace and the worker's mental health. Three types of change are possible: (a) the work setting could change from self-paced to machine-paced work (or vice versa); (b) there could be a change in the intensity of work pace in settings where the work is paced by machine; (c) workers could change to a new job which differed from their old job in whether the pace of work was controlled by machine. We consider each of these three changes separately.

(a) The first kind of change is associated with an event—a change in the conditions of work. As a result, all of the considerations raised earlier about the analysis of life event effects apply here. In particular, it should be relatively easy to determine why the conditions of work changed and whether this was unrelated to the worker's prior behaviour. If exposure is random, causal imputation is much more clear than it would be otherwise.

There are two complications to consider here. One is that some workers may decide to change jobs when the conditions of work change. It is likely that this attrition will be associated with the mental health effects of the change in job conditions, which means that failure to take drop-out into consideration will bias the estimate of mental health effects among workers who remain in the sample. This problem can be corrected by using the sample selection bias correction procedure already described (see the second section on Matching, above).

The second complication is that the analogy with a life event confounds the interpretation of chronic stress effects. It might be that short-term mental health effects of the transition to machine-paced work are due to the event—the transition and consequent *loss* of personal control over work—rather than to the condition of machine pacing. To guard against this kind of short-term effect, it is important to conduct long-term assessments of worker health. It is also useful in this regard to search for reverse changes across two types of setting—one which converted from machine-paced to self-paced work and another which converted from self-paced to machine-paced work. Consistent evidence of reversible processes which have the same patterns of change in health as a function of exposure-time would argue strongly for a causal interpretation.

(b) The first kind of change only exists when the stress under consideration is discrete—it either exists or does not exist. While this is true for some chronic stresses, there are others which exist in degrees for most people. Time-pressure, closeness of supervision, and interpersonal difficulty with colleagues are a few job stresses that could not be studied with the discrete approach.

When this is the case, intensity of exposure to the stress can be studied in a longitudinal framework. If a relationship exists between intensity of stress and ill health, then it should be the case that change in exposure intensity is associated with a parallel change in the health outcome. This might be estimated as an equation with the expectation:

$$H_t = b_0 + b_1 S_t + b_2 S_{t-1} + b_3 H_{t-1}, \tag{12a}$$

which can be reparametrized as:

$$\Delta H = b_0 + b_1 \Delta S + (b_1 + b_2) S_{t-1} + (1 - b_3) H_{t-1}. \tag{12b}$$

This reparametrization shows clearly that b_1 can be interpreted as the influence of change in S on change in H (Kessler and Greenberg, 1981, 16–17).

Several cautions are in order here. First, it is important to understand the determinants of change in S if one is to interpret Eq.(12) correctly. The mere existence of change does not guarantee that reciprocal influences between a pair of variables like S and H can be disentangled empirically. It might be that change in H affects change in S, in which case Eq.(12) cannot be estimated without bias (Greenberg and Kessler, 1982). Change only helps us separate complex causal relationships if we know enough about the determinants of change either to rule out the possibility of a particular causal path (like an influence of H on S) or to measure variables which can be used as instrumental variables in a more complex simultaneous equation system.

If we want to study the relationship between change in intensity of machine-paced work and change in mental health among workers, we would probably be on safe grounds to assume that change in the speed of the assembly line is due to factors independent of the workers' prior mental health, in which case we could estimate Eq.(12) and interpret $\hat{b}_1$ without fear of bias. Or, if we are concerned that the changed intensity of pace occurred partially in response to the workers' low morale, we could measure other determinants of the change across a variety of settings which could reasonably be assumed to be independent of H_t. Changing consumer demand for products might be one such determinant. This variable could be used as an instrument variable to estimate b_1 while adjusting for the possibility that ΔH affects ΔS (as in subsection B.1.).

Second, this entire scheme hinges on the assumption that a causal influence of S appears within a time period that is encompassed by the longitudinal analysis. We know that many relationships will not meet this requirement, especially those that involve serious health problems which are not affected by temporary variations in the intensity of stress exposure. It is therefore important when one uses this approach to focus either on acute health outcomes or on proximate outcomes which are sensitive to short-term changes in intensity.

Third, it is important to remember that analysis of the relationship between *intensity* of exposure and health has a clear meaning only when a dose–response relationship has been established previously. As noted above, machine-paced control of work is a qualitative feature of the work environment. It might be experienced as stressful because it takes away the worker's sense of personal involvement in the work process. If this is so, then there is no reason to think that the speed of the assembly line will be associated with health damaging effects. Failure to document an influence of change in intensity on change in mental health consequently should not be over-interpreted as meaning that the qualitative condition of being exposed to this stress situation is inconsequential.

(c) The third type of change is another event, in this case one in which the worker leaves the job setting we are studying rather than as in case (a) where the setting itself changes. All of the considerations in case (a) apply to this type of event, with the added complexity that the determinants of job change must be taken into consideration. These were discussed above (see the section: Multivariate control approach), where we concluded that it is extremely difficult to develop sufficiently precise controls for selection into the event to interpret the influence of the event on subsequent change in health. The same conclusion holds here and, indeed, is made even more convincing by the added difficulty of interpreting the event narrowly with respect to the influence of a change in one particular job condition.

The disaggregated time-series approach

As noted above, longitudinal analysis has only limited potential for studying chronic stress situations because these situations, by their very nature, do not change very much. Yet from a more focused perspective, there are better and worse days even in the most stressful of situations and some times of the day that are more stressful than others. This kind of variation can sometimes be used to study the effects of stress on health.

One of the most appealing features of a disaggregated approach is that fluctuation in stress exposure can often be considered random *within* individuals over time even though differences in average intensity of stress exposure *between* individuals is not random. For example, personal style is obviously involved in a person's decision to work at a high-pressure job, yet it is likely that day-to-day variation in how much stress there is on the job is independent of this selection factor.

A limitation to the approach is that the relationship between daily variations in stress and health can only be studied for health outcomes which change meaningfully from one day to the next. This means that most significant health outcomes cannot be studied directly. This limitation can be partly overcome by working with more proximal outcomes. For example, even though we could not directly study the relationship between cardiovascular disorder and daily variation in job stress, we could examine influences of the latter on heart rate, respiration rate and blood pressure.

Although there is as yet not a large literature on the disaggregated analysis of chronic stress, significant work has been done on the development of data collection strategies. A daily diary approach is the most common method for obtaining data (Stone and Neale, 1982). A sampling approach has also been developed to focus on stress and health symptoms at random moments in time (Larson and Csikszentmihalyi, 1983). Other methods of data collection have been developed to obtain daily (Bourne et al., 1968) or continuous time (Rubin, 1974) monitoring of physiological outcomes.

Two main approaches can be used to make causal inferences from disaggregated data of this sort. One is to treat the data as a time-series and to use conventional econometric methods for making causal inferences from lagged correlograms, time-series regressions and cross-spectral models (Chamberlain, 1982; Granger, 1969; Sims, 1972). These methods will not be discussed here. The second is to treat the data as a multi-level data array and use the comparative analysis of averages and residuals to make inferences about misspecification. As this approach is less readily accessible than the more conventional econometric approach, it will be discussed here.

The multi-level approach is appropriate when fundamental processes are thought to exist at the level of time disaggregation under investigation and when the more conventional analysis of the stress–health relationship in this domain uses measures which can be thought of as *averages*. This is the situation, for example, in much of the work on the relationship between marital stress and depressed mood, where both the stress and health measures are obtained by asking respondents to report retrospectively on typical levels of conflict in the marriage and typical levels of depressed mood (Ilfeld, 1982).

In a situation of this sort, the conventional survey approach uses measures which are essentially equivalent to averages of daily measures. This means that one could obtain the average H_i and S_i scores for each respondent over t days to estimate a model like:

$$\bar{H}_i = b_0 + b_1\bar{S}_i + b_2C_i + e_i, \tag{13}$$

where $\bar{H}_i$ and $\bar{S}_i$ are, respectively, the average H_{it} and S_{it} scores for respondent i over the t days of the time series, and C_i is some control variable which is a constant for person i across time but varies across respondents.

Note that this equation would probably be superior to one based on a conventional cross-sectional analysis because the kind of retrospective recall bias which creeps into self-reports about 'typical' levels of stress and symptoms is removed. Otherwise, this regression of average values is equivalent to the kind of model we would estimate in a cross-sectional analysis.

We already have seen above (see the section: Multivariate control approach), that there is a serious problem with models such as this: that we usually fail to measure C_i adequately and thereby introduce bias into the estimate of b_i. In the example considered here this misspecification would yield the equation:

$$\bar{H}_i = b_0^* + (b_1 + b_2b_{C_iS_i})\bar{S}_i + e_i^*. \tag{14}$$

Availability of multi-level data can help us make inferences about such misspecifications. This is true because Eq.(13) implies that for each individual there exists an equation:

$$H_{it} = b_0 + b_1S_{it} + b_2C_i + e_{it} \tag{15a}$$

where H_{it} and S_{it} are the observed scores for individual i at time t. Note that the product by b_2C_i is a constant for each individual. Therefore, this equation can be rewritten at the individual level as:

$$H_{it} = (b_0 + b_2C_i) + b_1S_{it} + e_{it}. \tag{15b}$$

In other words, we do not need to measure C_i in order to estimate b_1 without bias from an equation summed over t for individual i.[7]

The difficulty is that our estimate of b_1 would be an inefficient one if it were obtained in this way. In fact, we would obtain i separate estimates of b_1—one for each respondent. A more powerful way of estimating b_1 and still avoiding the bias that would exist in Eq.(14) is to disaggregate Eq.(15b) and estimate it over all i-times-t person-days simultaneously.

To demonstrate how this pooled estimate is made, we begin by noting the equalities:

$$H_{it} = \bar{H}_i + \Delta H_{it} \tag{16a}$$

$$S_{it} = \bar{S}_i + \Delta S_{it}, \tag{16b}$$

where ΔH_{it} and ΔS_{it} are residuals obtained by subtracting each individual's mean scores $\bar{H}_i$ and $\bar{S}_i$ from his scores at time t. These equalities can be substituted into Eq.(15b) to obtain:

$$(\bar{\mathrm{H}}_i + \Delta H_{it}) = (b_0 + b_2C_i) + b_1(\bar{S}_i + \Delta S_{it}) + e_{it}. \tag{17}$$

Then, noting that H_i and ΔH_{it} are orthogonal, we can subtract Eq.(17) from Eq.(13) to obtain:

$$\Delta H_{it} = b_1\Delta S_{it} + (e_{it} - e_i) \tag{18}$$

Eq.(18) can be estimated over all i-times-t residuals to arrive at an unbiased and efficient estimate of b_1.

It is also possible to estimate b_1 in an approach which simultaneously evaluates the magnitude of the specification bias in Eq.(14). To derive this estimate we sum Eq.(14) and Eq.(18) to obtain:

$$H_{it} = b_0^* + b_1\Delta S_{it} + (b_1 + b_2b_{C_i\bar{S}i})\bar{S}_i + (e_{it} + e_i^{**} - e_i) \tag{19a}$$

$$= b_0^* + b_1S_{it} + (b_2b_{C_i\bar{S}_i})\bar{S}_i + (e_{it} + e_i^* - e_i) \tag{19b}$$

Eq.(19b) can be estimated over all i-times-t observed values to arrive at the same estimate of b_1 as in Eq.(18) with the same standard error and also to obtain an estimate of the produce $b_2b_{C_i\bar{S}_i}$. The standard error of this product can be used to evaluate the significance of the specification bias.

Extensions are also possible. The most obvious is to investigate interactions between $\bar{S}_i$ and ΔS_{it} in predicting H_{it}, which would imply that typical intensities of stress modify the influence of particular changes. This is the kind of situation one would expect to find, for example, in highly stressful marriages where little irritations are capable of upsetting a fragile emotional equilibrium.

Other extensions might include the introduction of lagged effects or even a distributed lag structure. These would capture stress processes which set off emotional reactions that take several days to resolve. It is possible that the distributed lag structure of stress effects interacts with $\bar{S}_i$ as well. This is the kind of situation one would expect to find if a turbulent ongoing situation prolonged the time it took to recover from a particular daily stress.

All of the models developed in this section are based on the simplifying assumption that there is no systematic error component in the reports of a single individual at multiple time points. When this assumption is correct, simple regression analysis can be used to estimate these equations. When more complex error structures are expected an iterative estimation procedure is required. Such an approach is discussed by Mason et al. (1983).

SUMMARY

In this chapter, I have considered the most fundamental question which stress researchers address: whether stressful life experiences have adverse health effects. I examined a range of approaches available for making an assessment about this question from non-experimental data. My argument has been a simple one: that it is much more difficult to provide a clear answer to this seemingly simple question than one might think, that casual attempts to estimate causal effects are likely to yield biased estimates, and that a clear consideration of the various approaches available will often turn up a design or an analysis scheme which is capable of providing accurate information about causal influences.

I will not attempt to summarize the many technical points here, but several broad conclusions are obvious. It is usually much easier to make a causal interpretation of life event effects than of chronic stress effects. The clearest causal imputations are possible when the stress under consideration can be considered a random occurrence. The easiest way to generate a data set in which the assumption of randomness is plausible is to use matching. When this is not possible, a range of more tenuous approaches can be considered, but their appropriateness varies depending on a number of considerations. There are times when these other approaches can be used to obtain estimates which are equally as reliable as those obtained in an experiment. When the assumptions required to use these approaches are not met by the data, though, the estimates obtained will be biased. It is a serious limitation of current research on stress processes that the extreme sensitivity of these approaches to violation of their underlying assumptions is not generally recognized. If we are to make progress in mapping the links between stressful life experience and health, especially the subtle aspects of these relationships which are currently the focus of attention among stress researchers, it is vitally important that we do all we can to obtain optimally precise estimates of stress effects. Consideration of the various approaches exposited here should help facilitate this goal.

NOTES

1. This discussion assumes that the researcher is involved in a focused analysis of a particular event. In general population studies of many different events, the parallel strategy is to examine separately a subset of events which can be assumed to have occurred for reasons that are essentially random with respect to the outcome under consideration. Brown and Harris (1978) illustrate the use of this approach. When this restricted subset of events can be constructed accurately and all relevant structural determinants of event exposure are controlled, a revised version of Eq.(1) can be used to estimate the impact of life event exposure on the health outcome. Structural determinants of event exposure include role configurations which are definitionally related to risk of a particular event occurring. For example, one must be married to be at risk of widowhood. It is therefore necessary to control statistically for marital status in any aggregate life event analysis which includes widowhood as a component event and where the health outcome is related to marital status. In this analysis, all people who became widowed during the event period should be coded married on the control variable because they were married at the time the event occurred. This coding convention guarantees that the health outcome will be compared between stably married respondents and recently widowed respondents when the impact of widowhood is evaluated. In the more conventional coding, where recently widowed respondents are coded as widowed, their health would be incorrectly compared to widowed people whose spouses had died prior to the event period.
2. Note that because S totally determines exposure to LE, there is a perfect non-linear relationship between S and LE. This means that b_1 can be interpreted as the node of a spline regression. The correct parametrization of the non-linear functional relationship between S and H is critically important for estimation of this node. One refinement possible in this regard is to generate a separate estimate of the functional form linking S and LE in a sample of people who have not been exposed to the event in question. For example, in a study of job lay-off, the relationship between seniority and health could be assessed in a control plant where there was no lay-off taking place. The structural coefficients estimated in this control sample could then be applied to the data obtained from the plant experiencing lay-offs to generate a baseline set of predicted H scores. By pooling data from the two plants in a constrained model which estimates the S effects in the control sample it is also possible to separate the effect of being laid off (b_1) from the effect of working in a plant where lay-offs are occurring (b_4) in the following equation:

$$H_i = b_0 + b_1 LE_i + b_2 S_i + b_3 S_i^2 + b_4 P_i + e_i,$$

where P is a dummy variable defining whether respondent i is a member of the sample drawn from the lay-off plant or the control plant.
3. We could measure the job setting itself rather than its personality determinants and thereby sidestep this problem. Indeed, this would be a preferable strategy. To do this, though, would be to engage in an exercise which is equivalent to the matched comparison approach discussed above (see the first section on Matching). As noted in

that section, the use of matching often helps resolve problems of misspecification that are otherwise intractable. This is an example of a situation in which this is the case.
4. When the researcher has a time-series of observations for each unit of analysis, it is possible to use the empirical trajectory of H to generate a baseline model of expected H_t scores. These can be compared to the observed H_t scores to evaluate the impact of *LE*. This approach is known as interrupted time-series analysis (McDowell et al., 1979). Although a useful approach when explicit information about C_1 through C_n is absent, interrupted time-series analysis is insensitive to changes in the *C* variables which could not have been predicted from their earlier values and therefore generates a less accurate baseline than by using the *C* variables explicitly. These considerations will not be discussed here because time-series data are seldom available to the stress researcher. It is useful to note, though, that in the one case where a model of this sort has been used to study the impact of stress—in Brenner's time series analysis of unemployment and health—problems of insensitivity and time misspecification have been central points of criticism (Dooley and Catalano, in press).
5. I omit a discussion of the regression–discontinuity design for analyzing the effects of chronic stress because it seems infeasible to isolate a single variable which totally accounts for exposure to an ongoing stress. The only examples I can think of are situations where a life event leads to a change in one's ongoing life situation. For example, we could evaluate the health damaging effects of retirement in this way by studying people who work at jobs which have a mandatory retirement age. (Adjustment for the bias introduced by some people retiring early could be handled by using Heckman's hazard rate selection bias correction procedure.) One could even carry out a series of such analyses in sub-groups which differ in the mandatory retirement age, which is sixty-five in some job settings and seventy in others. This kind of parallel analysis would provide a strong test of whether retirement has health damaging effects, for one would expect the inflection point in the discontinuity curve to appear five years earlier in the sample of people who retired at sixty-five. (A related use of parallel analyses postulating the appearance of lagged inflections appears in Hennigan et al., 1982).
6. A critique of the multivariate job stress approach similar to the one developed here appears in Kasl (1981).
7. This result illustrates a point made in the literature on aggregation bias, that problems can arise in attempting to make inferences about the behaviours of individuals from more highly aggregated units of analysis. The classic case was Robinson's (1950) study of the relationship between being foreign born and illiterate. He demonstrated that the association between these two variables differs depending on whether individuals or states are taken as the unit of analysis. The discrepancy is due to other factors besides a person's country of birth affecting literacy, particularly the availability of schooling in a state. In the equation where individuals were the unit of analysis, education was *negatively* related to being foreign born, in Robinson's data. In the state-level equation, by comparison, access to education was *positively* related to rates of foreign-born residents because most of the latter lived in the north eastern states where educational services were greater than other areas of the country.

It has been demonstrated that the correct specification of this model in the aggregate data can yield an unbiased estimate of the individual-lever parameter if there are no interactions between context and individual-level processes (Hanushek and Jackson, 1977, 84–6). In other words, even though some new control variables are required at the aggregate level, it is still possible to estimate the individual-level equation with *additional* controls. Our result shows the opposite: that when one can use disaggregated data, *fewer* controls are necessary.

REFERENCES

Berk, R. A., and Rauma, D. (1983) Capitalizing on nonrandom assignment to treatments: A regression-discontinuity evaluation of a crime-control program, *Journal of the American Statistical Association*, **78**, 21–7.

Biderman, A. D., and Moore, J. C. (1980). *Report of the Workshop on Applying Cognitive Psychology to Recall Problems of the National Crime Survey*, Washington, D.C., Bureau of Social Science Research.

Bourne, P. C., Rose, R. M., and Mason, J. W. (1968). 17-OHCS levels in combat, *Archives of General Psychiatry*, **19**, 135–40.

Brown, G. W., and Harris, T. (1978). *Social Origins of Depression: A Study of Psychiatric Disorder in Women*, New York, Free Press.

Burgess, A. W., and Holmstrom, L. L. (1979). Adaptive strategies and recovery from rape, *American Journal of Psychiatry*, **136**, 1278–82.

Chamberlain, G. (1982). The general equivalence of Granger and Sims causality, *Econometrica*, **50**, 569–82

Clark, D. M., and Teasdale, J. D. (1982). Diurnal variation in clinical depression and accessibility of memories of positive and negative experiences, *Journal of Abnormal Psychology*, **91**, 87–95.

Converse, P. E., Alwin, D., and Martin, S. (1983). Marriage termination and felt well-being: Immediate impact versus ultimate effects. Unpublished paper, Institute for Social Research, The University of Michigan.

Cook, T. D., and Campbell, D. T. (1979). *Quasi-Experimentation: Design and Analysis Issues for Field Settings*. Chicago: Rand McNally.

Dohrenwend, B. S., Dohrenwend, B. P., Dodson, M., and Shrout, P. (1984). Symptoms, hassles, social supports and life events: The problem of confounding measures, *Journal of Abnormal Psychology*, **93**, 222–30.

Dohrenwend, B. P., and Shrout, P. E. (1985). 'Hassles' in the conceptualization and measurement of life stress variables, *American Psychologist*, **40**, 780–5.

Dooley, D. and Catalano, R. (In press) Do economic variables generate psychological problems? Different methods, different answers. In A. J. Macfadyen and H. W. Macfadyen (eds.) *Economic Psychology: Intersection in Theory and Application*, New York, North-Holland.

Duncan, O. D. (1975). *Introduction to Structural Equation Models*, New York, Academic.

Fisher, F. M. (1965). The choice of instrumental variables in the estimation of economy-wide econometric models, *International Economic Review*, **6**, 245–74.

Granger, C. W. J. (1969). Investigating causal relations by econometric models and cross-spectral methods, *Econometrica*, **37**, 424–38.

Gravelle, H., Hutchinson, G., and Stern, J. (1981). Mortality and unemployment: A critique of Brenner's time-series analysis, *The Lancet* (Sep. 26) **2(8248)**, 675–9.

Greenberg, D. F., and Kessler, R. C. (1982). Equilibrium and identification in linear panel models, *Sociological Methods and Research*, **10**, 435–51.

Hanushek, E. A., and Jackson, J. E. (1977). *Statistical Methods for Social Scientists*, New York, Academic Press.

Heckman, J. J. (1979). Sample selection bias as a specification error, *Econometrica*, **47**, 153–61.

Hennigan, K. M., Del Rosario, M. L., Cook, T. D., Wharton, J. D., and Calder, B. J. (1982). Impact of the introduction of television on crime in the United States: Empirical findings and theoretical implications, *Journal of Personality and Social Psychology*, **42**, 461–77.

Ilfeld, F. W. (1982). Marital stressors, coping styles, and symptoms of depression. In

L. Goldberger and S. Breznitz (eds.) *Handbook of Stress: Theoretical and Clinical Aspects*, New York, Free Press, pp. 482–95.

Jabine, T. C., Straf, M. L., Tanur, J. M., and Tourandau, R. (eds.) (1984). *Cognitive Aspects of Survey Methodology*, Washington, D.C., National Academy Press.

Kahn, R. L. (1981). *Work and Health*, New York, Wiley–Interscience.

Kasl, S. V. (1978). Epidemiological contributions to the study of work stress, In C. L. Cooper and R. Payne (eds.) *Stress at Work*. New York, Wiley, pp. 3–48.

Kasl, S. V. (1981). The challenge of studying the disease effects of stressful work conditions, *American Journal of Public Health*, **71**, 682–4.

Kessler, R. C. (1983). Methodological issues in the study of psychosocial stress: Measurement, design and analysis. In H. B. Kaplan (ed.) *Psychosocial Stress: Recent Developments in Theory and Research*, New York, Academic Press, pp. 267–341.

Kessler, R. C., and Greenberg, D. F. (1981). *Linear Panel Analysis: Models of Quantitative Change*, New York, Academic Press.

Larson, R., and Csikszentmihalyi, M. (1983). The experience sampling method. In H. Reis (ed.) *New Directions for Naturalistic Methods in the Behavioral Sciences*, San Francisco, Jossey-Bass.

Lazarus, R. S., DeLongis, A., Folkman, S., and Gruen, R. (1985). Stress and adaptational outcomes: The problem of confounding measures, *American Psychologist*, **40**, 770–9.

Lazarus, R. S., and Folkman, S. (1984). *Stress, Appraisal, and Coping*, New York, Springer.

Mason, W. M., Wong, G. Y., and Entwisle, B. (1983). Contextual analysis through the multilevel linear model. In S. Leinhardt (ed.) *Sociological Methodology 1983–1984*, San Francisco, Jossey-Bass, pp. 72–103.

McDowell, D., McCleary, R., Meidinger, E. E., and Hay, R. A., Jr. (1979). *Interrupted Time Series Analysis*, Beverly Hills, CA., Sage.

Nelson, R. E., and Craighead, W. E. (1977). Selective recall of positive and negative feedback, self-control behaviors, and depression, *Journal of Abnormal Psychology*, **86**, 379–88.

Price, R. H., Ketterer, R. F., Bader, B. C., and Monahan, J. (eds.) (1980). *Prevention in Community Mental Health: Research, Policy and Practice*, Beverly Hills, CA, Sage Publications.

Robinson, W. (1950). Ecological correlations and the behavior of individuals, *American Sociological Review*, **15**, 351–7.

Roos, P., and Treiman, D. J. (1980). DOT scales for the 1970 Census classification. In A. R. Miller, D. J. Treiman, P. S. Cain and P. A. Roos (eds.) *Work, Jobs and Occupations: A Critical Review of the Dictionary of Occupational Titles*, Washington, D.C., National Academy Press, pp. 336–89.

Rubin, R. T. (1974). Biochemical and endocrine responses to severe psychological stress. In E. K. E. Gunderson and R. H. Rahe (eds.) *Life Stress and Illness*, Springfield, Ill., C. C. Thomas, pp. 227–41.

Selye, H. (1982) History and present status of the stress concept. In Leo Goldberger and Shlomo Breznitz (eds.) *Handbook of Stress: Theoretical and Clinical Aspects*, New York, Free Press, pp. 7–20.

Silver, R. L., and Wortman, C. B. (1980). Coping with undesirable life events. In J. Garber and Martin E. P. Seligman (eds.) *Human Helplessness: Theory and Applications*, New York, Academic Press, pp. 279–375.

Sims, C. A. (1972). Money, income, and causality, *American Economic Review*, **62**, 540–2.

Stone, A. A., and Neale, J. M. (1982). Development of a methodology for assessing daily experiences. In A. Baum and J. Singer (eds.) *Advances in Environmental Psychology: Environment and Health* (Volume 4), New York, Erlbaum, pp. 49–83.

Trochim, W. M. K. (1984). *Research Design for Program Evaluation: The Regression Discontinuity Approach*, Beverly Hills, Sage.

Turkkam, J. S., Brady, J. V., and Harris, A. H. (1982). Animal studies of stressful interactions: A behavioral–physiological overview. In L. Goldberger and S. Breznitz (eds.) *Handbook of Stress: Theoretical and Clinical Aspects*, New York, Free Press, pp. 153–82.

PART TWO

Developments of Concepts and Measures in Stress Research

Chapter 6

The Family as a Context of the Stress Process

Leonard I. Pearlin and Heather A. Turner
University of California, San Francisco

Researchers into social stress, regardless of their orientations and disciplinary affiliations, must inevitably give serious thought and consideration to the family. It is unquestionably the institutional sphere that, more than any other, engages the stress process in intense and varied ways. There are many reasons why the family is so central to the study of stress. Foremost, the family is the arena in which relationships are formed at birth and continue through the entirety of life. Although one relinquishes many roles in moving across the life course, one does not cease being a son or daughter or a brother or sister; it is typically death alone that breaks these relationships. Clearly, relationships that begin with life itself and are terminated only by death, foster powerful emotional stakes. As a result, people are likely to be distressed by things that go badly in the family. Conversely, family relationships that go well are likely to be a source of profound reward. In either case, family attachments, created so early and typically tested over such a long period of time, are not experienced with emotional indifference.

Of course, the power of the family does not depend merely on the earliness or duration of its relationships. It is also central in people's lives because it is the place where crucial needs are both created and satisfied. Indeed, at the earliest stages of life and, occasionally, at the last stages, people depend on family for their very biological survival. It is the place, too, where conceptions of self, both as we are and as we would like to be, begin to take shape; and it is also to the family that we look for approval and approbation of what we are and what we are becoming. Ultimately, though, family attachments are strong not because they give people what they seek but simply for their own sake. Family ties are quintessentially what Cooley (1915) described as primary group attachments: they are prized and cherished in and by themselves, not for what can be gained from them.

Support for this work was provided by the W.T. Grant Foundation and by Grant MH38830 from NIMH

Research Methods in Stress and Health Psychology. Edited by S. V. Kasl and C. L. Cooper.

The family, then, is crucial to stress because it is crucial to social and emotional life itself. Although it shares its influence with other institutions, no other affects its members so pervasively nor reaches their inner lives so deeply. In fact, as we had occasion to observe in earlier work (Pearlin, 1983a), the family stands as a significant force at virtually every point along the stress process. First, it constitutes a fertile *source* of stress for people (Croog, 1970) and much of our effort in this chapter will be directed toward identifying familial origins of stress. Next, we shall be emphasizing that the family is not self-contained, it does not stand in isolation from surrounding institutional contexts. Its members work outside the family, have friends, go to church, attend school, participate in voluntary associations, and interact with neighbours. In the course of acting in these multiple outside roles, family members are likely to encounter situations that are stressful and these outside stresses, in turn, may find their way into the family domain. Thus, the family may act as a *conduit* for stresses as well as a primary source of stress. Finally, we shall consider the family as a *mediating force* in the stress process; that is, a place where the individual can find the resources to deal with stress, whatever its source. The resources to which we refer are social supports and coping repertoires, two constructs whose conceptual boundaries can become very fluid and obscure in the family. Indeed, the interface between coping and social support is increasingly coming to be recognized in the literature (Gore, 1985; Thoits, 1986; Pearlin and Aneshensel, 1986). Yet, the family can be distinctly seen as providing not only social support to its members but also a reservoir of coping dispositions. These dispositions, in part, are the products of a family screening system that encourages some coping modes and discourages others.

Thus far we have been referring to the family as though it were an institution about whose significant properties researchers are in agreement. The family, however, is a very complex and differentiated institution and its very complexity invites a variety of conceptual orientations and research questions. For example, it can be viewed as a system having properties that are different from the sum total of the attributes of its individual members (Fisher, 1982; McCubbin and Patterson, 1982; Reiss and Oliveri, 1980). Solidarity and flexibility, for example, are system properties not easily deducible from the actions or dispositions of individuals. To assess such elements, it is necessary to observe the functioning of the family unit, not its separate members. This is a difficult task at best and it is usually done under laboratory conditions. Strictly speaking, most studies that purport to be family studies are not. Instead, they are studies of the individual-in-family. This genre of investigation has produced much of what we know about 'family' stress. At this point in our research, we know more about the stress that individuals experience in the family than we do about families under stress, the goal of some early stress research (Hill, 1949).

Indeed, much of our own discussion will centre on individuals within the context of the family, not on the family as an integrated system.

We should emphasize that our interest in this chapter is less on *how* to measure family-related stressors than in suggesting *what* to measure. Thus, we are primarily concerned with identifying dimensions of stressors that have been or might be fruitful to measure. With few exceptions, we do not deal with concrete measures or with the mechanics of measurement. It is not that the development of reliable and valid scales and indicators having acceptable metric properties is unimportant; far from it. However, it is our strong conviction that the advance of stress research at this time depends much more on clarifying conceptual issues than on critiquing or promoting existing measures.

THE FAMILY AS A SOURCE OF STRESS

It is curious that in recent years much more attention has been given to the mediation of stress than to its social origins. As a result, we perhaps know less about the nature and source of stressors in the lives of people than about how they cope or benefit from social supports (Pearlin, 1982). This does not mean that nothing is known of family stressors. On the contrary, it would be possible to assemble a long list of such stressors that have been identified in a variety of studies. The loss of family function due to job loss (Elder, 1974), eruptive crises—such as premature death of a family member (Pearlin and Lieberman, 1978), status inequalities between husbands and wives (Pearlin, 1975) and the dissolution of marital ties (Pearlin and Johnson, 1977) are but a few examples of family stressors. But, despite the attention it has received, it can be stated accurately that knowledge about family stress is fragmented, largely because it is unguided by a clear conceptual framework. To achieve some of the conceptual clarity and unity the area needs, it is helpful to recognize that stressors found in the family do not necessarily originate there. As we pointed out earlier, family members have multiple roles and as a consequence, some of the stressors that appear in family relations can be traced to sources located outside the family. This is a phenomenon we shall consider later in the chapter. First, however, we shall treat the family as though it stands by itself, considering only those stressors that are likely to arise *directly* out of family functions and relationships.

In general, there are two types of stressors that arise within the boundaries of the family: one is represented by eventful change and the demands it imposes for re-equilibration and adjustment (Dohrenwend and Pearlin, 1982) and the other by the more persisent, chronic strains that are rooted in the relatively durable conditions of people's lives (Pearlin, 1983b). Among the changes embodied in life events are those events that arise out of normative or scheduled transitions and, very different, those that are unscheduled, more eruptive and often undesired (Pearlin, 1980a). Among the scheduled transitions are such events as marriage—marking the initiation of a new nuclear unit—birth(s), launching of children, retirement, and widowhood. With the exception of the 'timely' death of a spouse, these normative or scheduled changes have not been revealed as potent sources of stress (Pearlin, 1982; Menaghan, 1982). This is somewhat surprising, for some of the scheduled family transitions entail a rather fundamental restructuring of the family and household. The birth of a first child, for example, is hardly an event that goes unnoticed by parents. Why is it, then, that scheduled transitions in the family life cycle typically do not result in stress that can be detected through time?

Two explanations have been offered. One is that their very expectable character enables people to begin preparing for the changes anticipatorily (Pearlin, 1980b). Because these transitions are scheduled, one can begin adjusting to them far in advance of their actual occurrence. By the time the events finally take place, they require far less adjustment and re-equilibration than would be the case if people had to confront their reality *de novo*, without prior knowledge or preparation. This explanation seems plausible and, indeed, may account somewhat for the minimal stress created by scheduled transitional events. But the explanation is limited. Despite prior learning, a first-born infant defies anticipatory preparation; the new-born brings surprises and challenges for which no amount of prior socialization leaves the parent quite prepared. Similar surprises lie in wait for people engaged in other scheduled transitions. Foreknowledge of and early socialization to a future role help but prior preparation is always incomplete and frequently inappropriate.

An alternative explanation would suggest that there really are stressful readjustments occasioned by scheduled family transitions but that we fail to observe them because we are not looking at the right time for the right effects. That is, the stressful effects of role transitions, to the extent that they exist at all, might be most likely found immediately following the change, rapidly diminishing thereafter. If this is the case, it is notable that any anxiety or depressiveness that results from transitional change would be of an ephemeral nature, unobservable after a relatively brief lapse of time. It would be stress of a very episodic, short-lived type, not one that remains as a relatively durable state. To capture the fullest impact of these events, therefore, it is necessary that they be observed within a brief time frame following the event.

In addition to failing to time our observations in a way that enables us to appraise accurately the stressful effects of scheduled events, there may be another, more fundamental, deficiency in our research. We usually treat events as universal 'happenings'; that is, as occurrences whose relevance to people's lives need not be questioned. In fact, however, the relevance of an event and its stressful effects vary widely among people experiencing it. The birth of a first-born in a family where the parents are unemployed is likely to be experienced very differently from the household where it is part of the untroubled unfolding of a life-plan. Retirement may be taken as another example of this issue. By and large, research has revealed no stressful effects stemming from retirement (Sheppard, 1976). However, there might be some people who are distressed by this transition and others who are made euphoric by it. When the distressed and the euphoric are pooled together as a single group experiencing a common transition, they statistically appear as unaffected by it. Thus the pooling could obscure the possibility that some retirees experience the change as alienating them from their own skills, as a loss of status or as a separation from cherished friends while others relish it as a totally liberating experience.

Thus, we would argue that transitions cannot be treated separately from the past and present conditions that structure their meaning. The very scheduled transitions that appear to be innocuous might, in fact, have stressful consequences under some conditions. Until the conditions are recognized and incorporated into research, the consequences of the events cannot be fully recognized. Some of the relevant conditions reside in such circumstances as life stage, economic status, and gender, and others in the nature of the experiences people had in the roles or statuses being relinquished and, in still others, in the expectations and hopes for the roles newly acquired in the transitions. The major point is that we must be alert to the conditions that shape the meaning of the change and, therefore, influence whether it is experienced as rewarding or punishing. It is not the scheduled transition by itself that determines whether it will be stressful but whether the transition is experienced as a gain or loss.

Although the weight of current evidence does not reveal scheduled family transitions as being appreciable precursors of psychological stress, this is not the case with the more unscheduled, eruptive events that can arise in families. Changes propelled by events of this type have frequently been observed to have deleterious consequences. The serious injury or illness of a child, for example, is accompanied by considerable emotional distress and there is no event of any type that surpasses the death of a child in its stressful effects (Pearlin and Lieberman, 1978). Separation and divorce, the premature death of a spouse, illness or injury to a spouse or to one's self, the return to the household of a previously launched child, and change of family residence are all unscheduled events—that is, events not tied to the uncoiling of the family life cycle—that have the capacity to arouse considerable stress.

How do these unscheduled family events come to exert their forceful effects? In some instances, the answer to this query appears self-evident. The sudden death of a spouse, for example, invokes the loss of a relationship that can be deeply embedded in one's own sense of being. Therefore, events that involve the loss of important relationships can also involve the loss of important elements of one's very self. Another, more general, interpretation of the effects of events holds that change *qua* change, especially that which is undesired, underlies stress. This assumption, rooted in much of the early life-events research, views change as imposing a tax on the organism whereby the greater the change, the greater the tax (Holmes and Rahe, 1967). This argument, which we feel is difficult to substantiate either on theoretical or empirical grounds, has been giving way to still a different explanation. It is that disruptive events acquire much of their stressful character not by their own direct impact but by disrupting and dislocating the more structured elements of peoples' lives (Pearlin et al., 1981). Unscheduled events, in other words, can become transformed into chronic strains and it is these strains that then give rise to stress. Such events may also intensify pre-existing strains and exacerbate their stressful effects. To understand family stress, therefore, it is necessary to look not only at the events that happen to it, but also to how events become intertwined with the conditions that prevail within it.

In the attempt to identify the chronic strains that stand as sources of stress, we necessarily turn our attention away from that which is exotic, unusual, or episodic. The warp and woof of the fabric that makes up ordinary daily life often contains much that has the capacity to arouse stress. The structure of repeated experience within the context of our various social roles can contain a bountiful supply of conflicts and uncertainties, of frustrations and relentless pressures. Because they are built into the conditions of the roles that people play, these kinds of life problems are likely to be relatively dogged. Though they are certainly not immutable, such problems—or strains—can be quite durable, especially as compared to eventful upheavals. Their very chronicity calls attention to the tenacity of some life problems and to their resistance to ameliorative efforts. Their persistence, moreover, endows them with a power exceeding that of most life events to create and maintain stressful states, depression in particular.

The identification of strains in family roles is far from complete. However, beginning with qualitative interviews, we were able to develop measures of a number of dimensions of family strains and to use these in surveys of community populations (Pearlin and Schooler, 1978). Four types of strain have been conceptualized as occurring within the family and, for that matter, within other institutional spheres as well. One type concerns the level of demands and pressures that one encounters in one's family roles. This type of stressor is essentially the familial counterpart of job pressures, tapping the magnitude of one's tasks and the limits of time and energy that are available for performing the tasks. It is a dimension of family strain particularly relevant to homemakers, reflecting the relentless burdens they can experience in this role. Our own examination of homemakers' strains indicates that they are important—and somewhat overlooked—sources of stress in the family domain (Pearlin, 1975).

A much more common type of stressor, one that can embroil all family members, involves interpersonal conflict. It must be kept in mind that the family represents what is called a role set (Merton, 1957), a number of closely interrelated roles. A mother cannot be a mother without there also being a child and a husband must have a wife to be a husband. The very notion of role implies an interrelated role. Because roles are interrelated, it means that the actions, problems, and passions of one must affect those of the others in that role set. The inevitable ripples that actions initiate in a role set create a potential for conflict among its participants. This is perhaps particularly so in the case of family roles, for here interaction can be broad in its scope, very continuous and very intense. Indeed, given the number of relationships involved, even in small nuclear families, it is perhaps surprising that interpersonal conflict does not dominate family life.

Several dimensions of interpersonal conflicts, some involving husbands and wives and others parents and children, have been identified and measured in our past research. These have been described in various sources (e.g. Pearlin, 1983b) and need only brief treatment here. There are four areas of marital conflict. One involves the lack of *reciprocity*, a situation where a husband or wife appraises his/her contributions to the relationships as greater than those of the spouse. The conflict thus revolves around a lack of equity in the marriage. Second is the lack of *affective exchange*, found in instances where a marital partner feels either that there is insufficient affection given to him/her by the spouse or that the spouse does not accept the affection that the partner offers. A third dimension of interpersonal conflict in marriage is linked to the self. Specifically, there can be a failure of *authentication of the self*, a situation where the desired self-image of a person is not confirmed in the eyes of the partner. In effect, it is an alienating experience, one where the prized elements of one's self are felt to be inaccurately or incompletely recognized by the other. A final marital strain is the *frustration of role expectations*. Marital partners usually have a set of expectations of each other, many of them having to do with the household division of labour. Where there is a failure on the part of one or both to fulfil these expectations, disappointment and frustration can result. These four dimensions of marital strain certainly do not describe all conflict that can arise in marriage. Nevertheless, much of the stress-provoking marital conflict appears to cluster around one or another of them.

Turning now to a consideration of parent–child strains, we found in our research that the nature of these conflicts closely depends on the age of the child. Our own inquiries into parental stressors begin with children five years and older; thus we have little to observe concerning what are undoubtedly severe stressors parents may experience between the time their children are born and the start of their schooling. From the ages of five or six to sixteen years, however, parents are likely to confront a variety of circumstances that are potentially stressful: being treated disrespectfully by their children; being ignored as sources of guidance and advice; being disobeyed; and failure on the part of the child to perform household chores. Parents are also often concerned that their children's friends are exerting bad influences, that they are failing to acquire the social skills appropriate to their ages, that they are not devoting sufficient effort to their school work, or that they do not use their spare time appropriately.

Parents of older children, those between sixteen years and the time of launching—that is, the time when they leave the parental household—often face additional kinds of problems with their children. It is in this period that some parents become concerned about their children's adherence to what they consider as unacceptable moral beliefs and practices or to their susceptibility to the use of drugs or excessive drinking. It is in this time-span, too, that parents begin to judge whether their children's achievement trajectories are consistent with the aspirations they hold for their children's futures. Where parents judge that their children's current performance is likely to leave them short of the goals that parents envisioned for them, it can produce considerable anguish and recrimination.

Adult children, those living outside the parental home and, in many instances, having their own household and families, are sources of similar kinds of parent–child conflicts. Now, however, parents no longer only express uncertainty about future achievement but may have to confront either the great likelihood or the current reality of their children's 'failure'. Finally, parents of adult children may also be sensitive to symbols of abandonment, especially the neglect of children to visit, write or to phone.

Thus far, then, we have called attention to two types of family-based strains as potential sources of stress. One entails role pressure or overload, best exemplified by the burdens of homemaking. The other is that of interpersonal conflicts, of which there is a rich variety, some involving husbands and wives, others parents and children. Although we shall not consider them here, it should be noted that siblings and segments of the extended family can also be embroiled in family conflict.

We turn from interpersonal conflict to consider a third type of strain that can arise within the boundaries of the family (as well as in the occupational realm); it is what we refer to as *role captivity*. Briefly, role captivity exists where people are bound to one role while preferring another. Within the family context, this strain typically besets women more than men. Concretely, there are many women who are wives, mothers and homemakers who would like to be and to do other things, either in place of or in addition to what they are doing. However, they continue to play the unwanted role because they are unable, for a variety of reasons, to change or augment it. Role captivity, then, is defined by one's inability to move from an unwanted role to one that is desired, thus leaving one captive. Although most common among homemaking women, it is not limited to this group, for it can also surface among employed people who would prefer not to work or to non-workers, such as retirees, who would prefer to work but cannot. In whatever role it occurs, it is a dimension of strain associated with stress and one that deserves more attention than it has received.

The same can be said of a final type of family role strain, that which entails the *restructuring of established family role sets*. As we emphasized earlier, one of the distinguishing features of family relations is that once formed, they exist until disrupted by death. With the exception of marriage, which can be broken by divorce, relationships remain intact (albeit not necessarily active or harmonious) for the duration of life itself. We are always children, parents, sibs, nieces and nephews, aunts and uncles. Yet, although the family role set remains unchanged, the nature of interactions among the people constituting the set must inevitably undergo alterations as the set moves across the life course. If there is resistance to such alteration, conflict is likely to result. Thus, adolescents rebel if their parents persist in dealing with them as though they were still pre-adolescents; young mothers who are now responsible for their own infant may not tolerate their mothers treating them as being too immature to be responsible for themselves; and elderly parents who may have prided themselves on being able to help their children may resent having to be dependent on their children. Thus, although the family is made up of the same actors in the same status relations, there can be a profound and stressful restructuring of the ways in which participants deal with each other. The restructuring can entail the displacement of prior expectations by new ones, changes in patterns of deference, or alterations in claims to rights and privileges. These changes can stand as potential sources of severe strains and stresses. Obviously, in thinking about family stressors we need to adopt a developmental perspective, for the problems that exist at one life stage may be pushed aside with time and age, giving way to new problems. Some of these new problems, indeed, may be caused by developmental restructuring itself.

THE EXTRA-FAMILIAL SOURCES OF FAMILY STRESSORS

Thus far we have been focusing our discussions on those stressors that arise directly within the family and its criss-crossing interpersonal relationships. The events we considered, both scheduled and unscheduled, occur within the family domain. And the types of role strains we have considered also have their primary roots within the family. However, the family is certainly not an island unto itself—far from it. The multiple roles of its members are the channels through which the family becomes integrated with and influenced by other social institutions and arenas of social life. If we were simply to add the roles played by an ordinary nuclear family of four members, we would probably be surprised by the magnitude of the number. Some of these roles will be more important than others, of course, and, correspondingly, they will not have equal importance as sources of stress in the lives of the family members. Moreover, not everything that one experiences in extra-familial roles is necessarily relevant to what goes on in the family. Nevertheless, the conditions that people experience outside the family can have pronounced effects on the stress process within the family. These are the issues to which we now turn.

Essentially, then, we need to consider how circumstances outside the family result in the emergence of stressors within the family. Virtually any domain of social life can conceivably be a source of distress, although occupation has probably been the most intensely studied by stress researchers (e.g. House, 1974; Kasl, 1974; McLean, 1979). Unfortunately, there is little or no literature dealing with the issue that concerns us here; namely, the process by which stressors confronted in one realm, such as occupation, come to be transformed into family stressors. We think that stressors in an outside role can result in stressors in the family, and we shall detail three distinct mechanisms by which this happens.

One, perhaps the most obvious, begins with the arousal of emotional distress in an outside role—occupation, for example. We submit that the distress thus aroused may be carried into the household where it then becomes a disruptive force in ongoing family relations. The anger, frustration, anxiety or depression generated in the workplace creates a strain on family relations; these newly strained relations, in turn, become secondary but independent sources of stress. In this way, the stress of the worker is exacerbated and, in addition, his/her stress produces stress for other family members. We have recently completed a series of qualitative interviews with husbands and wives and the data from these interviews will help to illuminate this process, for in the interviews we questioned people directly about the transfer of occupational problems and stresses to the household.

One of the queries in these qualitative interviews was whether the subject talked to his/her spouse about bothersome problems at work. A surprising number of respondents, husbands and wives alike, indicated that they attempted to segregate stresses aroused in the workplace from the family domain. Several reasons were given: people feel that their own distresses would only distress their spouses and they would then be placed in the position of having to assuage and calm the other, something they did not want; others feared that their spouses would blame them for the problem, in effect withdrawing esteem; some anticipated that their spouses would give them unwanted or inappropriate advice that they would have to reject, thus inviting conflict; the spouses are already under stress for other reasons and would unnecessarily be further burdened; or the person wants to work the problem through before discussing it. Thus, there is a number of reasons why people attempt to barricade from the family domain the distress that is generated elsewhere.

However, they rarely, if ever, succeed. Invariably spouses informed us that they can tell when their partner is stressed, regardless of whether the partner talks about it. Mood changes, shifts in activities (such as immersion in television) and other behavioural clues alert the spouse to the fact that his or her mate is troubled, even though they do not know why. Of course, many people will sooner or later begin to talk about the trouble, the talk sometimes initiated by the puzzled spouse. Quite commonly, though, the uninformed spouse wonders whether he or she has unwittingly caused the distress or whether he/she is failing to do something that would ease it. Thus, attempts to screen outside stresses from the family and the uncertainty created by such attempts can themselves impose strain on marital relations. Where this is not a once-in-a-while episode but is a frequently occurring pattern, there can be a pronounced undermining of the marriage.

But, while silence can itself impact on family relations, the open expression of emotional distress created elsewhere can also have its deleterious effects. This is particularly the case when the distress is presented in a manner that makes the members of the family the displaced objects of anger and hostility, where a pervasive atmosphere of heightened anxiety is created or where the household is wrapped in the mantle of the stressed person's depression.

One way, then, that stress initiated in roles outside the family can beget stress within the family is through the disruptive transfer to the household of emotional disturbances aroused elsewhere, such as in the job setting. The disrupted marital relations, in turn, can become a source of stress in their own right. This can come about both in instances where people attempt to shield the family from the outside stress as well as where no such attempts are made. When the outside stress is either enduring or frequently repeated, the troubled family relations can themselves become chronic role strains and the antecedents of persistent stress. This represents one way in which family stressors come to be part of a larger cluster of stressors extending beyond the family boundaries.

A second way in which family stressors are interconnected to outside roles is through the competition between or incompatibility among the multiple roles played by family members. Some of the conflicts that are anchored to the competing demands of multiple roles are intrapersonal. That is, they leave the individual suspended in a running dilemma of simultaneous commitment to two or more roles. Satisfaction of one commitment is unavoidably at the expense of the other. Women who are employed outside the household are, in some instances, subjected to this kind of intrapersonal conflict, a conflict that typically results from investment in work, on the one hand, and obligation to children and homemaking on the other. Working-class women are especially exposed to these strains, for it is they who are more likely to have difficulty in making adequate caretaking arrangements for their young children. Middle-class women are often more able to avoid the dilemma by employing surrogates to stand in for them in household roles (Pearlin, 1975). However, although middle-class women may more easily deal with the logistical conflicts, they more often face the prospect of motherhood jeopardizing career goals.

Some of the conflicts resulting from outside, competing roles have more immediate and direct consequences for *interpersonal* than for intrapersonal conflict. This was very apparent in the reports given us in the qualitative interviews we conducted. A number of people told us, for example, that they were too fatigued by work to do the things at home that they felt they should do. Thus they felt unable to mobilize the energy to engage with children or with spouses in the kinds of activities that were expected of them and that they wanted for themselves. As a result, they failed at such activities as doing their fair share of household tasks or devoting time to playing with their children. This, in turn, leads to argument and remonstration as well as to guilt. Indeed, judging from what some of our respondents told us, fatigue from work can be a major inhibitor of the exchange of affection between spouses.

Not all interpersonal conflicts in the home result from fatigue created outside, of course. They can also result when one or both of the spouses have preoccupying involvements with their work such that they are unable to leave them behind them when they come home. This is illustrated in the unusual account of one woman who reported that she occasionally gets ideas about her work in the midst of having sex and, once this happens, the magic moment evaporates. There are less extreme indications that occupational involvements displace involvements with family and household. Such displacements can come to constitute stress-provoking strains in family relations. This particular type of conflict, that between outside commitments and family roles, we might note, is especially likely to occur among those in middle-class occupations.

Thus far, then, we have considered two ways in which the multiple roles of family members can create stressor conditions in their family relations. One is through the *emotional distress* that is generated outside but expressed in the actions and affect inside the family. The second is through the interconnections with *competing or incompatible roles*, where the duties, obligations, and investments in the outside role intrude on the expectations and performance of family roles. There is a third way in which family stressors surface in response to outside circumstances. This is where external conditions pose a *direct threat* to the functioning of family relations.

Perhaps the best documented illustration of such threats involves the involuntary loss of job by a breadwinner (Pearlin et al., 1981; Elder, 1974; Brenner, 1973; Catalano and Dooley, 1977; Kasl, 1979; Gore, 1978). The job loss can come about in different ways; it can be the result of a general economic downturn, the consequence of a plant closing, or the job displacement of an individual. Where one is unemployed for a length of time and prospects for future employment are unclear, certain processes are set in motion that can have an inimical impact on family relations. For example, there may be a loss of status of the unemployed breadwinner in the family, real or presumed. The unemployed person, usually the husband and father, can come to feel that he has let his family down and no longer merits their respect. Some of his functions and authority might shift to his wife, especially if she is employed (Elder, 1974), or to his older children. His own self-esteem will be bruised and he might deal with this by withdrawing from family relations, disinvesting his self from them. For example, there is some evidence from a study of Italian families that fathers who consider themselves occupational failures are less affectionate than the occupationally successful with sons, but somewhat more affectionate with daughters (Pearlin, 1971). Presumably, this selective expression of affection reflects something of fathers' own self-defined inability to serve as appropriate role models for sons.

Of course, occupational failure and economic deprivation do not always result in emotional withdrawal in the family. In place of—or in addition to—withdrawal there can be an increase in harshness and the punitive disciplining of children. These kinds of changes, moreover, can be reflected not only in the behaviour of the unemployed father but in the actions of the wife and mother as well (Elder and Liker, 1982). Prolonged and severe economic loss attendant upon job loss can obviously have a profound effect on family relations, turning the family into a reservoir of secondary stressors. We should note that while involuntary unemployment is the most extensively researched, there are other conditions that also stand as direct threats to ordinary family functioning. Seafaring, military service, or other occupations in which a spouse and parent is absent for prolonged periods can also threaten ordinary role definitions and expectations and can lead to severe strains (Hill, 1949).

Thus far we have distinguished stressors that arise directly within the family from those that are prompted by circumstances outside the family. Included among the former are (a) scheduled transitions in the family life cycle; (b) unscheduled or eruptive family changes; and (c) varieties of more chronic role strains. Family stressors triggered by experiences in outside roles are of three types: (a) where emotional distress aroused in other roles are injected into family relations in a way that taints the emotional climate of the family; (b) where the outside roles are uncongenial with the obligations and expectations of family roles; and (c) where the conditions of outside roles pose a direct threat to the meaning and functions of one's family role.

It should be emphasized that both *exposure* to these various stressors and the stressful *responses* to them may vary with people's social statuses, such as class position, race and ethnicity, and age. In general, research into such variations in exposure and vulnerability to stressors has lagged. However, we probably know somewhat more about gender than other statuses in this regard. Where the family is concerned, there is some indication that women may experience stressors more intensely than do men. Because women may have greater involvement in family affairs, they become more sensitive not only to the untoward events that they experience directly but also to those that have adverse effects on other family members (Kessler and McLeod, 1984). Their active engagement in a web of family relationships and the emotional stake they develop in the harmonious functioning of these relationships means that they are unlikely to remain passive witnesses to the life problems of family members. Indeed, even if they prefer to remain uninvolved in the problems of others it may be difficult, for they are more likely than men to be sought out as social supports.

There is, then, some indication that women might be more susceptible to the impact of stressors affecting family members (Dohrenwend and Dohrenwend, 1977; Kessler, 1979). Although the notion that women may be more vulnerable to life problems than men is not well established, it does appear that the relevance of the family as a direct source or as a channel for outside stressors is not the same for men and women. Clearly, research into family stress needs to be designed in a manner that searches for these kinds of patterned variations around key social characteristics.

COPING AND SUPPORTS

We have sought thus far to identify some of the major mechanisms by which the family and its relationships give rise to stressors. Although we have been more concerned with describing the mechanisms than with detailing the stressors, it should be amply evident at this point that the family is a rich and varied source of primary and secondary pain and stress. It is a place where the well-being of people can be seriously damaged. But, paradoxically, it is also the place where the injured can be nurtured and healed and from which they acquire strength for protecting themselves. Much more than as a source of suffering, the family is a primary source of survival and emotional nurtuing. It is a central context in which coping skills may be developed and honed and to which people usually turn in seeking various forms of support.

Coping can be thought of as the things that people do on their own behalf in confronting stress while social supports are the things that others do for them (Pearlin and Schooler, 1978). As noted earlier, in the family this distinction can become quite blurred and difficult to maintain. Indeed, within this context we are inclined to agree with Thoits (1986) that social supports can be viewed as coping assistance. All coping behaviour can be considered to involve efforts: (a) to change and alleviate a difficult situation; (b) to alter and reduce the perceived threats of the situation; or (c) to manage the symptoms of stress arising out of the situation (Pearlin and Schooler, 1978). The particular behaviours one adopts in engaging in his or her coping efforts may be learned in the family context in the same way that other normative behaviours are acquired. Thus, individual family members learn to deal with life problems in one or another manner by observing other members or by being explicitly taught. Behaviour that is consistent with family norms will presumably be further reinforced by the approval of significant family members.

The process by which children learn coping behaviour from parents is somewhat more subtle. In seven of the households in which we interviewed husbands and wives we also interviewed an adolescent-aged child in order to learn whether and how young people learn coping from their parents. A major proving ground for the adolescent's acquisition and testing of his/her coping seems to be in the repeated confrontations with parents around issues that arise between them, issues that might involve the quality of their school work, the choice of friends, the performance of chores, and so on. From the child's perspective, these confrontations force upon them the need to adjust to a parental relationship. That is, the child must deal not only with the problem that has arisen but also with the parental relationship that has been formed in response to the problem. Through successive efforts to deal with parents and the form of their alliance (or misalliance), adolescents begin to learn and develop their coping repertoires. This will become clearer as we illustrate the types of parental relationships with which the child might have to contend.

One form of the relationship that could be discerned from the interviews may be called a consensual united front. It exists where the parents are in agreement both about the gravity of the problem and how it should be dealt with. A second form is related to this in that it, too, shows a united front; however, it is a unity based not on a consensual view of the problem but on a commitment on the part of the parents to support each other when dealing with problems involving children, even where they might disagree about the problem or its remedy. This is a distinction that does not go unnoticed by the child. In still a third form, parents might feel as one with regard to the seriousness of the problem but be at odds over the most effective way to deal with it. There are frequent instances, too, where one parent (usually the father) may simply withdraw from involvement. In some of these instances, the withdrawn parent is subject to call by the other parent should the problem turn out to be difficult to handle. In other cases withdrawal is more unconditional.

One of the points to be underscored here is that a variety of relationships between parents can be formed as they face problems and conflicts with their child. A related point that also needs to be emphasized is that the child cannot successfully cope with these problems without at the same time finding a way to deal with the complex structures that his/her parents present. The ways which children learn to manage relationships with parents around problematic concerns become, in turn, important elements of children's coping repertoires that are acquired in the family context.

It is not possible at this time to specify in detail how particular parental alliances might lead to particular coping dispositions in children. However, our data at least suggest that the way the child learns how to negotiate, solve or ameliorate problems will vary with whether he/she is contending with parents united by consensus or by a commitment to mutual support, whether one parent is withdrawn and aloof or simply waiting in the wings. The readiness of adolescents to be yielding and compliant in the face of adversity, to be divisive and manipulative, to be rebellious, or to adopt other dispositions, will likely depend somewhat on the repeated encounters with their mothers and fathers, both as individuals and as parents bound to each other in various forms. Parents may not directly teach their children how to cope but, nevertheless, it appears that children indirectly learn how to cope in grappling with different forms of parental alliance.

Obviously, much remains to be learned both about the parental arrangements children characteristically encounter and the ways in which these arrangements might shape the learning and use of coping responses. Moreover, it cannot be assumed that the coping that is acquired in the course of dealing with family conflicts will necessarily be incorporated into people's repertoires for coping with conflicts and problems outside the family. But, while there are major issues surrounding coping and its family context remaining to be settled, it is clear that the family and its conflicts provide a crucial arena for the development and testing of children's coping repertoires.

More generally, the observation of coping within the context of the family underscores the social and interactive aspects of coping. Since most of the problems with which people cope arise within role sets, the ways in which any single participant copes will be constrained and influenced by the actions and reactions of the other participants in the role set. The family, of course, contains role sets of exceptional importance and durability. The modes of coping of an individual are bound to be formed here, at least in part; and it is also here that the acceptability of one's coping responses will be under close scrutiny.

Social support, too, inherently entails interactive processes, for there cannot be a recipient of support without there also being a donor. Curiously, however, the interactive aspects of support have been largely overlooked, with research typically centering only on the recipient. Thus, we know little of the behaviour of support donors, how donors and recipients exchange roles, the reciprocities between them, or the conditions that lead donors to withdraw support. However, our qualitative interviews of husbands and wives once again provide some illumination of the interactional character of support processes in the family.

Let us begin our description of these processes from the perspective of the spousal donor of supports. For the donor, the process is initiated with the recognition that there is a problem, however ill-defined it might be initially. As we discussed earlier, recognition can result either from a 'reading' of behavioural cues or from the spouse verbally relating a problem. Once recognized, the donor usually makes an appraisal as to whether support will be welcomed or rejected and, related to this, a judgement as to the most effective timing of the support. Once the donor-spouse decides whether and when to react, a decision—conscious or otherwise—then is made as to the most appropriate form of support. Here there are many possibilities, including instrumental help, advice, an attentive ear, redefining issues, developing alternative lines of actions, reaffirmation of affection and esteem, and so on.

Taking into account the perspective of the recipient, it cannot be assumed that what is given will be experienced as supportive. Whether or not actions are in fact supportive depends on many conditions, including what the recipient wants and expects: Thus, the recipient might want a sympathetic ear but get advice, or expect reassurance but receive an objective critique. Because behaviour is usually supportive only to the extent that it is subjectively perceived as such, discrepancies between what is given and what is wanted can lead one to feel abandoned and desolate, feelings that only create or add to conflicts and problems.

Whatever the nature of coping and support processes, it should be clear that the family constitutes a particularly powerful context for shaping and modifying them and, consequently, is important in mediating the impact of stress. Fortunately, people can also find supportive relations outside the family. However, the family usually stands as a highly available and dependable context for supports, especially those that rest on intimacy and trust. The continuity and quality of its supportive interactions make the family a powerful and often unique support system.

In addition to its importance as a context of coping and social support, the family is a crucial source of self-esteem and mastery, two elements of self-concept shown to function as stress buffers (Pearlin et al., 1981). Self-esteem is rooted in the feedback that individuals receive about themselves in their interactions with others. Since the earliest, most enduring, and strongest bonds are formed around family relations, the family context becomes particularly relevant for self-esteem. Mastery, the extent to which individuals perceive themselves as controlling their life outcomes, is also largely a function of the individuals' past successes and failures in influencing their social environment. A person's conviction that his/her life is under personal control as opposed to being fatalistically ruled, is linked, we believe, to the responsiveness of the person's family, in particular. Patterns of interaction in the family contribute importantly to one's perception of mastery since they will provide, or fail to provide a major test of one's ability to modify his/her social environment.

The family, then, is a powerful context for facilitating various patterns of coping, for providing effective social support, and for shaping the self-concepts and personal resources of its members. It seems apparent that within the family these processes are highly interrelated and difficult to disentangle. That is, one might learn how to cope in the course of receiving social support or one might acquire personal resources while successfully coping. Regardless of the overlap in these processes, it is clear that familial relationships can either provide relief from life problems or, depending on the character and quality of the give and take, can impose an added burden. Most salient, the family context has a double significance for health and emotional well-being, being crucial to both the origins and mediators of stress.

DISCUSSION

It should be evident that the study of family stress processes embodies a myriad of issues and challenges. Necessarily and purposively, a large number of problems has been omitted from consideration here. A few of them, however, need to be acknowledged.

One that needs to be addressed concerns the objective–subjective nature of stressors and their indicators. By and large, most of the stressors that we have described reside not only in the objective conditions of people's lives but in the way that these conditions are experienced as well. This can result in some uncertainty; largely because indicators of stressors based on subjective perceptions can easily become analytically entangled with and indistinguishable from the emotional stress the stressors are supposed to create. Take as an illustration marital reciprocity. The meaure of reciprocity, it will be remembered, is based on the individual's appraisal of the equality of give and take in the marriage. Let's say that we discover that reciprocity is inversely related to emotional distress in marriage. By itself, this finding leaves us in a state of uncertainty; that is, it is not clear whether it captures a cause and effect relationship or whether the subjective appraisal is simply another indicator of stress, such that the relationship merely reflects the correlation of different indicators of the same underlying state. This kind of uncertainty exists to some degree wherever measures of subjective dispositions are being related to psychological states.

How do we deal with this problem? One solution is to seek indicators of stressors that are more objective. Thus, we might develop a measure of reciprocity that does not rely on subjective appraisal. It might be based, for example, on a careful cataloguing of the husband–wife division of labour, to see if one contributes more than the other to household functions. However, even if we ignore the problems of devising such a measure, it simply will not by itself capture the *experiencing* of a stressor. A stressor is not a stressor until it is experienced as such, and similar objective conditions are dissimilarly experienced by people exposed to them. In our view, the best way to deal with the dilemmas posed by using either objective *or* subjective indicators is to use both. We propose this with the conviction that the stressors that are typically of interest to stress researchers do not grow out of objective conditions alone but in conjunction with the subjective dispositions people bring with them to those conditions. In most instances, the threat, hardship, or deprivation experienced when confronting objective circumstances is determined by those circumstances in combination with what people want, expect, or believe—in other words, with the *meaning* people attach those circumstances.

Many examples could be given illustrating this view but we shall present one from our work that deals with family stress (Pearlin, 1975). Early family theorists had speculated that spouses coming from unequal status backgrounds had marriages that were more susceptible to strains and instability than those coming from the same status echelons of the society. Inequality of status in marriage can be regarded as an objective indicator of a potential stressor; all that is needed is factual information about the couple's status backgrounds, nothing about their inner dispositions. When we examine the status mix in marriage in relation to a measure of marital stress, we find, indeed, that this objective stressor is related to stress.

However, not all inequality results in stress; it is specifically inequality involved in marrying a spouse of lower status than produces stress. That is, people whose partners are from a lower status background are *more* likely to experience marital stress than those equal in status; but those marrying up are *less* likely to be stressed. Why should people marrying down—the hypogamous—be more susceptible while the hypergamous are less susceptible to stress? It seemed reasonable to suppose that the hypogamous were more apt to feel loss and the hypergamous more likely to feel gain in their respective marriages. But gain and loss, we reasoned, would be most keenly felt by those to whom status was important. And, in fact, that is the case. People who rated status advancement as very important but who were hypogamous were most stressed, while the hypogamous to whom status was not important were no more stressed than status equals. Conversely, status strivers who married up were least stressed of all groups while their counterparts who were indifferent to status aggrandizement were the same as the equals.

Here is an instance, then, where both objective and subjective measures are important to stress, but their importance depends entirely on how they are combined with each other. The ideal strategy clearly is to devise, wherever possible, objective measures of stressors. In attempting to understand *who* is vulnerable to objective stressors and *how* the vulnerability arises, however, we need to bring into analysis appropriate measures of subjective dispositions. It is these that shape the meaning of the objective stressors and determine whether the stressors will actually be experienced as stressors. When patterned variations are found between the different combinations of objective–subjective factors, as in the example above, there is no longer any cause for concern that the measure of subjective disposition is but another indicator of emotional stress, thus eliminating the possibility that their relationship is merely tautological. At the same time, it becomes possible to understand more clearly the conditions under which a potential stressor is most likely to have a stressful impact. Looked at together, objective circumstances and subjective dispositions bring us closer to a dynamic specification of the stress process.

Quite aside from their objective–subjective character, it is difficult to identify stressors that are universally found in the family. One reason for this is the varied forms that the modern family assumes. Much of our discussion in this chapter took as a point of departure an intact nuclear family composed of a mother, father, and one or more children. In looking at the different parts played by the family in the stress process, it needs to be recognized that there is a very sizable number of households in this society that do not fit this model. There are, for example, families in which there is but one parent; others have step-parents, some of which might have merged children from the previous marriage(s); and still others are three-generational, with an elderly parent in residence or an adult child who has returned to the parental home with children of his/her own.

Our purpose in drawing attention to the many forms of family life in society is to emphasize that each may very well be host to stressors unique to it. For example, a three-generation family household gives rise to problems different from those experienced by a two-generation family. Or the legitimacy of authority exercised by step-parents may be questioned in ways that are absent in the case of natural parents; and so on. Even the ways in which the family functions as a conduit of problems that arise outside its boundaries might vary with the form of the family. And, finally, there is reason to expect that the contributions of the family to coping and social supports will differ among different types of families. In short, we cannot assume that the stress process as it is observed under one set of family conditions will be the same as observed under other conditions.

There is another kind of differentiation that must be made when examining the family as a source of stress or as a context of stress mediation. This involves the social and economic characteristics of the family members. Gender, of course, is an outstanding example of what we are referring to. As we discussed earlier, men and women have very different roles in the family, come to it with different expectations, look to the future with somewhat different dreams, are hurt by different things, and respond to their hurt in somewhat different ways. Therefore, the stress process, whether in the context of the family or other institutions, can be strikingly different for women and men.

Similarly, the location of the family and its members in the larger stratification order influences the kinds of stressors that are likely to be filtered through the family. People's positions within the surrounding social structures regulate the stressful experiences they have within particular institutional settings and, consequently, regulate those that will be brought into the family from outside. In order to conceptualize the stressors and mediators that are tied to family life, therefore, it is necessary to recognize that marriage and parenthood entail very different roles for people having different social and economic characteristics. The measures of stressors, of coping, and of support that we eventually construct should ideally be sensitive to this kind of differentiation.

There is a final issue whose importance is not reflected by the attention we have given it. This concerns the developmental changes in the nature of the stressors to which people are exposed. We have indirectly made some reference to this in discussing role restructuring, as where, for example, adult children come to assume responsibility for elderly parents. Quite obviously too, certain stressful events are closely associated with location along the life course, such as the loss of a spouse in old age. In general, however, little attention has been given to identifying the kinds of stressors to which people are likely to be exposed as they traverse the life course. In particular, little is known of young adults and the stressful effects of entering into a succession of new institutional roles within a relatively compressed time-span. Thus, the completion of training, marriage, having children, finding housing, establishing and advancing in occupational life all take place in a short period of time. Although there is some evidence that this takes an emotional toll, it has not been the focus of concerted study. We are suggesting, then, that the stressful conditions of life change their form with movement along the life course.

We would also emphasize that when people at different locations in their life course are exposed to similar conditions, the conditions might be experienced by them in very different ways. An involuntary job loss for a newly married man with a working wife, for example, is essentially a different experience than when the loss occurs in the life of a middle-aged man whose children are getting ready to enter college and whose wife is a homemaker. The life course is both itself a seedbed of potential stressful experiences and an important context that shapes the meaning and impact of the experiences on individuals and families. Research into family stressors could profitably address these life course issues.

In sum, it is somewhat misleading to speak of *the* family in relation to the stress process. Although the term directs attention to a central social institution, it should not obscure what is so very clear: there are many family forms that incorporate a web of criss-crossing relationships made up of people having varied attachments to other social institutions and bearing a multitude of achieved and accorded statuses. Moreover, the mix of these ingredients changes as the family and its members move from one stage to another along the life course. Given this very textured fabric of family life, it is understandable that the nature and range of the stressors that appear within it are themselves highly differentiated. Despite these complexities, the family is an accessible and exciting area of study for the stress researcher. In this chapter we have attempted to provide some conceptual order that will contribute to its study.

REFERENCES

Brenner, M. H. (1973). *Mental Illness and the Economy*, Harvard University Press, Cambridge.

Catalano, R. and Dooley, D. (1977). Economic predictors of depressed mood and stressful life events, *Journal of Health and Social Behaviour*, **18**, 292–307.

Cooley, C. H. (1915). *Social Organization*, Scribner, New York.

Croog, S. H. (1970). The family as a source of stress. In S. Levine and N. Scotch (eds.) *Social Stress*, Aldine, Chicago, pp. 19–53.

Dohrenwend, B., and Dohrenwend, B. (1977). Sex differences in psychiatric disorders, *American Journal of Sociology*, **81**, 1447–59.

Dohrenwend, B., and Pearlin, L. I. (1982). Report on stress and life events. In G. Elliott and C. Eisdorfer (eds.) *Stress and Human Health: Analysis and Implications of Research*, Springer, New York, pp. 55–80.

Elder, G. H. (1974). *Children of the Great Depression*, University of Chicago, Chicago.

Elder, G. H., and Liker, K. (1982). Hard times in women's lives, *American Journal of Sociology*, **88**, 241–69.

Fisher, L. (1982). Transactional theories but individual assessment: A frequent discrepancy in family research, *Family Process*, **21**, 313–20.

Gore, S. (1978). The effect of social support in moderating the health consequences of unemployment, *Journal of Health and Social Behaviour*, **19**, 157–65.

Gore, S. (1985). Social support and styles of coping with stress. In S. Cohn and L. Syme (eds.) *Social Support and Health*, Academic Press, New York, pp. 263–78.

Hill, R. (1949). *Families Under Stress*, Greenwood Press, Connecticut.

Holmes, T. H., and Rahe, R. H. (1967). The social readjustment rating scale, *Journal of Psychosomatic Research*, **11**, 213–8.

House, J. S. (1974). Occupational stress and physical health. In J. O'Toole (ed.) *Work and the Quality of Life*, M.I.T. Press, Cambridge, MA, pp. 145–70.

Kasl, S. (1974). Work and mental health. In J. O'Toole (ed.) *Work and the Quality of Life*, M.I.T. Press, Cambridge, MA, pp. 171–96.

Kasl, S. (1979). Changes in mental health status associated with job loss and retirement, In J. E. Barrett (ed.) *Stress and Mental Disorder*, Raven Press, New York.

Kessler, R. (1979). A strategy for studying differential vulnerability to the psychological consequences of stress, *Journal of Health and Social Behaviour*, **20**, 100–8.

Kessler, R., and McLeod, J. D. (1984). Sex differences in vulnerability to undesirable life events, *American Sociological Review*, **49**, 620–31.

McCubbin, H. I., and Patterson, J. M. (1982). Family adaptation to crisis. In H. I. McCubbin, A. E. Cauble, and J. M. Patterson (eds.) *Family Stress, Coping and Social Support*, Charles C. Thomas, Springfield, Ill., pp. 26–47.

McLean, A. (1979). *Work Stress*, Addison-Wesley, Reading, Mass.

Menaghan, E. (1982). Assessing the impact of family transitions on marital experience. In H. I. McCubbin, A. E. Cauble, and J. M. Patterson (eds.) *Family Stress, Coping and Social Support*, Charles C. Thomas, Springfield, Ill., pp. 90–108.

Merton, R. K. (1957). The role set: Problems in sociological theory, *British Journal of Sociology*, **8**, 106–20.

Pearlin, L. I. (1971). *Class Context of Family Relations: A Cross-National Study*, Little Brown & Co., Boston.

Pearlin, L. I. (1975). Status inequality and stress in marriage, *American Sociological Review*, **40**, 344–57.

Pearlin, L. I. (1980a). The life cycle and life strains. In H. M. Blalock, jun. (ed.) *Sociological Theory and Research: A Critical Approach*, Springer, New York, pp. 349–60.

Pearlin, L. I. (1980b). Life strains and psychological distress among adults: A conceptual overview. In N. J. Smelzer, and E. H. Erikson (eds.) *Themes of Love and Work in Adulthood*, Harvard University Press, Cambridge, MA, pp. 174–92.

Pearlin, L. I. (1982). The social contexts of stress. In L. Goldberger and S. Breznitz (eds.) *Handbook of Stress*, The Free Press, New York, pp. 367–79.

Pearlin, L. I. (1983a). Developmental perspectives on family and mental health. Unpublished Report, Behavioral Sciences Research in Mental Health, Dept. of Health and Human Services, Washington, D.C.

Pearlin, L. I. (1983b). Role strains and personal stress. In H. B. Kaplan (ed.) *Psychosocial Stress: Trends in Theory and Research*, Academic Press, New York.

Pearlin, L. I. and Johnson, J. S. (1977). Marital status, life strains and depression, *American Sociological Review*, **42**, 704–15.

Pearlin, L. I., and Schooler, C. (1978). The structure of coping, *Journal of Health and Social Behaviour*, **19**, 2–21.

Pearlin, L. I., and Lieberman, M. L. (1978). Social sources of emotional distress. In R. Simmons (ed.) *Research in Community and Mental Health*, JAI Press, Greenwich, Conn., pp. 217–48.

Pearlin, L. I., Lieberman, M. L., Menaghan, E., and Mullan, J. T. (1981). The stress process, *Journal of Health and Social Behaviour*, **22**, 337–56.

Pearlin, L. I., and Aneshensel, C. S. (1986). Coping and social supports: Their functions and applications. In L. H. Aiken, and D. Mechanic (eds.) *Applications of Social Science to Clinical Medicine and Health*, Rutgers University Press, New Brunswick, NJ.

Reiss, D., and Oliveri, M. E. (1980). Family paradigm and family coping: A proposal for linking the family's intrinsic adaptive capacities to its responses to stress, *Family Relations*, **29**, 431–44.

Sheppard, H. L. (1976). Work and retirement. In R. H. Binstock and E. Shanas (eds.) *Handbook of Aging and the Social Services*, Van Nostrand Rheinhold Co., New York, pp. 283–309.

Thoits, P. A. (1986). Social support as coping assistance, *Journal of Consulting and Clinical Psychology*, forthcoming.

Chapter 7

Measurement and Methodological Issues in Social Support

Roy L. Payne and J. Graham Jones

MRC/ESRC Social and Applied Psychology Unit
The University of Sheffield, U.K.

INTRODUCTION

Social support emerged as an important concept from attempts to mobilize families in dealing with personal crises (Caplan, 1976). Since then it has been incorporated into the stress process generally (Payne, 1980; Pearlin et al., 1981). This has been necessary because empirical studies have shown that good support helps people to cope with many kinds of stress. However, a little thinking soon reveals that support may not only be of value when people are stressed, and that lack of it may even be a source of stress in itself (Gore, 1978).

Let us imagine Mary, a married woman with two children, both at school. She copes well with the demands this makes, but gets help with baby-sitting from her parents and friends and her husband shares many of the household chores. She has no major problem but she depends on the support of other people. Mary is offered a chance to return to her professional career. Whilst this causes some problems with her present arrangements she is able to hire a housekeeper and her parents and husband are glad to put in a little more effort to help her cope with this exciting opportunity. Mary is challenged and with people's help and some reorganization of resources she accepts the challenge and enjoys the new experiences it brings. She is not stressed, even though she is challenged, but she depends on the support of others. Mary's husband is tragically killed in an accident. Doctors, the clergy, friends, and family rush to help and Mary is deluged with emotional support, practical help, financial help, advice and encouragement for her brave efforts. Some months after this tragedy Mary finds much of her friends' enthusiastic support has evaporated, or that their well meant advice is annoying and irritating. The loss of this support worries her, and although she remains dependent on some of these people whom she finds irritating, she begins to withdraw from them, and joins a singles club to seek out people in similar situations to her own. This causes some raised eyebrows, 'so soon after the event'. Mary has experienced a very

Research Methods in Stress and Health Psychology. Edited by S. V. Kasl and C. L. Cooper.

negative life event which has turned into a situation of chronic stress. Her dependence on the help of other people has increased considerably. She is stressed and she needs support, but maintaining what support she had, and seeking new sources of support, helps her to cope well enough to begin to build a new life.

The purpose of this vignette is to illustrate that social support takes place all the time for most people, not just when they are stressed; that it is part of a complex process that takes place in a context and over time; that it can have negative as well as positive meaning for the recipient; that one gives as well as receives support; that support may be emotional, practical, financial, and/or informational in character and it may come from family, friends, the community and specialist professionals; that it sometimes has to be sought out actively and that there are costs in seeking it. Such a complex process presents an enormous challenge to empirical social science. As we shall see, the measures and methods used so far have not succeeded totally in achieving what Ashby (1956) called the 'requisite variety' to match this complexity. Our concerns, however, are with questions like, how far have particular approaches gone? And what are the advantages and disadvantages of different methods of measurement and design? Consideration of such questions, however, must be preceded by an assessment of the measures used to study the quantity and quality of social support.

Reliability and validity of some major measures

Early measures of social support were very crude indices of social embeddedness (Stokes and Wilson, 1984), often equating the concept with marital status or the availability of a confidant(e) during a crisis (Wilcox, 1981). It is only relatively recently that measurement issues in social support have been considered seriously, though in 1977 Dean and Lin reported that they could find no social support scales with sufficient evidence of reliability or validity. Leavy's (1983) comments reflect the current *Zeitgeist*:

> There is currently no assessment instrument which comprehensively measures the central components of social support with acceptable levels of reliability and validity... Most support questionnaires are ad hoc measures with questionable reliability and unknown validity. Obviously, progress in understanding the role of social support in relation to stress and disorder is jeopardized if we cannot trust the data we generate. Reliability problems are also an obstacle to comparing and generalizing findings (p. 16).

This situation has partly emerged from the failure to agree on how social support should be conceptualized and operationalized. The conceptual issues discussed in the previous section demonstrate that the general notion of social support is extremely vague and broad in nature. This conceptual diversity is reflected in the diversity of instruments purporting to measure social support. Researchers have often devised their own instruments to answer specific questions instead of building systematically on past and tried, if not proven, methods and measures. The list of measures which have been incorporated in social support studies is a lengthy one and includes scales concerned with: subjects' confidants and acquaintances (Miller and Ingham, 1976); the availability of helpful others in coping with certain work, family, and financial problems (Medalie and Goldbourt, 1976); interpersonal assets and liabilities (Luborsky et al., 1973); individual's level of functioning in the community (Renne, 1974); and perceived availability and adequacy of social support (Henderson, 1980).

The variety of different measurement instruments has complicated the process of integrating the findings, which have sometimes been conflicting. In many cases, social support has been found to have a positive effect on stress (e.g. Eaton, 1978; Gore, 1978; LaRocco and Jones, 1978; Sandler, 1980; Wilcox, 1981). However, some studies have failed to find any effect of social support (e.g. Andrews et al., 1978; Gad and Johnson, 1980; Lin et al., 1979), while some researchers have even reported negative effects of social support (e.g. Goldstein, 1980). Sandler and Barrera (1981) believe that these discrepancies can only be resolved by adopting a multi-method approach, by examining the relationships between the distinctly different measures of social support used in many studies. An alternative solution is to ensure the repeated use of measurement instruments which are proved and tested.

This would introduce some degree of uniformity into future research by repeatedly using measures which are precise, reliable and valid scales of social support and which allow comparisons across heterogeneous samples. We acknowledge at this point that what we are stating is not original as such an approach has already been recommended by Tardy (1985) in a review of suitable devices for measuring social support. Tardy first addresses the need to clarify conceptual issues in order to, in turn, clarify the decisions facing researchers. He concludes that measures of social support potentially encompass five interdependent primary elements:

(1) Direction: Is social support provided to others, or received from others, or both?
(2) Disposition: Is social support available (i.e. quantity or quality of support to which people have access) and/or enacted (i.e. the actual utilization of these resources)?
(3) Description/Evaluation: Is the quality and nature of the social support described and/or evaluated?
(4) Content: Does the content of the social support available focus on emotional, instrumental, informational or appraisal issues? (House, 1981).

(5) Network: What are the sources of support? Do they include family, close friends, neighbours, co-workers, community, and/or professionals?

Tardy assumes that all research on social support makes assumptions about these elements so that this provides a suitable theoretical and operational framework for decisions concerning social support studies. He then identifies seven instruments which are capable of measuring these components. Only five of these scales are discussed here. The Social Support Network Interview (Fischer, 1982) is omitted from this discussion as no reliability estimates are reported for this scale, whilst the Social Support Vignettes instrument (Turner, 1981) is not discussed due to inherent uncertainty about disposition and content in this measure.

Arizona Social Support Interview Schedule (ASSIS)

The ASSIS was developed by Manuel Barrera (1980, 1981) as an instrument to measure several aspects of support, including procedures for identifying support network membership and subjects' satisfaction with and need for support. The ASSIS requires subjects to identify individuals (by names or initials) who provide support in the following areas: private feelings; material aid; advice; positive feedback; physical assistance; and, social participation. Following each of six such questions, the subject is asked further questions concerning whether the people identified have provided support in the past month (i.e. enacted) and whether the support received was sufficient (i.e. evaluated). An illustrative example of a set of questions is presented below concerning the topic of social participation:

(1) Who are the people that you get together with to have fun or relax? These could be new names or ones you listed before.
Probe: Anyone else?

(2) During the past month, which of these people did you actually get together with to have fun or to relax?
Probe: Ask about people who were named in 1 but not 2.

(3) During the past month, would you have liked:
1—a lot more opportunities to get together with people for fun and relaxation?
2—a few more?
3—or was it about right?

(4) How much do you think that you needed to get together with other people for fun and relaxation during the past month?
1—not at all
2—a little bit
3—quite a bit

(Barrera, 1981, p. 92)

The interview schedule includes questions concerning negative interactions which require the subject to identify people with whom they have had personal conflict in the past month. Finally, the subject is asked a series of questions about the personal characteristics of individuals identified as providing support, such as age, sex and ethnicity.

The data obtained from the ASSIS allow the evaluation of (a) total network size; (b) conflicted network size; (c) unconflicted network size; (d) support satisfaction; and (e) support need. The test–retest reliability of the instrument was measured using a sample of forty-five university students and total network size produced a correlation coefficient of 0.88 over a period of two or more days (Barrera, 1981). Test–retest correlations were 0.54 for size of conflicted network, 0.33 for satisfaction and 0.52 for support need. Given the short time periods involved these data suggest affective judgements about support are quite labile. The predictive validity of the ASSIS was assessed in a study of pregnant adolescents ($N = 86$) (Barrera, 1981) in which conflicted network size correlated significantly with depression (r = 0.23) and anxiety (r = 0.30), satisfaction correlated with depression (r = −0.49) and anxiety (r = −0.34), and need correlated significantly with depression (r = 0.48), anxiety (r = 0.51) and somatization (r = 0.28). It can be assumed that life events will have an impact on social support networks, and, as we shall see later, Thoits (1982) has argued that many life events directly alter the network (e.g. loss of spouse, or job). Relationships between life events and measures of social support can, therefore, be construed as evidence for construct validity. In the study referred to above, life events were found to be correlated with unconflicted network size (r = 0.25), need for support (r = 0.36) and dissatisfaction with support (r = 0.38). These correlations represent modest support for the construct validity of ASSIS, though one might speculate about why conflicted network size does not correlate with life events.

Inventory of Socially Supportive Behaviours (ISSB)

The ISSB is another measure devised by Barrera (1981) and was designed for use with a wide variety of community populations. The ISSB asks subjects to state how people have helped them in the last month and to respond to each of the forty items as: not at all; once or twice; about once a week; several times a week; or about every day. This instrument, therefore, measures the receipt and enactment of social support but does not specify the source of the support. The ISSB measures four types of social support: emotional; instrumental; information appraisal; and socializing (Stokes and Wilson, 1984). Items assessing emotional support include ‘Expressed interest in your well being’, ‘Listened to you talk about your private feelings’, and ‘Was right there with you (physically) in a stressful situation’. Instrumental appraisal support is covered by such items as ‘Provided you with a place to stay’, ‘Loaned you over $25’, and ‘Provided you with some sort of transportation’. Informational appraisal support includes such items as 'Gave you some information on how to do something', 'Gave you feedback on how you were doing without saying it was good or bad', and 'Helped you understand why you didn't do something well'. Two items relate to socializing: 'Talked with you about some interest of yours'; and 'Did some activity together to help you get your mind off things'.

A test–retest reliability coefficient of 0.88 was obtained over at least two days and internal reliability coefficients of 0.93 and 0.92 were revealed with college students (N = 71) and pregnant adolescents (N = 86) respectively. The construct validity of ISSB is indicated by significant correlations with a measure of negative life events in studies by Barrera (1981) ($r = 0.41$) and Sandler and Barrera (1984) ($r = 0.38$).

Perceived Social Support from Family and Friends (PSSFA-FR)

The PSSFA-FR was devised by Procidano and Heller as a measure of perceived social support. This instrument primarily measures support receipt, both enacted and available, particularly with respect to emotional support. The instrument comprises two twenty-item self-report measures, one for family and the other concerning friends. Responses to every question require a simple 'yes', 'no' or 'don't know'. Illustrative items from PSS-FA are: 'I rely on my family for emotional support'; 'My family is sensitive to my personal needs'; and 'My family gives me the moral support I need'. The PSS-FR scale includes such statements as: 'My friends enjoy hearing about what I think'; 'I have a deep sharing relationship with a number of friends'; and, 'I feel that I'm on the fringe of my circle of friends'. A few of the items also refer to support provision, such as, 'My friends come to me for emotional support' and 'Certain members of my family come to me when they have problems or need advice'.

Measurement of the internal reliability of the two scales yielded alpha coefficients of 0.88 for PSS-FR and 0.90 for PSS-FA (N = 222 university students) (Procidano and Heller, 1983). Test–retest reliability was 0.83 over a one-month interval. Procidano and Heller (1983) also found these scales to correlate with measures of psychopathology and distress illustrating the scale's predictive validity.

Social Relationship Scale (SRS)

The SRS was developed by McFarlane et al. (1981) as part of a more extensive home interview. The subject is asked to identify (by initials and relationship) those individuals with whom they have had discussions about six potential areas of life stress: work; money; home and family; personal and social; health; and, general social issues. The subject is asked to rate the helpfulness of the discussion on a seven-point scale ranging from 'makes things a lot worse' to 'makes things a lot better'. Tardy views the SRS as providing more information than most measures of social support. It measures both the provision and receipt of support as well as providing information about sources of support, support content, the availability and satisfaction with support. This instrument also provides for negative outcomes so that the researcher is able to assess both positive and negative aspects of social support in the six potential areas of life stress.

The reliability of the SRS was measured using a sample of college students ($N = 73$) over a one-week period. Correlations on the number of individuals in each category ranged from 0.62 to 0.99, with a median of 0.91. The average helpfulness measure also demonstrates reasonable reliability, with the correlations in each category (i.e. work, money, home, health, personal, society) ranging from 0.54 to 0.94, with a median of 0.78. Criterion validity was demonstrated by the ability of the instrument to differentiate significantly between a sample of parent therapists ($n = 18$) and parents soliciting psychiatric counselling ($n = 15$). The latter group reported inferior levels of social support.

Social Support Questionnaire (SSQ)

The SSQ is a self-report questionnaire and was developed by Sarason et al. (1983) to measure the availability of and satisfaction with social support. The instrument comprises twenty-seven items, each of which require the subject to identify people who they can turn to in specific situations and to indicate their satisfaction with these supports. Illustrative items are: 'Whom can you really count on to listen to you when you need to talk?'; 'With whom can you totally be yourself?'; and, 'Whom can you count on to console you when you are very upset?'. An availability index is calculated by summing the number of persons listed and dividing by the number of items. Most of the items are concerned with emotional support so that this scale is probably most appropriate to assess emotional support (Tardy, 1985).

An examination of available psychometric data suggests that the SSQ is a viable measure of social support. Reliability coefficients over a four-week period were 0.90 for the availability measure and 0.83 for satisfaction using a sample of university students ($n = 105$). The alpha coefficients for internal reliability were 0.97 for availability and 0.94 for satisfaction, again using university students ($n = 602$). Predictive validation studies revealed significant negative correlations between both measures and depression scores. Correlation coefficients for availability were −0.24 for men ($n = 100$) and −0.31 for women ($n = 127$), and −0.22 for males and −0.43 for females in the case of satisfaction measures. A positive relationship between the availability of social support and positive life events and a negative relationship between support satisfaction and negative life events (Sarason et al., 1983) ($n = 295$) demonstrated construct validity, and is consistent with other studies already mentioned.

These five measures have been demonstrated, therefore, to have acceptable test–retest reliability and internal homogeneity. They are also quite successful on predicting psychological symptoms, indicating useful predictive validity. There is much less data on construct validity but relationships with life events are encouraging. It is important to emphasize that construct validity contrasts sharply with empirical approaches in which the validity of a measure is gauged purely by its success in predicting a criterion (Kerlinger, 1973). Apart from life events, there is little evidence provided to demonstrate the construct validity of these scales, although the ISSB was found to correlate significantly with another measure of social support, Cohen and Haberman's Interpersonal Evaluation List: the correlation was 0.46 in a sample of ninety-two undergraduates (Cohen et al., 1984). Nevertheless, provided that one is aware of inherent limitations, these measures may be used to study a wide range of issues concerning social support. The details of these five scales are summarized in Table 1.

A further measure of social support which is not discussed by Tardy (1985) but which is particularly worthy of mention here is the Interview Schedule for Social Interaction (ISSI) (Henderson et al., 1980). The ISSI is a rather long interview schedule comprising fifty-two questions concerned with the availability and adequacy of persons in specified roles. The questions are mainly concerned with the availability of and satisfaction with the six provisions proposed by Weiss (1974), which are: attachment, provided by close affectional relationships; social integration, provided by membership of a network of persons having shared interests and values; the opportunity for nurturing others; reassurance of personal wealth; a sense of reliable alliance; and, obtaining help and guidance from informal advisors in times of difficulty. The questions are two-part in nature, with a question about the availability of a specific provision immediately followed by a question concerning adequacy. Although the items cover all six provisions proposed by Weiss, a much greater emphasis is focused on attachment than the remaining five. This is due to Henderson et al.'s belief that attachment theory leads to the prediction that it will have the strongest association with the development of psychiatric symptoms. Illustrative items are:

> 'How many friends do you have whom you could visit at any time, without waiting for an invitation. You could arrive without being expected and still be sure you would be welcome.'

None	1
1–2	2
3–5	3
6–10	4
11–15	5
More than 15	6

Table 1: Summary of Social Support Measures (Amended from Tardy, 1985)

Scales	Direction	Disposition	Description/ evaluation	Content	Network	Additional features
Arizona social support interview schedule (Barrera, 1981)	Received	Enacted and available	Described and evaluated	Multiple	Supporters listed by respondents	Contains separate negative items
Inventory of socially supportive behaviours (Barrera, 1981)	Received	Enacted	Described	Multiple	Not measured	Can be labelled to measure network
Perceived social support from family and friends scale (Procidano and Heller, 1983)	Mostly received	Part enacted and part available	Described	Emotional	Friends and family	None
Social relationship scale (McFarlane et al., 1981)	Received	Enacted	Described and evaluated	Multiple	Supporters listed by respondent	Contains a negative support item
Social support questionnaire (Sarason et al., 1983)	Received	Available	Described and evaluated	Mostly emotional	Supporters listed by respondent	None
Interview schedule for social interaction (Henderson et al., 1980)	Received	Available	Described and evaluated	Multiple	Supporters listed by respondent and/or others	Contains negative emotional contacts

'Would you like to have more or fewer friends like this, or is it about right for you.'

Less	1
About right	2
Depends on the situation	3
More	4

This scale yields four main scores for each respondent: availability of attachment (AVAT); perceived adequacy of attachment (ADAT); availability of social integration (AVSI) (by combining acquaintance, friendship, reassurance of worth, and reliable alliance); and, perceived adequacy of social integration (ADSI). It is also possible to calculate two further indices. Three items enquire about unpleasant interactions. An illustrative item is: 'How many people whom you have to see regularly do you dislike?' These items yield a score for the number of attachment persons with whom the respondent has recently been having rows or unpleasant interactions (ATTROWN). In addition, it is possible to calculate a score for the number of facets of attachment relationships which the respondent says he has not got but can do without (NONAT).

Test–retest reliability scores for the four principal indices over an eighteen-day period using a general population sample (n = 51) were 0.76 for AVAT, 0.71 for ADAT, 0.75 for AVSI and 0.75 for ADSI. Correlations over a twelve-month period (n = 221) were 0.85, 0.69, 0.85, and 0.66 for AVAT, ADAT, AVSI, ADSI respectively (Henderson et al., 1980). Internal reliability scores (n = 756) were 0.67 for AVAT, 0.69 for ADAT, 0.71 for AVSI, and 0.79 for ADSI.

The validity measures for the ISSI are also reasonably impressive. A measure of construct validity is presented by Henderson et al. (1980) in which they considered the four principal ISSI indices in relation to the more enduring personality traits of neuroticism and introversion–extraversion as measured by the Eysenck Personality Inventory (Eysenck and Eysenck, 1964). The ISSI and EPI were administered to a general population sample (n = 225) at the beginning and end of an eight-month period. The results are presented in Table 2. In the case of neuroticism, there is a negative relationship with both the availability and satisfaction measures. This is in line with logical expectations as one would predict that a highly neurotic individual would have problems in forming and maintaining social relationships and would consequently be dissatisfied with these relationships. In the case of extraversion, the moderate correlation (r = 0.31) with AVSI and the marginal relationship (r = 0.15) with ADSI would be expected as an individual scoring high on extraversion presumably has a wide range of social contacts. However, extraversion is not related to the availability and adequacy of attachment.

Table 2: Correlations of ISSI Scores with Personality Dimensions ($N = 225$) (from Henderson et al., 1981)

	Trait neuroticism	Extraversion
AVAT	−0.18	0.03
AVSI	−0.24	0.31
ADAT	−0.29	0.06
ADSI	−0.31	0.51

The predictive validity of the ISSI can be extracted from a study carried out by Henderson et al. (1981) to examine the relationship between neurosis and the social environment in a sample of residents of Canberra, Australia. The strong predictive validity of the ISSI can be demonstrated by examining its relationship with two measures of psychiatric disorder used in the study: The General Health Questionnaire (Goldberg, 1972) and the Zung Self-Rating Depression Scale (Zung, 1965, 1967). Correlations between the three measures are presented in Table 3.

Table 3: Correlations between GHQ and Zung SDS and the ISSI (amended from Henderson et al., 1981)

	GHQ ($n = 754$)	Zung SDS ($n = 751$)
AVAT	−0.96*	−0.151†
ADAT	−0.294†	−0.318†
AVSI	−0.96*	−0.230†
ADSI	−0.280†	−0.245†
ATTROWN	0.324†	0.206†

*$p < .01$
†$p < .001$

As expected, the availability and adequacy of both attachment and social interaction correlated significantly and negatively with psychiatric disorder and depression. In addition, unpleasant interactions (ATTROWN) correlated significantly and positively with the two symptomatological scores.

Other unusual validation evidence is available for ISSI. Henderson et al., have shown that scores differ for different social groups in predictable ways e.g. married couples versus widows, divorced people etc. They have also shown that individuals who have recently moved to Canberra have less developed support networks.

The ISSI was also adopted so that it could be administered to persons who knew the focal respondent well, and could provide information about their perceptions of his/her social activities. All correlations between the scores of the focal respondent and the informant were significant beyond 0.01 level and ranged from 0.26 to 0.59. The correlations were higher for availability measures than adequacy measures as might be expected.

Finally, the ISSI was related to the Lie Scale of EPI and the Crowne-Marlowe Inventory (Crowne and Marlowe, 1960, 1964) to assess the effect of social response set. Combinations of these measures accounted for only 6–11 per cent of the variance in these principal ISSI measures. Whilst these are not negligible given the size of predictive validity and construct validity coefficients, they are certainly not large enough to obscure other effects.

In summary, the ISSI has been demonstrated to be a particularly adequate measure of social support in terms of both internal and test–retest reliability and construct and predictive validity. This measure together with the five measures discussed earlier provide the basis for reliable and valid research on social support in the future. They are certainly more desirable tools than the simple ratings of single items used in some of the earlier studies of social support (e.g. Caplan et al., 1975; Pinneau, 1975). It must not be forgotten, however, that studies using such scales stimulated interest in the topic itself and are an important part of its history.

If one were to distinguish between work-related and home-related support, stronger relationships would be hypothesized within each type than between them (i.e. convergent versus discriminant validity). Seers et al. (1983) studied a sample of 104 predominantly female respondents working for a large government agency. Relationships between work-related sources of support were relatively strong, with unit manager support correlating with branch manager support (r = 0.39) and co-worker support (r = 0.29), and co-worker support correlating with branch manager support (r = 0.23). However, correlation coefficients, although significant, were lower between family and friends support and branch manager support (r = 0.19) and unit manager support (r = 0.19). On the other hand, support from family and friends correlated highly with co-worker support (r = 0.56). House and Wells (1978) found similar results using a sample of 1809 white male rubber workers. Co-worker support correlated moderately with supervisor support (r = 0.30), whilst there was a strong relationship between wife support and friend and relative support (r = 0.62). However, friend and relative support was only marginally related to supervisor support (r = 0.16), whilst support from friends and relatives again correlated moderately with co-worker support (r = 0.32).

One possible explanation for these sorts of relationships is that the workers' friends were also co-workers. Another explanation for the correlations between these two major sources of support concerns the personality, and hence popularity, of the individual. A person who is popular is likely to attract support from both home-related and work-related sources.

Such studies of convergent and discriminant validity do, however, serve to increase confidence in the ability of support measures to discriminate between different sources of support.

So far we have more or less taken for granted that social support is an important determinant or mediator of psychological health and well-being and some of the predictive validity data supports this. We examine this more systematically by looking at the size of the relationship between social support and measures of psychological health/illness and measures of stress. Before reviewing this, however, it is necessary to understand the theoretical perspectives that have directed such studies.

Theoretical perspectives in social support research

These have been explicated by House (1981) and elaborated by Thoits (1982) and the following draws heavily on their contributions. The central issues can be presented diagrammatically as in Figure 1. The underlying assumption is that stress has an acute, and/or chronic effect on both psychological and physical health. The underlying question is, does social support in any way protect the person's health? The specific questions are: if it does, is it because:

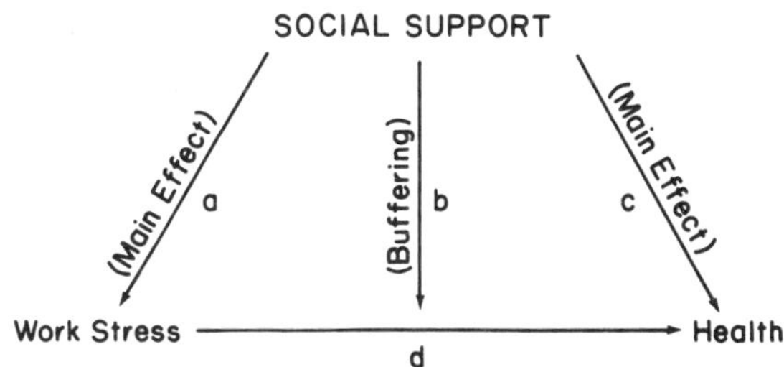

Figure 1: Potential Effects of Social Support on Work Stress and Health

(1) Social support has a direct effect on health (arrow c) by providing emotional comfort which reduces the effects of symptoms, promotes recovery etc. or perhaps because people provide timely help and advice which treats the symptoms more effectively? Or perhaps social support meets an important human need anyway, and lack of it causes psychological damage directly.

(2) Social support directly reduces the stressors affecting the individual? (arrow a). Support providers might for example lend a person money, solve the problem, remove the person from the stressors, or convince the person the stressors are not really dangerous.

(3) Social support disturbs or mitigates the relationship between stressors and health (arrow d): this has come to be known as the buffering hypothesis (arrow b). This hypothesis assumes that there are no direct effects of social

support on either health or stressors but the relationship between them is in some way altered. To clarify the sorts of empirical relationship involved we follow House and present graphs depicting the expected relationships for each of these three hypotheses under conditions of high, medium and low social support.

Figures 2(a), (b), and (c) are taken from House (1981) and show the expected empirical relationships between stress and poor health under different degrees of social support for the direct effects of health hypothesis (a), the buffering hypothesis (b) and the combined direct effect on health and buffering hypothesis (c). As the figures show, the main difference between the direct effect on health and the buffering hypothesis is that in the direct effect case, social support always has a positive effect on health. In the buffering case,

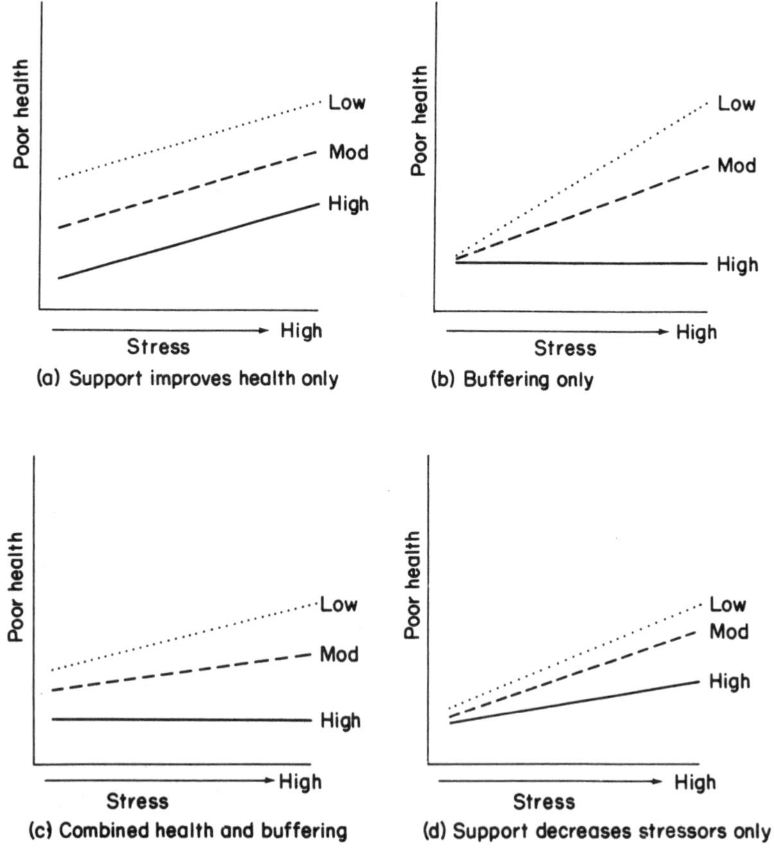

Figure 2: Possible Relationships between Social Support, Stress and Health

social support only influences health under conditions of stress. For the combined case the main difference is under conditions of low stress, where social support is shown to have a positive effect on health, though not as strongly as it would in the direct effects case. For some reason, House has not included the direct effects on stress hypothesis. We have added this as figure 2(d). We have assumed that high social support will not totally remove the negative consequences of high stress, though it would work to keep the stress within manageable proportions in most cases. Thus even under high support, symptoms of illness increase under high stress, and this is the main difference from the buffering hypothesis which assumes that high social support pretty well prevents the relationship between stress and ill-health occurring.

On the face of it this is a pretty unlikely assumption: even the most well loved, socially supported individuals get physically ill, and this in itself probably leads to at least minor symptoms of anxiety and depression. Similarly, well loved, socially supported people still have accidents and failures which may cause loss of confidence etc. Perhaps more importantly, however, neither House, nor Thoits, nor anyone else we can think of, defines the socio-psychological mechanisms by which the buffering hypothesis works. House uses the analogy of a chemical catalyst which modifies the effect that one chemical has on another. But how would social support affect the relationship between stress and health without having direct effects on either stress or health?

Most theories of stress would assume it involves a complex set of psychophysiological processes taking place over time and that the process involves something like the following:

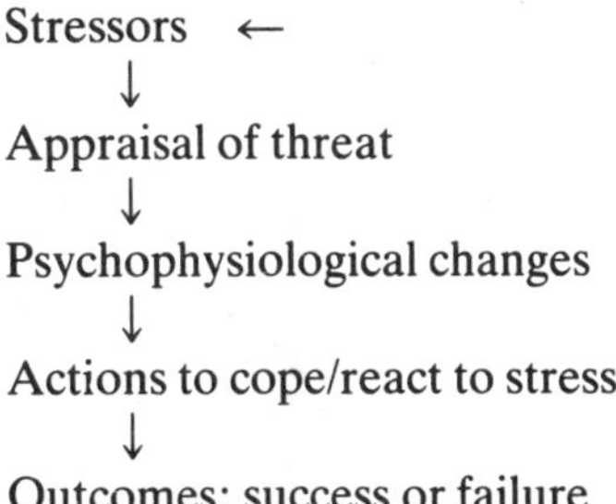

If this process occurs frequently enough, or for long enough, the psychophysiological changes are assumed to damage bodily organs and/or ego functioning leading to illness and perhaps disease. The question for the buffering hypothesis is, how can social support alter this process without acting directly on health or stressors? Accepting House's (1981) useful breakdown of social support into emotional, instrumental, informational, and appraisal, it is possible to argue that emotional support might intrude into the above process particularly at the point of appraisal. A supportive person may help the individual to decrease his/her emotional arousal, deny the strength of the stressors etc. or provide the comfort which helps the person to feel less anxious because they are not alone. This decrease in emotional arousal may then inhibit physiological mechanisms and reduce physical damage to heart, arteries, kidneys etc. In the long run this may protect the immune system which is more and more believed to be suppressed by stress (Cooper, 1984). Informational support may help at the action stage to improve decision-making, and instrumental support may help to allow decisions to be implemented by providing financial and other forms of practical assistance. Appraisal support may help at the outcome end of the above process by providing realistic feedback on the efficacy of the actions taken and the person's role in putting these actions into effect.

This seems plausible and the catalytic analogy might even be pursued further by arguing that with a lot of social support a stressful situation is turned into a developmental opportunity, the interaction thus changing the nature of the psychological situation. We are not at all sure ourselves whether this proposition really avoids the potential claim that there are still direct effects of social support on both the stressors and health. Since the buffering hypothesis has been so vital an issue in this literature we will assume that theoretically this sort of catalytic process can occur and that it is different from the direct effects of support on stress and health. Since the buffering hypothesis has largely been tested statistically by using the interaction term (stressor × support) to predict symptoms, we do wish to signal a concern that statistical possibility might have driven research rather than conceptual clarity.

Having briefly described the major perspectives we can now look at the empirical support for each of them.

Main effects: social support and psychological symptomatology

Several reviews of the literature on social support (Payne, 1980; Thoits, 1982; Kessler et al., 1985) almost take for granted that there is a strong association between social support (however measured) and psychological symptoms (however measured), though Leavy (1983) does caution that the size of the association is weak. Given the recent prominence of the topic, Leavy's caution comes as something of a surprise, though none of the reviews details the actual size of the relationships, but rely more on reporting that there is a 'significant' association.

In Table 4 we report a sample of relationships. The studies all use psychological symptoms as the dependent variable. These are measures such as the Beck Depression Inventory, the Langner Scale, and the General Health Questionnaire. Some well known studies used other indices such as job satisfaction and illness (e.g. House and Wells, 1978) and these have not been included. The selection of studies includes large and small samples from different countries and a range of measures of social support including social network indices.

It is difficult to draw reliable generalisations from the data in Table 4. The largest relationships tend to arise from measures of support which tap feelings about it, rather than its availability. The studies by Turner (1981) and Lin et al. (1979) are the two which show up to 15% of variance is shared between support and symptoms. However, the very largest relationships are found in the Cohen et al. (1984) study where a measure of availability accounts for 26% of the variance in both depression and general symptomatology. In the same study tangible aid and the presence of emotional support account for less than 2% of the variance. On the other hand availability of support accounts for only 2.8% of the variance in the study by Bell et al. (1982), and less than 2% in the papers by Pearlin et al. (1981) and Ullah et al. (1985).

The studies using indices about the social network also contain differences. Size of network accounts for about 7% of the variance in the Phillips (1981) study, but less than 2% in the Griffith (1985) study. Within the study by Etzion (1984), availability and quality of support at work, and in life in general, account for 10% of the variance in a measure of burnout, but support at work accounts for only 1.0% of the variance in work stress.

Pursuing the line of reasoning that larger samples give more reliable estimates of the true relationship between variables, Table 4 does show that the larger samples tend to produce the smaller relationships. Considering those studies with more than 500 in the sample, the Etzion (1984) study shows that availability of support accounts for 10% of the variance in burnout, and the Phillips (1981) study shows that some network indices account for 7–9% of the variance. Other than these, however, the percentage of variance in the large studies lies between zero and 4%.

Main effects: social support and stressors

Table 5 contains examples of studies showing the size of the relationship found between perceived stressors and measures of social support. The stressors are dominated by life events indices and measures of role conflict and ambiguity. The data in the table show clearly that the size of the relationship between life events and social support is much lower than it is for role measures, particularly role ambiguity. Role ambiguity and support share more than 10 per cent of the variance in four out of five studies. The direction of these relationships indicates that those who perceive less ambiguity in their roles report more/better social support. There is an implicit assumption here that role ambiguity is a stressor. In at least one study (Fineman and Payne, 1980) many technical staff in a nuclear power station reported high ambiguity, but actually liked it. More important for present purposes, however, is to ask why such stressors would be expected to correlate with measures of support. The

Table 4: Size of Effects: Social Support and Psychological Health Illness

Authors	N	Sample	Type of support measure	% Variance	
House & Wells (1978)	1809	US male workers	Availability of support	0.01	
Lin et al., (1979)	132	Chinese—US adults	Feelings about support	13.0	
Pearlin et al., (1981)	604	US adults	Availability of emotional support	T1 1.9	T2 0.08
				Anx.	Dep.
Turner (1981)	292	Canadian family volunteers	Feelings about support	14	15
	65	Maladaptive parents	Feelings about support	0.8	11
	430	Hearing impaired adults	Feelings about support	6	9
				Men	Women
Phillips (1981)	1050	18+ Californian adults	– size of network	7.8	6.3
			– density of network	0.4	0.0
			– number of confidants	1.4	0.0
			– number of contexts	4.0	9.0
Bell et al., (1982)	2029	US adults	Availability of support	2.8	

Abdel-Halim (1982)	89	Middle-lower managers	– work group climate	14	
			– leader consideration	5	
Kaplan et al., (1983)	1600+	Young US adults	Felt rejection by peers	2.9	
			Felt rejection by family	4.4	
				Anx.	Dep.
Jayaratne and Chess (1984)	553	Social workers	Emotional support	0.08	0.05
Cohen et al., (1984)	92	College undergraduates		Beck	Langner
			– tangible aid and emotional	1.9	1.4
			– availability of support	26	26
Etzion (1984)	567	Israeli managers		Burnout	
			– availability and quality at work	10	
			– life in general	10	
Quast and Schwarzer (1984)	602	US university students		Depression	
			– no supportive persons	9	
			– satisfaction	14	
Ullah et al., (1985)	1150	Unemployed 17 year olds in UK		Dep.	Anx.
			– availability	1.9	0.02
Griffith (1985)	361	US adults		Dep.	Anx.
			– network size	1.9	0.02
			– reciprocity	0.4	0.4

Table 5: Size of Effects: Social Support and Stressors

Authors	N	Sample	Type of support measure		% Variance
House and Wells (1978)	1809	US male workers	Availability	Role Conf.	3.9
				Responsib.	1.2
				Quality	8.9
				Workload	1.0
Lin et al., (1979)	132	Chinese—US adults	Feelings	Life events	0
Pearlin et al., (1981)	604	US adults	Availability emotional	Job disruption	0
Abdel-Halim (1982)	89	Middle managers	Group climate	Role Conf.	4
				Role Ambig.	15
			Leader Consid.	Role Conf.	10
				Role Ambig.	11
Bell et al., (1982)	2029	US adults	Availability	Life events	2

Seers et al., (1983)	104	Bank clerks	4 measures of availability from role set	Role Conf. Role Ambig.	1.5* 1.5*
Cohen et al., (1984)	92	College students	– tangible aid and emotional	Neg. Events	6.5
			– Availability	Neg. Events	0.0
Etzion (1984)	567	Israeli managers	– Availability at work	Work Stress	1.7
			– Availability in life	Life Stress	12.0
Jayaratne and Chess (1984)	553	Social workers	Emotional from co-workers	Role Conf. Role Ambig.	3.2 13
			Emotional from supervis.	Role Conf. Role Ambig.	3.5 17
Quast and Schwarzer (1984)	602	Students at US University	Number of supportive persons Satisfaction	Negative life events	0

**mean over 4 relationships*

assumption for role ambiguity, we assume, is that good interpersonal relationships will allow people to clarify their roles and reduce ambiguity, or that people who are supportive strive to reduce ambiguity for others anyway. Similar arguments can be applied to role conflict, and the similarity of the patterns for these two variables shown in Table 5 suggests there are common processes involved. It must also be noted that the two measures correlate themselves; Fisher and Gitelson (1983) report a correlation of 0.37 based on their meta-analysis of studies of these two variables. Whilst Fisher and Gitelson do not report on relationships with social support, they do report those with satisfaction with supervisor and satisfaction with co-workers, which might be considered indirect measures of emotional support. The meta-analysis shows correlations of about 0.33 with each variable which is similar to the 10% reported for other measures of social support in Table 5. The evidence is reasonably good, therefore, that social support does reduce perceived conflict and ambiguity, and assuming that these are stressful, that support has a direct effect on such stressors.

The evidence that social support is related to life events is much weaker. The Cohen et al. (1984) study reports 6.5% of common variance between tangible aid/emotional support and negative life events. Availability of support, however, has no relationship and this is true for the studies by Lin et al. (1979) and Quast and Schwarzer (1984). The very large study by Bell et al. (1982) found that negative life events and availability share 2% of variance. These results are somewhat surprising in that it has been suggested by Thoits (1982) and others that negative life events often remove sources of social support. This is obviously true for death of spouses, friends or relatives, and is presumably true in many divorces. Job changes and house moves also often involve the loss of valued friends and organizations. Since life events measures ask the respondent to look back over a given period and report the number of events, one would have expected them to have had time to influence social supports which are measured after the events, but there is little evidence in the coefficients quoted that this is actually happening.

An even better test of the relationship between social support and life events appears to occur in Lin and Ensel (1984). This is a longitudinal study where negative life events, support and depression were measured on large samples ($N = 871$) at two points in time. The researchers calculated change scores from T1 to T2. This permits a test of the general proposition that changes in negative life events will affect social support. The two change scores correlate −0.23. Unfortunately, the authors do not comment on this negative relationship, because it appears to indicate that the greater the change in negative life events the less the change in strong social ties. This is exactly the opposite to what Thoits would have predicted. This study failed to find statistical significance for interaction terms and thus for the buffering hypothesis, but both main effects were significant. However, we now turn to a more detailed consideration of the evidence relating to the buffering hypothesis.

Interaction effects: the buffering hypothesis

Since most of the studies testing the buffering hypothesis use beta weights in multiple regression tables to indicate the size of the effect of interaction terms it is not easy to reproduce a table for the buffering hypothesis which indicates the percentage of variance accounted for by the interaction term(s). Wilcox (1981) quotes support for the buffering effect reporting that the interaction of support with life events adds 12% of the variance. In their reply to the criticism of their analyses of data on the buffering hypothesis made by Schaefer (1982), House et al. (1982) quote that those tests which were significant, and which they argued were beyond chance levels, accounted for between 5 and 15% of the variance. Table 6 lists some studies which provide support for the buffering hypothesis and Table 7 contains some which do not.

The studies in Tables 6 and 7 illustrate the range of samples and situations which have been used to test the buffering hypothesis. They are by no means exhaustive. Studies by Aneshensel and Stone (1982), Schaefer et al. (1981), LaRocco and Jones (1978) have also failed to support the buffering hypothesis, whilst Revenson et al. (1983) and Beehr (1976) provide support for it. The balance, however, tends to be with studies that fail to support the buffering hypothesis. Husaini (1982), in an editorial on a special issue on social support as a buffer published in the Journal of Community Psychology, points out that, 'While the independent effects of these variables on distress (i.e. lower support, higher distress) is reported consistently, only two papers (out of eight) have found evidence for the buffering effect'. (p. 291).

Since a strict interpretation of the buffering hypothesis involves no main effects of support on stress or health, then it would seem appropriate only to accept studies which have shown no main effects but significant interaction effects. As the quotation from Husaini implies, and as Tables 6 and 7 demonstrate, the finding of main effects is very common. This strikes us as an overly conservative view. In an issue of such complexity, it is almost certain that main effects of both types occur and interactions do sometimes. The questions of interest are what conditions facilitate each sort of effect? Or, are there really only main effects and the interactions found merely those that would occur by chance? Only a thorough meta-analysis of published and unpublished studies would provide an answer to this. We know of one Ph.D student who has tested 250 interactions involving social support and a range of psychological and physical health measures and found only a chance level of significant relationships (Glowinkowski, 1985, personal communication).

Even the modest support cited here, however, probably overestimates the evidence favouring the buffering hypothesis as Thoits (1982) has so brilliantly argued. The details of her argument are presented later.

Table 6: Some studies supporting the buffering hypothesis

Author	N	Sample	Comments
Cobb and Kasl (1977)	100	Males facing plant shutdown	'The negative effects of unemployment on depression are completely eliminated by adequate social support'
LaRocco, House and French (1980)	636	Males from varied jobs	Support for mental and physical health but not job strains
Wells (1982)	1830	Blue collar males	5 out of 9 tests support buffering of job strains
Turner (1981)	750	3 very different groups (see Table 4)	Effects vary by social group
Billings and Moos (1982)	329	Male and female community sample	Work and family sources of support
Cohen et al., (1984)	92	College students	Differed by pos. v. neg. life events
Etzion (1984)	567	Israeli managers	Sex differences work stresses
Ullah et al., (1985)	1150	Unemployed 17 yr olds in UK	Varied by type of support and dependent variable

Table 7: Some studies showing lack of support for buffering hypothesis

Authors	N	Sample	Comments
Pearlin et al., (1981)	604	US sample	No support for depression b[illegible] some for job disruption; longitudinal
Lin et al., (1979)	132	Chinese adults	Strong main effects but no interaction
Abdel-Halim (1982)	89	Middle/lower managers	No support for anxiety but some for positive job outcomes
Seers et al., (1983)	104	Mixed levels in US Government agency	No support for either role conflict or role ambiguity
Jayaratne and Chess (1984)	553	Social workers	Emotional support only measured
Kaplan et al., (1983)	1633	Young US adults	Only 1 of 6 tests support buffering: longitudinal study
Parry and Shapiro (1985)	193	Working class mothers in UK	Instrumental and expressive support measured

However, a more optimistic interpretation of the evidence supporting the buffering hypothesis can be found in the extensive review by Cohen and Wills (1985), though they limit their claims to studies employing measures of availability of social support, and ones that enhance broadly useful coping capacities such as raising self-esteem and providing information.

Many of the studies referred to in Tables 6 and 7 contain only cross-sectional data, and though many of them show a correlation between social support and symptoms, such studies are open to the criticism that the symptoms a person has may either determine the quality of support he or she receives, or they may affect the person's perceptions of the quality of support they are getting. That is, a depressed person may say they get poor support due to the fact that they are depressed. Thus, many authors have called for longitudinal studies to avoid this sort of measurement contamination and to increase confidence in the causal relationships between social support and changes in symptomatology. By now several longitudinal studies have been completed and the following section considers their contribution.

Longitudinal Studies

Gore (1978) reports one of the earliest studies to assess support before the stressor (job loss and unemployment) occurred and to measure symptomatology before, during, and after loss of the job. Her data are taken from the classic study of Cobb and Kasl (1977) where 100 men were studied at five points in time. At time 1 the men were anticipating job loss due to closure of their plant. At time 2 they lost their jobs, at time 3 they were readjusting either to a new job or to unemployment. The men were then studied one year after the plant closure and then again a year later. Availability and satisfactoriness of support were measured at time 1 and the Gore paper looks at the effect of support on those men who remained unemployed at time 3. The unemployed who were supported came out better on three of the four dependent measures. Indeed, their scores were actually better than the sample of men who obtained immediate re-employment. Whilst this can be considered as evidence that support has buffered the men against the stress of unemployment, Gore herself preferred the explanation that the fact that the men were not receiving support was itself a source of stress. This is partly because these men scored higher on depression and number of illnesses even before they lost their jobs. Since support itself was only measured once, this study still leaves uncertainties about the causal role of support in stressful situations.

Pearlin et al. (1981) investigated the psychological effects of job disruption examining the mediating effect of available emotional support. Two waves of data were collected on a sample of over 2000 adults in the Chicago area. There was four years between the two sets of data. Because of the longitudinal data set they were able to look at changes in depression and the other three dependent variables they measured (economic strain, felt mastery, and self-esteem). They found that social support did not mediate the effects of job disruption on depression, though it did on economic strain and mastery. Pearlin et al., also calculated interaction terms to examine the buffering hypothesis and found limited support in that the interaction terms which were significant related to self-esteem and mastery, but not economic strain or depression. In terms of the model they were proposing these two variables are regarded as antecedents to depression, so this study illustrates one way in which the psychosocial mechanisms underlying the buffering process could work (see the discussion above pp. 181–182). The study also shows that supports are most effective for those most in need (those with job disruption) which is also indirect support for the processes inherent in the buffering hypothesis, as opposed to the direct effects model.

Holahan and Moos (1981) not only looked at changes in psychological health they also looked at these in relation to changes in support. They did this by controlling for initial levels of psychological health, social support, and stress. The study involved 245 male and 248 female adult family members who were interviewed twice, one year apart. When initial levels of maladjustment, social support and life events were controlled, six out of ten tests were significant beyond the five per cent level. The largest significant partial correlation was 0.27 and the results showed that the relationship held for both work and family environments. When there were decreases in support in either of these two environments during the year, then there were increases in psychological maladjustment over the same time period.

One of the most impressive longitudinal studies is that carried out by Henderson et al. (1981). It is impressive because of the range of measures used (several measures of psychological health), a very thorough assessment of availability and adequacy of social support (as described above at pp. 174–178), and finally because the data were collected four times over a period of one year. The sample was drawn from the electoral rolls of the city of Canberra, Australia. Around 200 people were interviewed over the four waves. In the longitudinal analysis they selected out those individuals who had a certain level of symptoms at time 1 so that they could then investigate factors influencing the development of symptoms over time.

Since they carried out both cross-sectional and longitudinal analyses, the study demonstrated the different findings of the two methods. In the cross-sectional analyses they found that adequacy of social support rather than availability protected the person from experiencing neurotic symptoms. They also tested the buffering hypothesis and found the interaction of stress (adversity) × adequacy of support added about 5% of the variance, the two main effects being of a similar size (see page 149 of their book for details). Support was particularly effective for those who had had most adversity, as Pearlin et al. (1981) found, again providing support for the buffering hypothesis. Indeed, they were able to account for 30% of the variance in symptoms for those with high adversity and only 4% for those with low adversity. However, this finding only became apparent in the longitudinal analyses and is the main difference between the two sets of analyses: the authors state their greater confidence in the longitudinal findings.

The conceptual water is muddied, however, by other analyses carried out. The authors also measured trait neuroticism using the Eysenck Personality Inventory (Eysenck and Eysenck, 1964). When this is entered into a multiple regression it explains 69% of the variance in their combined illness measure. Indeed, neuroticism not only predicts illness, it also predicts social support and adversity. After controlling for neuroticism and adversity, the relationship between support and illness disappears as does any interactive effect and thus support for the buffering hypothesis. To quote the authors, '... the conclusion we have arrived at is that the actual availability of social relationships has little to do with the causes of neurosis. The perceived adequacy with which others meet the individual's requirement, especially under adversity, seems much more important. What we do not yet know is how much lies in the actual performance of others, and how much is the product of some intrapersonal attribute.' (p. 197). This finding and the recent review of the ubiquitous effect of general negativity by Watson and Clark (1984) indicate that one methodological improvement that researchers in the stress field need to make is the inclusion of measures of stable traits such as neuroticism and optimism–pessimism in their designs.

Williams et al. (1981) provide more methodological sophistication by dividing their sample into two and cross-validating their findings. Since the data were gathered from a sample of 2,234 persons living in Seattle, this still left large samples for model fitting and then validation. Once again the data were collected one year apart. The support measure measured availability of contacts and satisfaction with them. The cross-validation matched the model fitting analysis very closely indeed. Mental health at time 1 accounted for 34 per cent of the variance in mental health at time 2, but life events and social support also contributed significantly. There was no evidence of interaction effects, however, and thus no support for the buffering hypothesis.

Another study which assessed variables at four points in time over a one year period is that by Aneshensel and Frerichs (1982) who studied 740 adults using depression as the dependent variable. They tested a series of latent variable causal models over time spans of four, eight and twelve months. Depression and support (socio-emotional and instrumental) were found to be relatively stable over these time periods, but stress (life events) was much less so. The experience of recent stressors was found to increase depression and the availability of support was found to decrease the severity of depression, though depression itself had a small relationship with subsequent stress. The authors conclude, 'The results are consistent with the viewpoint that social support has a direct (modest) positive impact on the individual's psychological well-being irrespective of the level of stress, without negating an interaction effect.' (p. 375).

In her paper reassessing studies of the buffering hypothesis, Thoits (1982) reanalysed data from the New Haven Panel data (Myers et al., 1971). Data were collected from 720 adults two years apart. By using this longitudinal data, Thoits was able to avoid using measures of support which were taken after stressful life events had occurred (and which might have altered support itself). When this is done the results show that lack of support does leave the individual more vulnerable to life events, but the results show little support for the buffering hypothesis, and demonstrate clearly that results of cross-sectional studies are biased in favour of the buffering hypothesis when support level is measured after life events have taken place.

To find that social support affects mental health over periods of four months or a year is not too surprising, but to find main effects over ten years is somewhat unexpected. Kaplan et al. (1983), however, found that felt rejection by family and/or peers (i.e. emotional support) during 7th grade was related to psychological distress ten years later. Not surprisingly, the effects were not huge and measures of self-derogation and negative life events over the ten years added more to the 13% of the variance accounted for than did the measures of social support. One out of six support stress interactions was significant. The sample size was 1,633.

Finally, Lin and Ensel (1984) carried out an interesting analysis of 871 adults interviewed at two points in time and one year apart. Four groups of subjects were created: those who were not depressed at either time 1 or time 2 (73%), those who had recovered from a depression by time 2 (10%), those who became depressed by time 2 (10%), and those depressed both at times 1 and 2 (7%). They carried out a sequential analysis looking at changes in depression, life events, and social support over time and showed that social support had a protective effect in all situations. They found no support for statistical interactions, but did warn that social support does mediate the effects of life events and that interaction terms may not be the only way to understand the processes by which support affects mental well-being.

As a whole, these longitudinal studies provide strong evidence for the causal effects of both social support and life events on psychological symptoms. They also show that the size of effects shown in the cross-sectional studies were reasonably accurate estimates, and that up to 30 per cent of the variance in symptoms can be predicted for certain groups of individuals (those who are vulnerable, stressed, and lacking in support) whilst it is very much more difficult to predict the psychologically stressed in the 'normal' population.

The results on the buffering hypothesis are also consistent with the cross-sectional studies in that some studies find interactions and some do not. Our own feeling about these results, however, is that the longitudinal studies are better tests and that support for the buffering hypothesis is weak, and probably not greater than would be expected by chance.

Clinical, intervention, and experimental studies

Many of the studies referred to so far have been correlational in design. Other designs have been used to investigate the effects of social support on health and well-being. These include studies in clinical samples, comparison of cases with controls, and evaluations of studies where support has been deliberately incorporated into a treatment programme. Broadhead et al. (1983), Levy (1983) and Kessler et al. (1985) contain reviews of these areas.

In studies of clinical groups with psychological disorders such as anxiety and depression, it has been shown that their social networks differ from those of normals. Psychotics tend to have restricted family-oriented networks, but the networks of neurotics tend to be loose and sparse. Just what causal routes lead to these differences is highly problematic, and little is known about the social dynamics that create them. There is evidence that reducing the level of expressed emotion among the families of schizophrenics improves their relapse rate (Boyd et al., 1981). Brown and Harris (1978) and others have shown that having the support of a close confidant protects women from vulnerability to depression. The literature to date suggests that emotional support is the major feature of the support given and the balance of the evidence is reviewed by Kessler and McLeod (1984), though it is readily apparent from much of the data presented in Tables 4 and 5.

A range of studies has now been carried out on groups who have experienced specific unpleasant events such as loss of spouse, criminal attack, loss of a business or employment. Most of these have followed up the subjects over time and found that poor levels of support early in the crisis are associated with distress over periods as long as two years (Gore, 1978; Vachon et al., 1982). Whilst such studies convince one of the practical benefit of social support they have done little to enhance understanding of what is happening amongst people in these 'support transactions' (Coyne, et al., 1984). Kessler et al. (1985) make the critical point nicely:

> To date, studies of specific life crises have not realized their potential, either as a means of increasing our basic understanding of fundamental support processes or as a foundation on which interventions can be built. Most studies of this sort have simply attempted to show that support is associated with subsequent adjustment without linking support to other variables that might help elucidate causal processes. For progress to be made, the advantages of this research design will have to be more fully exploited in the future. (p. 545).

In addition to these studies of adjustment to traumatic occurrences, there has been a growing attempt to intervene in the adjustment process by increasing support amongst the victims. Studies of adjustment to surgery are reviewed by Mumford et al. (1982) and the review by Levy (1983) includes studies of chronic health problems. Not surprisingly, most of these have involved support from the professional groups involved in treatment and care, and given they have largely been experimental studies their evidence is encouraging in that the experimental groups have usually shown less severe symptoms and made more rapid recovery than the controls. Since many have focused on reducing the stress (e.g. pre-operative anxiety) and the outcomes (e.g. post-operative recovery) they are not able to distinguish between these two competing explanations, and unfortunately, as it is pointed out by Kessler et al. (1985), they do not inform us much about the processes which are leading to the desirable achievements they effect.

All such attempts will be significantly improved if the measures of support are thoughtfully designed to fit the different sorts of circumstances to be studied. We offer some thoughts on how this might proceed.

Some thoughts on measures

Tardy (1985) has usefully identified the major facets and elements (Foa, 1965) of social support measures as we indicated earlier. We believe, however, that these may be more usefully used to design measures of social support by reordering the facets. Figure 3 outlines a sort of decision-tree for different kinds of measures. The first facet to be considered is *source* of support. This has six elements. The researcher might identify immediately that he/she is only interested in two of them. The second facet is *content* which has the four elements suggested by House (1981). The researcher again may decide that they wish to focus on emotional and instrumental support, but not informational or appraisal. It is our view that the next most important/logical question follows from what Tardy called *disposition*. That is, is the support just potentially available (which is what is identified in many network studies) or is it actually enacted? The next important question becomes, do we want to know what the support is like (description) or how the person feels about it (evaluation)? i.e. *description/evaluation*. Finally, the researcher might be interested in *direction* of the support: is it received or given? The vast majority of studies have been about support which is received, but studies of both types from the perspective of givers versus receivers might have potential in understanding the dynamics of social support.

This approach is suggested for the very practical reason that the framework in Figure 3 implies the potential existence of 192 different measures. It is unlikely that researchers will wish to use them all. Thus Figure 3 is offered as a decision-making aid at one level, but also as a systematic tool for designing

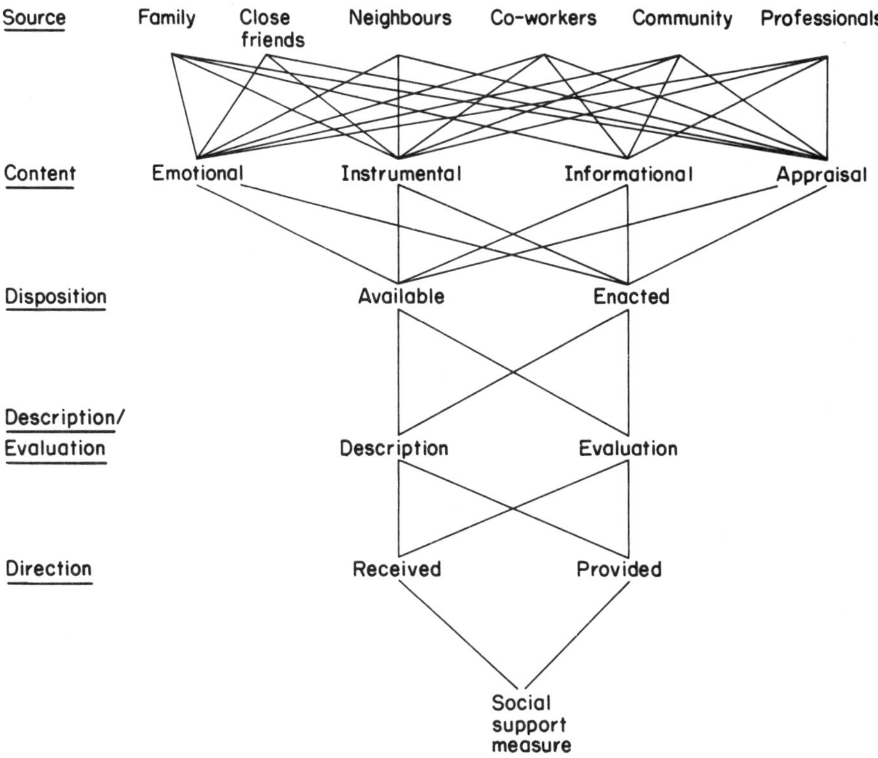

Figure 3: Decision Tree for Designing Social Support Measures

questions about social support issues. Researchers might decide to ignore a facet, for example, but hopefully Figure 3 will enable them to see what they are ignoring and the implications it may have. Finally, it has value in comparing different measures.

Some thoughts about future studies

Whilst we have doubts about the strength of the evidence for the buffering hypothesis, it has been a major theoretical issue in the field and focuses attention on the value of competing hypotheses such as those outlined in Figure 2. The most insightful comments on the buffering hypothesis and tests of it have been provided by Thoits (1982). We now wish to use Thoits' arguments to lead us into consideration of what sort of studies would be needed to test the buffering hypothesis and the other major hypotheses in the field.

Testing competing hypotheses

Thoits' argument is centred on the fact that social support is confounded with negative life events, because many life events involve changes in social support. Not only does divorce of a spouse remove the support of the third most frequently used support person (Griffith, 1985), but it may also alienate other central persons such as in-laws, friends and even parents. Thoits points out that in cross-sectional studies, or even longitudinal studies where support has been measured after a change in stressors, there may be fewer social supports because their loss is directly associated with the life events themselves. Thus those who are most stressed by negative life events are also more likely to have worse social support systems. This biases results in favour of the buffering effects of social support for those with higher levels of stress (see Figure 2b). Thoits continues her criticism of previous tests of the buffering hypothesis by arguing that what is important is changes in the level of stable support normally available to the individual. Her refined buffering hypothesis is: 'the higher the initial level of support and the greater the degree to which this level is maintained throughout the crisis period, the less impact life changes will have upon psychological state'. This implies that social support needs to be measured before a change in stressors, during the crisis, and at some period after when the stressors are judged to have decreased in severity. This would appear to be the absolute minimum number of observations.

Let us pursue the implications of Thoits' observations. To understand the effects of social support on mental health we need to know (a) the person's ongoing mental health; (b) the quantity and quality of ongoing social support; (c) the nature and strength of changes in life circumstances (life events; increases or decreases in stressors); (d) the extent to which social support is maintained during the crisis; finally, (e) the change to the person's mental health having faced the crisis. To simplify the problem let us assume that each of the first four variables can take only two or three values. Ongoing mental health is assumed to be simply good or poor. Similarly ongoing social support is allowed to be either good or poor. Changes in stressors is allowed to take three values: more, same or less. This is because we are going to use this framework to generate predictions about future mental health from each of the three main competing hypotheses shown in Figure 2: i.e. the stressors only, the health only, or the buffering hypothesis. Since the buffering hypothesis involves the assumption that support does not affect mental health under conditions of low stress, it is important that we consider situations where stress has decreased or remained the same. This is why the 'same' category is utilized for change in stressors. The final variable also has three values. It is assumed that support can be maintained at a given level, or it can actually get better, or it can get worse.

This 'oversimplified' framework creates thirty-six different possible situations. To save space and facilitate communication we will focus on the implications of two subsets of these. Table 8 contains nine of the possible thirty-six conditions where in all nine ongoing Psychological Health is good and ongoing Social Support is good. Below each of the nine columns are three

Table 8: Predictions of Health Change in Differing Situations For 3 Competing Hypotheses: Ongoing Health is Good

Ongoing Psychological Health					GOOD				
Ongoing Social Support					GOOD				
Change in Stressors		More			Same			Less	
Support Maintenance	*B	S	W	B	S	W	B	S	W
Column No.	1	2	3	4	5	6	7	8	9
Predictions of:									
Direct Stress Hypothesis	†I	S	D	I	S	D	S	S	S
Direct Health Hypothesis	S	S	D	I	S	S	I	S	S
Buffering Hypothesis	S	S	D	S	S	S	S	S	S

*Key: B = *Better*
S = *Same*
W = *Worse*
† I = *Improvement in psychological health*
S = *Stability in psychological health*
D = *Deterioration in psychological health*

predictions about the *change or stability* in mental health of individuals located in each of these sets of circumstances. The first prediction is derived from the Stressor hypothesis, the second from the Health hypothesis and the third from the Buffering hypothesis. As the key to the table indicates, the predictions relate to changes in mental health as a result of being in each situation. There are some necessary assumptions: First, that mental health is not so good or so bad that it cannot either improve or deteriorate; secondly, that social support is positively valued by most individuals and lack of it is stressful. The predictions also assume 'all other things are equal' such as personality, coping capacity etc: unlikely, but necessary.

Table 9 describes nine situations for individuals who start out with poor mental health and poor ongoing social support. It is worth noting that in some situations our reasoning suggests that all three hypotheses would make the same predictions (e.g. 2, 5, 8 and 9 in Table 8). In other columns different predictions are made by different hypotheses. In column 7 of Table 8 the prediction from the Direct Stressor hypothesis is that health will stay the same. This is because stressors have decreased and even though support has got better it will not affect the person's health because the stressors are already low and support was good to begin with. The Direct Health hypothesis has a different prediction. Since health is improved by social support it predicts that health will improve in a situation where stressors have also gone down. Since the Buffering hypothesis predicts that support will only buffer the person when there is stress, then no change is predicted in health under column 7.

There is no difference for the three hypotheses under column 2 of Table 8 where health is expected to remain the same. For the Stressor hypothesis this is because although stress has increased since support is good and remains good there will be no change in health. For the Health hypothesis this is because good support improves health and even under stress its effects will be maintained. For the Buffering hypothesis support only buffers under high stress but even though stress has increased, the high level of support will continue to buffer the individual. Note that in column 3 when support has decreased in the face of increased stress, all three hypotheses predict a deterioration in health.

If column 2 of Table 8 is compared to column 2 of Table 9 then the predictions of all three hypotheses are consistent within each table, but different between the tables. In column 2 of Table 9 our reasoning for the Stressor hypothesis is that this is because stress has increased and support has not changed but since support was low to begin with it will mean the person is more stressed and health will deteriorate. For the Health hypothesis, health will deteriorate because support is low. In the case of the Buffering hypothesis, stress has increased but there is low support, so the person will not be buffered from the increased stress: again health will deteriorate.

It is perhaps worth noting that the predictions in Table 9 for column 8 differ for the Health hypothesis because under conditions of poor ongoing social support, health will deteriorate even if stressors are lower as long as social support remains static or worsens.

Some other features of Tables 8 and 9 are worth observing. First, that the Buffering hypothesis does not appear to predict improvements in health at all. It largely predicts that health will be protected under stress if supports are adequate. In three cases we argue it predicts deterioration. This small proportion of predicted differences for the buffering hypothesis is of course consistent with the relatively small number of significant findings in the literature.

As we have already seen it is sometimes impossible to distinguish between the predictions of the three hypotheses, and quite often difficult to distinguish the Stressor from the Health hypothesis. This sort of thinking, however, would appear to indicate what sorts of situations are more likely to lead to different

Table 9: Predictions of Health Change in Differing Situations For 3 Competing Hypotheses: Ongoing Health is Poor

Ongoing Psychological Health					POOR				
Ongoing Social Support					POOR				
Change in Stressors		More			Same			Less	
Support Maintenance	*B	S	W	B	S	W	B	S	W
Column No.	1	2	3	4	5	6	7	8	9
Predictions of:									
Direct Stress Hypothesis	†S	D	D	I	S	D	S	S	S
Direct Health Hypothesis	S	D	D	I	D	D	I	D	D
Buffering Hypothesis	S	D	D	S	S	S	S	S	S

*Key: B = *Better*
S = *Same*
W = *Worse*
† I = *Improvement in psychological health*
S = *Stability in psychological health*
D = *Deterioration in psychological health*

outcomes and competing tests of these three hypotheses. It is also worth reminding ourselves that these all require longitudinal studies which are looking at dynamic changes in variables, including changes in the dependent variables. The nearest empirical example we can think of which approaches the problem from this sort of perspective is that of Lin and Ensel (1984). Their sequential analysis looking at predictions of the percentage changes in the number of depressed people as a result of changes in life events and changes in social support follows this sort of analytical process. As they point out themselves, two waves of data are insufficient to properly test the propositions they offer, and this is consistent with the three waves of data inherent in the analysis presented in Tables 8 and 9.

CONCLUSIONS

Even given the sometimes *ad hoc* measures of social support so far used the evidence from cross-sectional and longitudinal studies is good enough to claim with reasonable confidence that social support can influence the severity of stressors and the psychological experience of individuals. In the long run it probably affects physical health too. There are main effects though the effect size is modest. What we are still ignorant about is which aspects of support work best for whom, under what conditions. We know little about the psychosocial processes involved in the giving and receiving of social support. Thus future studies need to focus on revealing the nature of these processes. This almost certainly means they will be longitudinal in design whether they are intervention studies, experimental studies or large-scale survey studies. Further cross-sectional studies are probably valueless, unless they are used to design and test new measures of support which might be used in longitudinal and other designs.

REFERENCES

Abdel-Halim, A. A. (1982). Social support and managerial affective responses to job stress, *Journal of Occupational Behaviour*, **3**, 281–95.

Andrews, G., Tennant, C., Hewson, D. M., and Vaillant, G. E. (1978). Life event stress, social support, coping style, and risk of psychological impairment, *Journal of Nervous and Mental Disease*, **166**, 307–16.

Aneshensel, C. S., and Frerichs, R. R. (1982). Stress, support, and depression: a longitudinal causal model, *Journal of Community Psychology*, **10**, 363–76.

Aneshensel, C. S., and Stone, J. D. (1982). Stress and depression: a test of the buffering model of social support, *Archives of General Psychiatry*, **39**, 1392–96.

Ashby, W. R. (1956). *Introduction to Cybernetics*, London, Chapman and Hall.

Barrera, M. (1980). A method for the assessment of social support networks in community survey research, *Connections*. **3(3)**, 8–13.

Barrera, M. (1981). Social support in the adjustment of pregnant adolescents: assessment issues. In B. H. Gottlieb (ed.) *Social Networks and Social Support*, Beverly Hills, Sage.

Beehr, T. A. (1976). Perceived situational moderators of the relationship between subjective role ambiguity and role strain, *Journal of Applied Psychology*, **61**, 35–40.

Bell, R. A., Leroy, J. B., and Stephenson, J. J. (1982). Evaluating the mediating effects of social support upon life events and depressive symptoms, *Journal of Community Psychology*, **10**, 325–40.

Billings, A. G., and Moos, R. H. (1982). Work stress and the stress-buffering roles of work and family resources, *Journal of Occupational Behaviour*, **3**, 215–32.

Boyd, J. L., McGill, C. W., and Falloon, I. R. H. (1981). Family participation in the community rehabilitation of schizophrenics, *Hospital and Community Psychiatry*, **32**, 9, 629–32.

Broadhead, W. E., Kaplan, B. H., James, S. A., Wagner, E. H., Schoenbach, V. J. et al. (1983). The epidemiologic evidence for a relationship between social support and health, *American Journal of Epidemiology*, **117**, 521–37.

Brown, G. W. and Harris, T. O. (1978). *Social Origins of Depression: A Study of Psychiatric Disorder in Women*, Free Press.

Caplan, G. (1976). The family as a support system. In G. Caplan and M. Killilea (eds.) *Support Systems and Mutual Help*, New York, Grune and Stratton.

Caplan, R. D., Cobb, S., French, J. R. P., Van Harrison, R., and Pinneau, S. R. (1975). *Job Demands and Worker Health*, National Institute of Occupational Safety and Health, US Dept. of Health, US Government Printing Office, Washington DC.

Cobb, S. and Kasl, S. V. (1977). *Termination: The Consequences of Job Loss*, Cincinatti, US Department of Health, Education and Welfare.

Cohen, L. H., McGowan, J., Fooskas, S. and Rose, S. (1984). Positive life events and social support and the relationship between life stress and psychological disorder, *American Journal of Community Psychology*, **12(5)**, 567–87.

Cohen, S. and Wills, T. A. (1985). Stress, social support and the buffering hypothesis, *Psychological Bulletin*, **98**, 2, 310–57.

Cooper, C. L. (1984). *Psychosocial Stress and Cancer*. Chichester, Wiley.

Coyne, J. C., Kahn, J., Gotlieb, I. H. (1984). Depression. In T. Jacob (ed.) *Family Interaction and Psychopathology*, New York, Plenum.

Crowne, D. P. and Marlowe, D. (1960). A new scale of social desirability independent of psychopathology, *Journal of Consulting Psychology*, **24**, 349–54.

Crowne, D. P., and Marlowe, D. (1964). *The Approval Motive: Studies in Evaluative Dependence*, New York, Wiley.

Dean, A., and Lin, N. (1977). The stress buffering role of social support, *Journal of Nervous and Mental Disease*, **165**, 403–17.

Eaton, W. W. (1978). Life events, social supports, and psychiatric symptoms: a re-analysis of the New Haven data, *Journal of Health and Social Behaviour*, **19**, 230–4.

Etzion, D. (1984). Moderating effect of social support on the stress–burnout relationship. *Journal of Applied Psychology*, **69**, 4, 615–22.

Eysenck, H. J. and Eysenck, S. B. G. (1964). *Manual of the Eysenck Personality Inventory*, London, London University Press.

Fineman, S., and Payne, R. L. (1980). Role stress: a methodological trap? *Journal of Occupational Behaviour*, **2**, 51–64.

Fisher, C. D., and Gitelson, R. (1983). A meta-analysis of the correlates of role conflict and ambiguity, *Journal of Applied Psychology*, **68**, 2, 320–33.

Fischer, C. S. (1982). *To Dwell among Friends: Personal Networks in Town and City*, Chicago, University of Chicago Press.

Foa, V. G. (1965). New developments in facet design and analysis. *Psychological Review*, **72**, 4, 262–74.

Gad, M. T., and Johnson, J. H. (1980). Correlates of adolescent life stress as related to race, SES, and levels of perceived support. *Journal of Clinical Child Psychology*, **9**, 13–16.

Goldberg, D. P. (1972). *The Detection of Psychiatric Illness by Questionnaire*, Oxford, Oxford University Press.

Goldstein, M. B. (1980). Interpersonal support and coping among first year dental students, *Journal of Dental Education*, **44**, 202–5.

Gore, S. (1978). The effect of social support in moderating the health consequences of unemployment. *Journal of Health and Social Behaviour*, **19**, 157–65.

Griffith, J. (1985). Social support providers: who are they? Where are they met? and the relationship of network characteristics to psychological distress. *Basic and Applied Social Psychology*, **6**, 1, 41–60.

Henderson, S. (1980). A development in social psychiatry: the systematic study of social bonds. *Journal of Nervous and Mental Disease*, **168**, 63–9.

Henderson, S., Duncan-Jones, P., Byrne, D. G., and Scott, R. (1980). Measuring social relationships: The Interview Schedule for Social Interaction. *Psychological Medicine*, **10**, 723–34.

Henderson, S., Byrne, D. G., and Duncan-Jones, P. (1981). *Neurosis and the Social Environment*, London, Academic Press.

Holahan, C. J. and Moos, R. H. (1981). Social support and psychological distress: a longitudinal analysis. *Journal of Abnormal Psychology*, **90**, 4, 365–70.

House, J. S. (1981). *Work, stress, and social support.* Reading, Massachusetts, Addison-Wesley.

House, J. S., and Wells, J. A. (1978). Occupational stress, social support, and health. In A. McLean, G. Black and M. Colligan (eds.) *Reducing Occupational Stress: Proceedings of a Conference*, DWEH (NIOSH) Publication No. 78-140, 8–29.

House, J. S., LaRocco, J. M., and French, J. R. P. (1982). Response to Schaefer, *Journal of Health and Social Behaviour*, **23**, 98–101.

Husaini, B. A. (1982). Stress and psychiatric symptoms: personality and social support as buffers: special editor's comments. *Journal of Community Psychology*, **10**, 291–292.

Jayaratne, S. and Chess, W. A. (1984). The effect of emotional support on perceived job stress and support. *Journal of Applied Behavioural Science*, **20**, 2, 141–53.

Kaplan, H. B., Robbins, C., and Martin, S. S. (1983). Antecedents of psychological distress in young adults: self-rejection, deprivation of social support, and life events. *Journal of Health and Social Behaviour*, **24**, 230–44.

Kerlinger, F. N. (1973). *Foundations of Behavioral Research*. New York, Holt, Rinehart and Winston.

Kessler, R. C., and McLeod, J. (1984). Social support and psychological distress in community surveys. In S. Cohen and L. Syme (eds.) *Social Support and Health*, New York, Academic Press.

Kessler, R. C., Price, R. H., and Wortman, C. B. (1985). Social factors in psychopathology: stress, social support, and coping processes. *Annual Review of Psychology*, **36**, 531–72.

LaRocco, J. M., and Jones, A. P. (1978). Co-worker and leader support as moderators of stress-strain relationships in work situations. *Journal of Applied Psychology*, **63**, 629–34.

LaRocco, J. R., House, J. S., and French, J. R. P. jun. (1980). Social support, occupational stress and health, *Journal of Health and Social Behaviour*, **21**, 202–18.

Leavy, R. L. (1983). Social support and psychological disorder: A review. *Journal of Community Psychology*, **11**, 3–21.

Levy, R. L. (1983). Social support and compliance: a selective review and critique of treatment integrity and outcome measurement. *Social Science and Medicine*, **17**, 8, 1329–38.

Lin, N., Simeone, R. S., Ensel, W. M., and Kuo, W. (1979). Social support, stressful life events, and illness: a model and an empirical test. *Journal of Health and Social Behaviour*, **20**, 108–19.

Lin, N., and Ensel, W. M. (1984). Depression-mobility and its social etiology: the role of life events and social support, *Journal of Health and Social Behaviour*, **25**, 176–88.

Luborsky, L., Todd, T. C., and Katcher, A. H. (1973). A self-administered social assets scale for predicting physical and psychological illness and health. *Journal of Psychomatic Research*, **17**, 109–20.

McFarlane, A. H., Neale, K. A., Norman, G. R., Roy, R. G., and Streiner, D. L. (1981). Methodological issues in developing a scale to measure social support, *Schizophrenia Bulletin*, **7**, 90–100.

Medalie, J. H., and Goldbourt, V. (1976). Angina pectoris among 10,000 men: II. Psychosocial and other risk factors as evidenced by a multi-variate analysis of a five-year incidence study. *American Journal of Medicine*, **60**, 910–21.

Miller, P. and Ingham, J. G. (1976). Friends, confidants, and symptoms. *Social Psychiatry*, **11**, 51–8.

Mumford, E., Schlesinger, H. J., and Glass, G. V. (1982). The effects of psychological intervention on recovery from surgery and heart attacks: an analysis of the literature. *American Journal of Public Health*, **72**, 2, 141–51.

Myers, J., Linderthal, J. J., and Pepper, M. (1971). Life events and psychiatric impairment, *Journal of Nervous and Mental Disease*, **152**, 3, 149–57.

Parry, G., and Shapiro, D. A. (1985). Social support and life events in working class women: stress buffering or independent effects? *Archives of General Psychiatry*, in press.

Payne, R. L. (1980). Organizational stress and social support. In C. L. Cooper and R. L. Payne (eds.) *Current Concerns in Occupational Stress*, Chichester, Wiley.

Pearlin, L. I., Lieberman, M. A., Menaghan, E. G., and Mullan, J. T. (1981). The stress process, *Journal of Health and Social Behaviour*, **22**, 337–56.

Phillips, S. L. (1981). Network characteristics related to the well-being of normals: a comparative base. *Schizophrenia Bulletin*, **7**, 1, 117-24.

Pinneau, S. R. (1975). Effects of Social Support on Psychological and Physiological Stress. Unpublished Ph.D Thesis, University of Michigan, Ann Arbor.

Procidano, M. E., and Heller, K. (1983). Measures of perceived social support from friends and from family: three validation studies. *American Journal of Community Psychology*, **11**, 1–24.

Quast, H. H., and Schwarzer, R. (1984). Social support and stress: theoretical perspectives and selected empirical findings. In R. Schwarzer (ed.) *The Self in Anxiety, Stress and Depression*, Amsterdam, North Holland.

Renne, K. S. (1974). Measurement of social health in a general population survey, *Social Science Research*, **3**, 25–44.

Revenson, T. A., Wollman, C. A., and Felton, B. J. (1983). Social supports as stress buffers for adult cancer patients. *Psychosomatic Medicine*, **45**, 4, 321–31.

Sandler, I. N. (1980). Social report resources, stress and maladjustment of poor children, *American Journal of Community Psychology*, **8**, 41–52.

Sandler, I. N. and Barrera, M. (1984). Towards a multimethod approach to assessing the effects of social support, *American Journal of Community Psychology*, **12**, 37–52.

Sarason, I. G., Levine, H. M., Basham, R. B., and Sarason, B. R. (1983). Assessing social support: The Social Support questionnaire, *Journal of Personality and Social Psychology*, **44**, 127–39.

Schaefer, C. (1982). Shoring up the 'buffer' of social support, *Journal of Health and Social Behaviour*, **23**, 96–8.

Schaefer, C., Coyne, J. C., and Lazarus, R. S. (1981). The health-related functions of social support, *Journal of Behavioural Medicine*, **4**, 381–405.

Seers, A., McGee, G. W., Serey, T. T., and Graen, G. B. (1983). The interaction of job stress and social support: a strong inference investigation, *Academy of Management Journal*, **26**, 2, 273–84.

Wilcox, B. L. (1981). Social support, life stress, and psychological adjustment: a test of the buffering hypothesis. *American Journal of Community Psychology*, **9**, 371–86.

Williams, A. W., Ware, J. E. Jun., and Donald, C. A. (1981). A model of mental health, life events, and social supports applicable to general populations, *Journal of Health and Social Behaviour*, **22**, 324–36.

Zung, W. W. K. (1965). A self-rating depression scale, *Archives of General Psychiatry*, **12**, 63–70.

Zung, W. W. K. (1967). Factors in influencing the self-rating depression scale, *Archives of General Psychiatry*, **13**, 508–15.

Chapter 8

Meaning and Measurement of Stressors in the Work Environment: An Evaluation

John M. Bailey and Rabi S. Bhagat

The University of Texas at Dallas

There is a distinct lack of agreement among experts on any particular definition of the concept of stress. Although many observations and studies are classified under the heading of stress, the work of Hans Selye is most responsible for explaining the concept and ushering it into the scientific vocabulary. Selye offered a definition which stimulated research efforts in the clinical and medical sciences (Selye, 1936). His definition describes an internal condition of an organism which is the result of the organism's response to evocative agents (stressors) and internal conditions (stress reactions). According to Selye (1936), stress is the 'state manifested by a specific syndrome which consists of all non-specifically induced changes within a biological system'.

Although Selye first introduced the concept of stress, the work of Joseph McGrath has recently adapted Selye's definition into a working definition which addresses the sets of conditions that are required before stress is considered present. According to McGrath (1976), stress is the result of an interaction of person and environment which forces on the person a demand, a constraint, or an opportunity for behaviour. The individual's perception of the stressful demand is the catalyst in McGrath's definition, i.e. the extent to which a demand upon a person is stressful depends upon whether or not it is perceived as stressful by the person. It must also be interpreted by him, with respect to his ability to confront the demand, circumvent, remove, or live with the constraint, or effectively use the opportunity. Finally, McGrath's (1976) definition contends that the stressee must perceive the potential consequences of successfully coping with the demand as more desirable than the expected consequences of leaving the situation unaltered.

McGrath eloquently describes and applies the multiphasic nature of his definition in the following passage:

> A potential for stress exists when an environmental situation is perceived as presenting a demand which threatens to exceed the person's

The authors would like to thank Sally McQuaid for her many useful suggestions.

Research Methods in Stress and Health Psychology. Edited by S. V. Kasl and C. L. Cooper.

capabilities and resources for meeting it, under conditions where he expects a substantial differential in the rewards and costs from meeting the demand versus not meeting it.

(McGrath, 1976, p. 1352)

McGrath's definition has the following implications built into it. First, it implies that the demand from the environment versus the capability of the individual, as perceived by the individual, must be substantially out of balance for stress to exist, and that this imbalance can be stressful in either direction. In other words, an underload of environmental demand may be just as stressful as an overload, although with different consequences. Secondly, it implies that the consequences anticipated from meeting the demand versus failing to meet the demand must be substantial and that these consequences are a result of the stressee's perceptions of high versus low rewards and/or low versus high costs (McGrath, 1976).

McGrath's (1976) working definition of stress has played a major role in job stress research. His definition has guided research resulting in empirical support for several general themes or propositions that represent a pragmatic set of working hypotheses. These generalizations are:

HYPOTHESIS 1: Cognitive Appraisal. Subjectivily experienced stress is contingent upon the person's perception of the situation.
HYPOTHESIS 2: Experience. Past experience, in the form of familiarity with the situation, past exposure to the stressor condition, and/or practice or training in how to deal with the situation, can operate to affect the level of subjectively experienced stress from a given situation, or to modify reactions to that stress.
HYPOTHESIS 3: Reinforcement. Positive and negative reinforcements can operate to reduce or enhance the level of subjectively experienced stress from a given situation.
HYPOTHESIS 4: The Inverted U. There is a non-linear, inverted U-shaped relationship between degree of stress and level or quality of performance. For example, at a low level of arousal where performance is minimal, an increase in stress results in enhanced performance. However, further increases in stress beyond an optimal level will lead to a decrease in performance.
HYPOTHESIS 5: Task Difference. The nature of the tasks in which the person is involved, and the relationship of those activities to the stressor conditions, influence the direction and the shape of the relationships between subjectively experienced stress, task performance, and consequences.
HYPOTHESIS 6: Interpersonal Effect. The presence or absence and the activities of other persons in the situation influence both the subjective experience of stress and behaviour in response to stress (McGrath, 1976, p. 1353).

McGrath's stress definition has provided researchers with a tool for rigorous empirical research. It is the basis for exploring a growing number of variables that can be considered major psychological demands of the work environment. Many psychological demands can be extremely powerful and threatening. If we lose our job or get passed over for a promotion that we felt we deserved, the demands for adjustment are powerful indeed. These sometimes abrupt, always powerful, catalysts from the workplace demand an adjustment that can originate from within or from outside of ourselves. Unlike our very specific reactions to ordinary demands made upon us, our response to stress, regardless of its nature or origin, is basically the same.

A physiological stress reaction has two stages. The first is the shock stage, which reflects our initial reaction to a severe, unexpected demand for action. Signs of injury appear: heart beat is irregular, blood pressure falls, muscle tone is lost, and body temperature drops. Then, in the second, or countershock stage, the body reactions are reversed and defense mechanisms are mobilized. The adrenal cortex is mobilized and enlarged, and the production of carticoid hormones is stimulated. Heart rate, blood pressure, and body temperature increase, muscle tone is restored, and we are prepared for either 'fight or flight'.

Our psychological reaction to stress follows a similar course. When we first hear bad news or good news, we are stunned, not really able to take in the information that has been revealed to us. After the initial shock of disbelief, the defence reaction follows. If we failed to get a much desired promotion, we may rationalize that it would entail too much work anyway or deny that we really wanted it or blame the decision on politics and the successful candidate's strategy of playing up to the boss. If the news is good, we reassess ourselves and the boss in a new and more favourable light. In victory, we may even be gracious to the unsuccessful candidate.

The way our body and mind mobilize for action in response to excessive demands of any kind is clearly a carry-over from our evolutionary heritage as hunters and gatherers in the wild. Such mobilization was essential if human beings were to survive in a world where most of the dangers came from without and were difficult, if not impossible, to anticipate or prepare for. For most people today, however, the body mobilizes its defenses in response to psychological rather than physical danger. Thus, psychological stress, since it comes from ourselves or from other people, is in many cases foreseeable. Stress has become a basic fact of life, and, since we tend to operate in habitual and predictable ways, we are in a better position to manage it than were our ancestors who had to cope with the pressures of the unforeseeable.

Thus, stress measurement is essential in our moden society as we can rarely resort to the physical action for which a stress response prepares us. In many cases, the mobilized energy is discharged through one or another body organ, and we experience a stress symptom such as headache, stomach ache, or nervous tension. If the stress continues and we have no other outlet, chronic stress diseases may result, such as migraine, ulcers, or colitis.

Stress can be either temporary or long-term, mild or severe, depending on how long its causes continue, how powerful they are, and how strong the individual's recovery powers are. If stress is temporary and mild, most people can handle it, or at least recover from its effects rather quickly.

Importance of measurement issues

In view of these facts, the importance of the accurate measurement of stress in modern society is apparent. The effects of stress touch our lives daily in both the work and non-work domain. The study of job stress in the work domain has increased in significance as stress in organizations is recognized as a pragmatic contributor to the success or failure of the organization. There is also emerging evidence that in some situations, an organization can be legally liable for the emotional and physical impact of job stress on employees. Poor working conditions, sustained conflicts with supervisors, traumatic events, or intentional harassment of employees sometimes results in anguish, neurosis, or even suicide. If liability is established, employees could possibly claim benefits under workers' compensation laws, as well as sue for financial damages. However, legal liability is just one of the concerns that plague organizations trying to cope with job stress. Lower productivity from the employee, absenteeism, turnover, poor quality of workmanship, and a decrease in employee morale are also major concerns of organizations coping with job stress.

The importance of studying stress in the work domain has been established. Although research investigating the effects of job stress on performance and productivity began in the early 1950s (Haiberg, 1982), programmes to improve employee relations, and health and to reduce the effects of stressors began much later. Nevertheless, a significant trend toward greater corporate involvement in promoting employee health through a variety of stress-reduction programmes has recently been on the increase (Fielding, 1984; Murphy, 1984). Also under recent scrutiny have been the conditions in the workplace that are stressful. The objective properties of the environment that are stressful in a job setting combined with the subjective assessment of conditions by the worker make up the overall conditions of the workplace. Government studies estimate a $17 billion annual decrease in United States industrial productivity due to stress-induced poor health (Rosen, 1984). However, putting a price tag on job-related stress is extremely difficult. It is hard enough to determine how much time was lost from the workplace and how many dollars of productivity were lost due to specific illness or deaths of employees, but attributing those illnesses or deaths to stress is basically speculation. While we can assert the importance of job stress by invoking dollar figures, there is usually little more than speculative assertion behind the figures. Nevertheless, researchers in the field of job stress, and increasingly, company managers, do contend that some aspects of stress are widespread, chronic, and worth trying to reduce. Thus, the development of work-based stress-management programmes are considered to benefit both employers and employees, but this is of course true only if the programmes are effective. In order for stress measurement programmes to be effective, they must be grounded in valid theoretical models that utilize reliable instruments for measuring job stress. This should be the primary reason for conducting research in the area of job stress. The importance, need and impact of such research from the organizational perspective has been established, However, methodological and definitional problems with conducting job-stress research seem to continue, posing a threat to rigorous research.

Differentiation between episodic and chronic stressful events

One basic problem with job-stress research instruments is a tendency for most instruments to regard and label job stress within a generic category while not taking into consideration the temporal nature of the phenomenon. Conceptually, theoretical models addressing job stress should consider both the chronic and episodic nature of stress. This differentiation has not been conceptually articulated in job-stress research and should be basic to sound theoretical research in the area.

Another basic problem with job-stress research instruments is the subjectivity that is inherent in self-report instruments. It is obviously not possible to develop an objective measurement instrument as long as researchers ask individuals to express their own opinions and attitudes, but there is a need to establish and develop an objective normative standard on which these opinions and attitudes can be based. Researchers have given little priority to developing a normative standard (e.g. one work group might be affected by job stress to a greater degree than another work group) because of its obvious biasing effect, but if the validity of such a normative standard could be achieved, more objectivity could be implanted into the subjective heart of job stress research.

A review of the literature on job stress suggests that researchers are primarily concerned with episodic events that produce stressful consequences for an employee (Bhagat and Beehr, 1985). Episodic stressors are the events that are temporary in nature and are characteristic of constantly changing types of environments. Relatively little attention is paid to the role of chronic or ongoing situations that might plague an individual employee day in and day out. One possible reason for the emphasis placed on episodic events might be the transient, ever-changing nature that characterizes many organizations. In other words, organizations seem to be primarily concerned with episodic events because their temporal, changeable environment makes an episodic event more evident and brings more attention to it. On the other hand, chronic stressful situations which are more permanent or long-lasting in nature may simply be viewed as a necessary part of the corporate culture. The recognition of these chronic situations may tend to be blurred during the daily routines of the organization, but their impact over time can be as damaging as that of episodic events.

Some chronic situations are transient, but others are of a recurring nature. For example, a demanding manager who insists on perfection in trivial tasks, a subordinate who constantly complains about inadequacies of the organization as the cause for poor performance, or a persistently sick child at home could produce stressful effects on an employee which obviously have important adaptive consequences (Kanner et al., 1981; Delongis et al., 1982). Lazarus and his associates (1983), termed these chronic situations 'daily hassles' and cited that they have been found to be better predictors of health outcomes than episodic life events. Delongis and others (1982) have suggested that 'hassles' or chronic situations, are more proximal measures of stress, whereas episodic events reflect distal measures. Beehr and Bhagat (1985) pointed out that one can make a strong case for the argument based on evidence found in recent clinical literature indicating that chronic situations are more powerful predictors of important stress-related outcomes than episodic events.

Lazarus (1983) suggested that the counterpart of chronic sources of stress, which he labelled daily uplifts, have also been found to be effective in predicting stress outcomes. For example, a complimentary remark from one's colleagues, an in-basket free from unnecessary paperwork, and a smile from one's spouse have such a pleasurable effect that they contribute to one's overall sense of emotional well-being on a daily basis. Klinger (1975, 1977) has noted that hassles and uplifts are likely to be associated with an individual's current concerns and commitments. In addition, since these concerns tend to shift across one's life span (Ryff and Boltes, 1976), the variability and the meaningfulness of these hassles and uplifts also change during the course of one's life.

As pointed out earlier, chronic situations or hassles are distinguishable from traumatic life event changes in the sense that hassles are more commonplace and accepted as part of a routine. While it is tempting to think of hassles as being by-products or outcomes of life events, many hassles have little or almost no relationship to life events and the correlation between life events and daily hassles is relatively weak. Therefore, DeLongis et al. (1982) argued that the construct of chronic situations or hassles makes an independent contribution to adaptational outcomes and experience of illness. It is this separate contribution that is important to recognize in job-stress research. Most instruments in job-stress research today do not emphasize the importance of differentiating between episodic events and chronic situations when addressing the problem of job stress within an organization. Thus, it is obvious that a more rigorous quality of research should be designed around this differentiation.

Severity of the stress outcome

The basic conceptual model of stress incorporates the idea of the duration of perceived uncertainties (Beehr and Bhagat, 1985) as an important variable in the stress formula. Like the differentiation needed between episodic and chronic stress, most stress research needs to employ differentiation within the duration variable. The duration variable is closely linked to the severity of the stress outcome, whether it be episodic or chronic in nature. The concept of duration helps in distinguishing between coping and adaptive skills that demand mobilization of new resources when confronted with an acute, situationally determined stressful event, as opposed to coping and adaptive skills that require continuous monitoring of various kinds of resources when confronted with a gradually developing stressful event (Beehr and Bhagat, 1985). However, to date, most research in job stress has focused attention on stressful events of a short-term duration and research on stressful events of long-term duration have been relatively rare. Kasl's work (1980) on job loss and plant shutdown and recent work in the area of job transfer (reviewed in Brett, 1980) are examples of work that involves looking at stressful events that require longer periods of time to be resolved fully or coped with adequately.

The differentiation between low time duration and high time duration can be linked directly with high of low severity of an episodic or chronic stressful situation. Low time duration correlates with low severity and high time duration correlates with high severity. For example, Jick (1985) noted that multiple, timed budget cuts have stronger effects than single cuts in generating chronic or persistent stress. This is an example of high severity with high duration and low severity with low duration. The inability of most job-stress research measures to differentiate between low and high time duration when integrating this variable into job-stress formulas can only lessen the rigor of research in this area.

Table 1 indicates a few examples of instruments used for measuring stress in the work environment. It also shows that the preponderance of measures are used to look at chronic stress of low severity and episodic stress of high severity. At present, there is a need to develop more instruments to measure chronic stress of high severity and episodic stress of low severity.

Up until this point, this chapter has dicsussed theoretical recommendations for changes in instruments used for measuring job stress, i.e. the basic differentiation between episodic and chronic stressors and the basic differentiation into high or low duration which should correlate with the high or low severity of the stressful event. These recommendations are made primarily because of a concern for the general nature of most job-stress instruments and a

Table 1: Conceptual scheme for classification of instruments used for Measuring Stress in the Work Environment

CHRONIC STRESS	EPISODIC STRESS	
Examples: 1. Job-related Tension (Khan, Wolfe, Quinn & Snoek, 1964) 2. Tension Index (Lyons, 1971) 3. Anxiety-Stress Questionnaire (House & Rizzo, 1972) 4. Depressed Mood at Work (Quinn & Shepard, 1974) 5. Self-Esteem at Work (Quinn & Shepard, 1974)	*Examples:* Lacking instruments—Need to develop Measures of episodic stressors that are triggered by minor changes in the work place (e.g. constant change of supervisors).	LOW SEVERITY
Examples: Lacking instruments—Need to develop measures of stressors that are triggered by major changes in the work place (e.g., major budget cuts)	*Examples:* 1. Life stress, organizational stress, & job satisfaction (Sarason & Johnson, 1974) 2. Total Life Stress (Bhagat, McQuaid, Lindholm, & Segovis, 1985) 3. Schedule of Recent Experiences (Holmes & Rahe, 1967).	HIGH SEVERITY

need to discover the diversities within the general category of job stress. With these theoretical concerns addressed, it is necessary to scrutinize further the problematic areas that currently exist with many instruments used to measure job stress today.

Validity in job-stress research

One concern with job-stress research is that many researchers, when assessing their results, do not attempt to demonstrate the validity of their research. Actually, the validity of job-stress research should be examined in three phases: pre-study research activities, research activities, and post-study research activities. Pre-study validity issues are those concerned with criteria or standards and the values used in identification and selection of elements and relations. During the actual research process, the concerns of validity are with the correspondence among a number of sets of elements and relationships among the domains. Post-study validity concerns are with the robustness or generalizability of the meanings inferred from the study outcomes (Brinberg and McGrath, 1982). These three phases of research integrate and utilize the multiphases of the basic meaning of validity. The first phase of this basic meaning looks at validity as value; that is, it suggests that the value of research needs to be established in the methodological domain and is most applicable to pre-study research activities. The next phase of the validity meaning couples the idea of correspondence between two sets of things, whether they be two sets of constructs, a set of concepts and set of observations or two sets of measures, and is most applicable to the actual research process. The last phase addresses the idea of robustness, dependability or generalizability. This post-study process is concerned with the degree to which a set of concepts or finding will stand up when generalized into areas beyond the actual research study (Brinberg and McGrath, 1982).

When considering the validity of job-stress research, it is essential to understand that a framework for organizing research designs is related to various types of validity. Generally, research validity can be defined as the informativeness of a specific study for the development and support of hypotheses (Campbell and Stanley, 1963). Although numerous kinds of validity have been defined, traditionally, four specific types have been considered essential to good research: internal validity; external validity; construct validity; and conclusion validity.

Internal validity is the extent to which the detected relationship between the independent and dependent variables is causal. External validity can be broadly lined to the issue of generalizability, that is, the extent to which samples represent the population. Construct validity is the degree to which the theoretical treatment, outcome, population, and setting have been successfully operationalized in the research. It refers to the extent to which the independent and dependent variables in a study successfully represent the theoretical constructs. Finally, conclusion validity is the extent to which the research design is sufficiently precise or powerful enough to detect relationships between the independent and dependent variables. In other words, conclusion validity refers to the extent to which the statistical conclusions of a research study are accurate (Cook and Campbell, 1979).

Thus, the multiphasic meaning of validity, the integration of validity into the three phases of research activity, and the four different types of validity should all be conceptually understood and pragmatically implemented to build the framework of a theoretically rigorous research design.

During the last few years, empirical studies on job stress and outcome relations have followed some systematic theoretical models (e.g. the Kahn et al. (1964) role stress model, and the French et al. (1974) P-E fit model) and we have some reliable sources of information based on research conducted within this social psychological mode. Like the Kahn et al., and the French et al., models, many of the models in job-stress research are theoretically sound, but the instruments used to measure the job-stress variables usually fall into a single-method category. Historically, research in this area has been carried out almost solely through the utilization of interviews and questionnaires.

Methodological problems of single-method job-stress research

Folger and Belew (1985) illustrate the methodological problems of single-method research by relating the story of an experimental psychologist studying classical conditioning in grasshoppers. Voltage passing through an electrified grid induced a grasshopper to jump, and the shock was paired with the sound of a tone. After conditioning had been successfully established, the grasshopper would reliably jump with presentation of the tone alone. The psychologist continued to study that response while systematically removing the grasshopper's legs, one at a time. Finally, after all the legs had been removed, tone presntation failed to elicit jumping behaviour. The psychologist concluded that grasshoppers hear with their legs.

With this anecdote, Folger and Belew (1985) emphasize that over-reliance on a single type of measure seriously jeopardizes sound interpretation and rigorous research. Research on job stress is all too prone to fall into this single-method trap. To base research solely upon survey methodology (questionnaires and interviews producing self-report data) is to fall victim to a methodology that is the easiest or most convenient to obtain. Webb and his colleagues described this type of methodology in the following passage (Webb et al., 1981, pp. 1–2): 'Interviews and questionnaires intrude as a foreign element into the social setting they would describe, they create as well as measure attitudes, they elicit atypical roles and responses, they are limited to those who are accessible and will cooperate.'

In this passage, Webb et al. (1981) are emphasizing that interviews and questionnaires influence the respondents' awareness of the measurement process. Thus, if the respondent is motivated to provide information that differs from what would be obtained when awareness of the measurement process is absent, the contaminating effects would be felt in the research results.

Threats to validity associated with the single-method approach to job-stress research

Because researchers in the area of job stress continue to use the convenient methods of interviews and questionnaires, it is essential to consider some of the basic problems or threats to validity associated with a single-method self-report measurement approach. Response styles, or the individual's habitual way of answering questions that is not influenced by the question's content, is one consideration. Some people tend to mark items at the extremes of a continuum while others are more apt to mark items at a neutral or middle of the road level. In addition to response styles, there may be a decreasing number of people willing to cooperate with interviews and questionnaires (Bryant and Hansen, 1976; Feldman, 1976; Frankel, 1976).

Reactivity is another basis for error in self-report measures. Reactivity describes the alteration of a response by a respondent because of his or her knowledge of being observed or assessed. Reactivity involves crystallization, cues, and response sets. Attitudes are said to become crystallized when the person being questioned is brought to a high level of awareness about the issue being studied. As a result of this new level of awareness, new attitudes tend to be created by the interviewing act, with subsequent changes in actual behaviour (Folger and Belew, 1985).

A study by Bridge et al. (1977) illustrated how the phenomenon of crystallization can affect behaviour and subsequently, validity. Two randomly chosen groups were questioned, one group about cancer and one about burglary. Integrated into the questionnaire on the first survey were items concerning the individual's opinions of the personal importance of good health and safety from crime. Several weeks later, all respondents were given the identical survey questions concerning both crime and cancer. The two groups did not differ on pre-tested attitudes towards crime and health, but there were some significant differences in ratings following implementation of the experimental manipulation. Respondents who initially had been surveyed on cancer attitudes subsequently considered good health to be of more importance that did those interviewed on burglary attitudes (Folger and Belew, 1985).

Further evidence of attitude crystallization (new attitudes created by the interviewing act) on behaviour was cited in a study of the phenomenon by Kraut and McConahay (1973), in which half of the sample of prospective voters were randomly chosen to be interviewed prior to the 1964 presidential primary. This group showed a significantly higher voter turnout (48 per cent) than did the non-interviewed group (21 per cent).

Another source of reactivity is that of cueing, either overt of covert, that directs a subject's response. If an interviewee is inclined to give the interviewer answers that the interviewee deems favourable, overt cues such as items that associate the interviewer with a particular cause or organization may signal a desired response. Often overt cues include letterheads on surveys, badges, buttons, or uniforms worn by the interviewer, as well as distinguishing characteristics of the interviewer such as age, gender, race, or style of dress (Folger and Belew, 1985).

A third source of reactivity has been labelled response sets. Often when people are aware that they are being studied and their responses are being investigated, their responses may be slanted to create impressions based on their assumptions about how the data will be used. A person's interest in creating a good impression is a common source of biased responses whenever anonymity is absent. The reason for such biased responses during an interviewing session is obvious. People are often distrustful of the interviewer's promises that their responses will remain confidential. Employees, not wanting to place their jobs and careers in jeopardy, are unlikely to risk doing so with a favourable survey response. Employees also view a self-report interview or survey as an opportunity to make a good impression with a supervisor who just might have access to the responses. Thus, responses to items concerning job satisfaction, absenteeism, punctuality, and projectivity may all elicit responses that are less honest or objective than would be elicited in an unobtrusive measurement situation (Folger and Belew, 1985).

Even if respondents believe in the anonymity of the self-report instrument or interview, true feelings are still often not expressed, which directly affects the validity of research. Orne (1962) pointed out that people sometimes falsify responses in the desire to be helpful to the interests of science by providing 'good' data that confirm what they believe is the investigator's hypothesis. Also, respondents sometimes falsify data if they are convinced they know how the data might be used. For example, if workers like a supervisor who is lacking in leadership skills, they might falsify self-report responses if they feel the supervisor will be adversely affected by truthful responses (Folger and Belew, 1985).

Threats to validity associated with an established model

Salancik and Pfeffer's (1977) examination of need-satisfaction models of job attitudes reveal further examples of methodological problems that can threaten research validity. They point to the phenomenon of response consistency which refers to the organization of information in consistent ways by individuals when interviewed about their attitudes and beliefs. Consistency effects come from an individual's awareness of his own responses to questions and while answering questions, he presents to himself as well as to the researcher, information that may not have been as salient before. With an awareness of the past questions, the person tends to answer questions so as to be consistent with past answers and in doing so, creates a consistency effect. This phenomenon is one of interpretation between attitudes and behaviours when the attitude is explored after the behaviour has occurred. That is, if persons are reminded of their past behaviour, their attitudes are more consistent with this past behaviour than in those cases in which past behaviour is not made known to them. The same phenomenon is true concerning the questioning process. The initial survey or interview requires answers from the respondent, which subsequently became salient information for the respondent and act as a constraint for later responses (Salancik and Pfeffer, 1977).

Another threat to validity revealed in Salancik and Pfeffer's (1977) examination is that of priming. The phenomenon of priming is sometimes seen, when in questioning a person about his activities or beliefs, the interviewer orients or alerts the respondent's attention to certain information. The priming effect is similar, but somewhat different from the consistency effect. A consistency effect presupposes a person's tendency to be logical in his statements about things and is concerned with how he processes information; the priming effect occurs in the questioning process when various aspects of the situation are made more salient than they might otherwise be. The priming phenomenon is based on the idea that an individual's attitude is derived from whatever information is available when asked about that attitude.

In the interviewing process, the researcher causes the respondent to concentrate on certain features of the situation. Priming, along with tendencies toward consistency, can be a powerful influence on shaping attitudes. As Salancik and Pfeffer (1977) point out, studies of job attitudes based on need-satisfaction theories are likely to introduce priming effects by using standard research interviewing methods. Questionnaires typically ask the individual to recall information about his job situation. This information is related to the investigator's own model of needs and job characteristics as these relate to attitudes. Thus, if a person is asked to describe his job in terms that are of interest to the investigator, he can do so. But if the individual is then asked how he feels about the job, he has few options but to respond using the information the researcher has made available. The correlation between job characteristics and attitudes from such an approach is not only unremarkable, but provides little information about the need-satisfaction model being tested (Salancik and Pfeffer, 1977).

Reactivity of measurement with mechanical devices

Another important issue is the reactivity of the measure even if it is an electronic recording instrument. Surely, an electronic recording device should produce results that are valid and unbiased. But this is true only when the reactivity of the measure is considered by the researcher. For example, when electronic recording instruments are used (e.g. EMG training), a period of time may be required for the respondents to adapt to the measuring device. Sallis and Lichstein (1979) reported a study in which subjects needed approximately eleven minutes to obtain a stable EMG recording level. In other words, after sensory electrode placement, EMG reading decreased for eleven minutes before the physiological adaptation stabilized. Obviously, experiments employing this type of training should allow time for adaptation to occur, but in their review of twenty-five articles, Sallis and Lichstein report that 44 per cent clearly permitted no time for stabilization. If within-subjects designs are used, significant results could be due to the adaptation response rather than to the treatment. Control groups in which participants were also attached to the electronic recording machine could be one way to eliminate this problem (Beehr and O'Hara, see this volume).

Naturally, constructors of self-report measures are uniquely aware of the many potential reactivity biases and as much as possible, efforts are made to eliminate those problems. However, it is obvious that because of the very nature of self-report instruments, it is impossible to eliminate all such biases. Because of these inherent biases characteristic of self-report measures, Webb et al. (1966, 1981) advocated the supplementation of surveys and interviews with additional, less reactive measures to give a convergence aspect to rigorous job stress research.

Measurement scales used in job-stress research

Stress must be defined and assessed from someone's viewpoint, and it is important to understand the convergence that exists among several possible operationalizations of a stress-related construct. Measurement related issues in job-stress research vary considerably. As discussed earlier, the major problem is that both independent and dependent variables are measured with the same method, usually a self-report instrument. This is not to say that self-report measures do not contribute to sound, theoretically correct, and rigorous job stress research. Such instruments as the Job-Related Tension Index (JRT), developed by Kahn, Wolfe, Quinn, Snoek, and Rosenthal (1964) and the Job-Related Strain Index (JRS) developed by Indik, Seashore and Slesinger (1964) are examples of instruments that have been used extensively in job stress research. Each scale was intended to measure a wide range of job characteristics, in particular role conflict and ambiguity, incompatibility between job demands and available resources, and work overload. Several researchers such as Burke and Belcourt (1974) and MacKinnon (1968) have examined the factor structure of the JRS and JRT and used subscales to measure facets of job stress. Typically, the factors that are derived relate to role ambiguity, role conflict, role overload and resource inadequacy/uncertainty about acceptance. Also, several papers have employed revised versions of the JRS (Berger-Gross, 1982), or used the JRS as a core for the development of a new instrument (e.g. Administrative Stress Index, Tung, 1980; Kock, Tung, Emelch and Swent, 1982), or used a subset of questions from the JRT for the development of a tension index (Lyons, 1971). The Administrative Stress Index (ASI) (Tung, 1980) contains measures of role-based stress, conflict-mediating stress and boundary-spanning stress. Another scale utilizing items from the JRT and other sources consists of both macro and micro work dimensions, and variants of the SDS have been used to discriminate among managers, nurses and medical technologists. Thus, the JRS and JRT have been used to stimulate research, but the employment of these scales alone, without the use of a multi-method approach, needs to be considered a theoretically weak approach to measurement in job stress research.

Use of the multi-method approach to improve methodological robustness

The validity of self-report instruments, such as the JRS and JRT, is not being questioned in this chapter. However, it is proposed that job stress research utilizing a multi-method approach to measurement would add considerable methodological robustness to strategies in job stress research.

As this chapter has pointed out, the effects of psychological treatments have traditionally been evaluated in a relatively restricted fashion with a heavy reliance upon rating scales and self-report inventories. Together with the limited range of assessment devices used, assessment conditions usually have been obtrusive. Because the respondents are aware that their behaviour is being assessed, perhaps performance under obtrusive conditions does not resemble performance under conditions where clients are unaware of the assessment procedures.

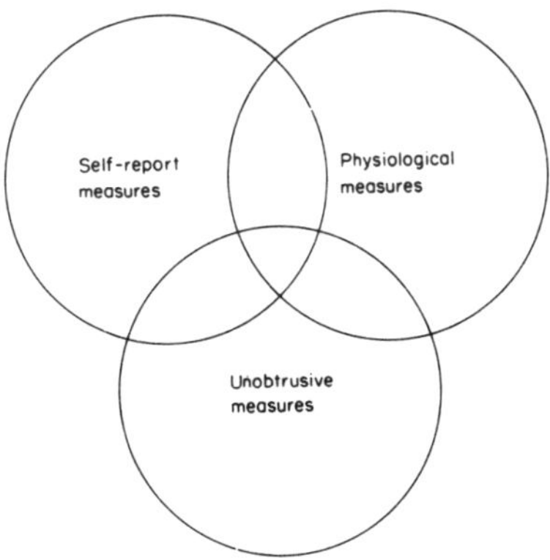

Figure 1: Proposed scheme for improving measurement strategies in job stress research

The use of unobtrusive measures is one way to create a multi-method approach to job stress research. Unobtrusive measures remove or greatly reduce awareness, and therefore minimize the biasing effect that is present in self-report instruments. In other words, unobtrusive measures constitute a subset of non-reactive measures (Folger and Belew, 1985). Historically, non-reactive measures are described by the categories devised by Webb et al. (1966): physical traces—erosion and accretion; archives—the running record; archives—the episodic and private record; simple observation; and contrived observation—hidden hardware and control.

Folger and Belew (1985) cite absenteeism as an example of an archival non-reactive measurement. Absenteeism data is a potential indicator of attitudes toward work, and such data might positively supplement data from self-report instruments about work. Other researchers using non-reactive measures as support for self-report instruments have also found archival data on absenteeism useful. Steers and Mowday (1981) found evidence that absences from the workplace could possibly be substitutes for quitting when resignation is not feasible; Blacker and Brown (1975) found that absences from the workplace correlated with worker boredom; and Nicholson, Wall and Lischeron (1977), found correlations between absenteeism and basic job dissatisfaction. The use of absenteeism as an unobtrusive archival measure, however, is not without problems of interpretation for the researcher. As Folger and Belew (1985) point out, absenteeism measures are probably less reactive than self-report measures but more reactive than other kinds or archival records. One obvious problem is that virtually no information about the recording process exists and many organizations lack any systematic record-keeping system for absenteeism. Also, when assessing the degree of reactivity, researchers must consider that if attendance is regularly checked and publicly recorded, absenteeism might be lower than if attendance is assessed sporadically without employees' knowledge.

The other two categories of unobtrusive measurement, physical traces and observation, require more creativity to prove worthwhile. Physical traces of ashtrays with piles of cigarettes in some departments and few, if any, in other departments could be an indication of job-related stress. Worn carpet that leads to the employee lounge may sound like a trivial observation, but it could be a possible indication of job dissatisfaction. Posters hanging in an office or cubicle are also examples of trace indicators that can illustrate a general feel for the prevailing work atmosphere. 'Friday is Coming', 'You Want It When?', and 'Have You Hugged Your Boss Today?' are examples of posters that could perhaps reveal a tense working environment. Observations, simple or contrived, may sound straightforward, but care must be taken if the researcher is going to be successful. In other words, it is difficult to observe employee behaviour without being obvious that observation is the primary reason for the researcher's presence. A co-worker approach to observation is usually the least obvious method, but it is also time consuming, especially when the researcher has to learn a particular skill to be effective as a worker.

Physiological indicators as measures of job stress

Thus far, this chapter has discussed the use of self-report instruments as the principal method for assessing job-related stress in the work place. The pitfalls of the single-method approach to measurement were discussed and the use of unobtrusive measures was introduced as one means to achieving a multi-method approach to measurement. Along with self-report instruments and unobtrusive measurements, a third measure—the use of physiological indicators of job stress—should be employed in order to achieve an integrated multi-method approach to measurement.

The use of physiological indicators as measures of job stress, of course, like the unobtrusive measures, is not as convenient nor as straightforward as self-report data to gather and interpret. For example, it is generally assumed that anxious persons recover more slowly in their physiological reactions to stress than non-anxious persons, yet anxiety levels are difficult to pin down objectively because of individual differences. Typical stressful situations studied in the social sciences involve eletric shock, sudden loud noises, and fast-paced, difficult tests of ability. What has been found in such studies is that persons respond differently to different physiological indicators. For example, while one person may typically respond to difficult stressful situations with increased blood pressure but not with increased rate of breathing, the reverse may be true for another person.

Threats to validity associated with physiological measures

Recent job stress literature indicates the importance of three major categories of factors that could affect the validity of physiological stress measurement. These factors are categorized as stable or permanent factors, transitory factors, and procedural factors (Fried, et al., 1984).

Stable or permanent factors are simply the differences inherent in individuals and groups with regard to their susceptibility to certain physiological symptoms. Physiological symptoms that vary with sex, race, age, or familial or genetic tendency must be accounted for when physiological measurement is used. For example, people with a familial tendency to high blood pressure appear to develop higher levels of blood pressure under stress than people who do not have such a familial tendency (Light, 1981).

Transitory factors are time- and situation-specific, including such variables as room temperature, humidity, time of day, physical exertion of the subject and consumption of caffeine and nicotine prior to the measurement (Fried et al., 1984). For example, an individual's level of cholesterol tends to be higher when standing than when sitting (Statland, Bokelund and Winkel, 1974) and drinking coffee or smoking before or during measurement tends to increase the level of cardiovascular activity (Siddle and Turpin, 1980).

Procedural factors are concerned with the procedural problems of measurement, such as the number of times physiological measures are made or the amount of time between measures. For example, blood pressure is not a static measure since there is a natural variation in the cardiovascular system which prevents a single measure of blood pressure from being a reliable indicator. Therefore, truly reliable measures of blood pressure would require subjects to make several visits to a measurement point and several measures per visit would be required for accurate assessment (Rosner and Polk, 1979, 1981).

The confusing nature and unconscious effects of physiological measurement, coupled with the inconvenience imposed on the subject and a common reluctance among subjects to allow physiological measurements, offers partial explanation why physiological measures are not widely used as a supplement to self-report instruments when gathering data on job stress.

Physiological measurement in job-stress research

Many physiological functions have, however, at some time or other, been measured and correlated with emotional reactions to stress. For example, a rough measure of muscular tonus can be obtained with a variety of mechanical recorders such as strain gauges. Electromyographic techniques are generally more convenient and allow a fairly precise measure of local muscle activity. Skin temperature can be determined by vasomotor activity, temperature of the blood, and general body temperature, and can be recorded simply by applying a sensitive thermocouple to the skin surface. Measures of metabolic rate generally depend on indices of oxygen consumption and carbon dioxide release. The nitrogen content of the urine as well as chemical analyses of other bodily waste products have been used in some studies (Grossman, 1967).

McGrath (1970, 1982) pointed out that non-reactive measures are extremely relevant to physiological indices. For example, archival data, such as the examination of medical records, could provide an unlimited source of information. Medical records that would be of most value are those that yield information about diseases and symptoms presumably precipitated by stress (e.g. arthritis, ulcers, and other digestive ailments). Also, accretions of bodily substances that can be biochemically analyzed, such as blood or urine samples, have value as physiological true measures.

Glass (1977) illustrated that catecholamine levels are associated with heart disorders in a variety of ways. The heart muscle is strained when epinephrine and norepinephrine make the heart pump faster. They also contribute to a rise in blood pressure, which makes the heart work harder and puts additional strain on the blood vessels.

The use of trace measures in job-stress research does pose unique interpretive problems, and thus, the importance of checking for relationships among stress-related variables is apparent (Folger and Belew, 1985). For example, Baade et al.'s (1978) study of parachute trainees measured levels of epinephrine and cortisol in blood plasma where studies of Frankenhaeuser and Gardell (1976) utilized urine samples. The difference in the procedures is that blood samples must be obtained by methods that might bring on a certain amount of stress and thus a degree of reactivity, whereas, obtaining a urine sample is usually stress free.

In Cox's (1980) review of studies on repetitive work, he examined studies which utilize trace measures for longer periods of time and thus this review is an appropriate source for obtaining data regarding the relationship between performance and physiological trace measures. An example from this review was O'Hanlon's (1978) study in which subjects were assigned a simulated inspection task that lasted an entire day. Although this length of time presents methodological problems due to diurnal fluctuations in the physiological measures, it is a positive change from the usual brevity of other laboratory measures. In this study, O'Hanlon found positive correlations of both epinephrine and triglycerides with performance efficiency. Cox (1980) also noted that triglycerides are the result of epinephrine-elevated free fatty acids that become converted when not used by the body and that 'there is a recognized positive relationship between elevated triglyceride concentration and the occurrence of cardiovascular disease, involving artherosclerosis' (Cox, 1980, p. 32).

Observation of ongoing physiological processes is another type of non-reactive stress measure in the physiological domain and is usually accomplished by using sophisticated biomedical equipment. Webb et al. (1966, 1981) defined 'contrived observations' as those involving the use of specialized hardware. Usually, the research conducted on job stress utilizes biomedical instruments that measure cardiovascular activity. For example, Manenica (1981) reviewed physiological indices utilized in looking at physical workload. He demonstrated that the caloric equivalent of oxygen is constant, and thus information about the level of oxygen intake allows for an objective measurement of physical workload.

Ursin and Ursin (1979), on the other hand, looked at the physiological indicators of mental workload. These researchers were instrumental in solving the dilemma regarding cardiovascular measures, i.e. whether an accelerated heart rate represents increased physical or muscle requirements or a generalized activation associated with mental and psychological requirements, such as concentration or anxiety (Folger and Belew, 1985). Ursin and Ursin's method required prior laboratory measurement of the workers under 'aerobic steady state muscle work' (Ursin and Ursin, 1979, p. 355) for calibration of the relationship between heart rate and oxygen intake. Then, in subsequent situations, these two researchers were able to determine how much heart rate acceleration was due to the tasking of the heart muscle and how much could be attributed to psychological activation (Ursin and Ursin, 1979, p. 355).

Objectivity of physiological measures

Physiological measures of stress are considered by many researchers to be a more objective approach to measurement than the subjective nature inherent in self-report measures. This objectivity, if actually present, adds considerable substance to a multi-method approach to measuring job stress. In other words, it is essential for researchers to understand that adequate procedures for the measurement of physiological processes are important to both the internal and external validity of job stress studies.

Most studies of job stress utilizing physiological indicators focus on (a) cholesterol in the blood; (b) blood pressure and cardiac activity (heart rate and ECG); (c) urinary catecholamines; and (d) peptic ulcer, In order for these different physiological symptoms to be measured correctly and thus be valid objective measures, the potentially contaminating factors (permanent, transitory, and procedural) need to be considered (Fried et al., 1984). There is sufficient evidence regarding the potential effects of these confounding factors on physiological measures to suggest maximum caution by researchers who use physiological measures as criteria to assess job stress.

When considering these confounding factors, researchers should strive to improve the validity of their results by using physiological criteria which are appropriate for measuring episodic versus chronic job stressors. For example, urinary catecholamines are less sensitive to transient events than plasma catecholamines, and thus make better criteria for chronic stressors than for episodic stressors. On the other hand, cardiovascular symptoms are highly sensitive to transient events and resemble the characteristics of plasma catecholamines. Past research has shown inconclusive or vague evidence connecting the effects of chronic stressful events with cardiovascular reactions. Thus, it seems that cardiovascular symptoms should be used primarily as criteria for identifying episodic, rather than chronic, job stressors (Fried et al., 1984). And finally, gastrointestinal symptoms, such as peptic ulcer, which develop over several months or years, would not be appropriate as criteria for episodic stressors, but should be used for identifying evidence of chronic stress.

Thus, the objectivity in the physiological measurement of job stressors depends solely on the validity of the measurement utilized. Presently, researchers should attempt to combine and integrate physiological and psychological measures that are appropriate to the assessment of chronic and episodic stressors. This integration can only be created with a more informed understanding of the physiological manifestations of job stress.

Conclusion

It is obvious from the discussion of both unobtrusive measures and physiological measures that creativity is an absolute necessity in producing measures that will contribute to rigorous job-stress research. However, it is also obvious that the integration of unobtrusive measures and physiological measures with self-report measures is a much needed positive step to attaining the best possible methodology for achieving reliable results in job-stress research. This should be coupled with the awareness that all job-stress situations should not be lumped together, but rather should be viewed in the diversity which they represent (e.g. episodic and chronic in nature). Furthermore, this differentiation into categories of job-stress needs to be supplemented by a differentiation into severity levels which are directly correlated to the time duration variable of the basic stress formula.

This integration will provide a multi-method approach and help eliminate the pitfalls of the self-report instruments that are so widely used in job-stress research. The differentiation between severity levels and type of stress will further complement the sophistication needed for research methodology robustness in the area of job-stress research.

REFERENCES

Baade, E., Ellertsen, B., Johnson, T. B., and Ursin, H. (1978). Physiology, psychology, and performance. In H. Ursin, E. Baade, and S. Levine (eds.) *Coping Men: A Study in Human Psychology*. San Francisco, Academic Press.

Beehr, T. A., and Bhagat, R. S. (1985). *Human Stress and Cognition in Organizations: An Integrated Perspective*. New York, John Wiley and Sons, pp. 401–15.

Berger-Gross, V. (1982). Difference score measures of social perceptions revisited: A comparison of alternatives. *Organizational Behaviour and Human Performance*, **29**, 279–85.

Blacker, F. H. M., and Brown, C. A. (1975). The impending crisis in job redesign, *Occupational Psychology*, **48**, 185–93.

Brett, J. (1980). Effects of job transfer on employees and their families. In C. L. Cooper and Roy Payne (eds.) *Current Concerns in Occupational Stress*, New York, Wiley, 99–136.

Bridge, R. G., Reeder, L. G., Kanouse, D., Kinder, D. R., Nagy, J. T., and Judd, C. M. (1977). Interviewing changes attitudes sometimes. *Public Opinion Quarterly*, **41**, 56–64.

Brinberg, D., and McGrath, J. E. (1982). A network of validity concepts within the research process. In D. Brinberg and L. H. Kidder (eds.) *Forms of Validity in Research*, San Francisco, Jossey-Bass.

Bryant, E. C., and Hansen, M. H. (1976). Invasion of privacy and surveys: A growing dilemma. In H. W. Sinaiko and L. A. Broedling (eds.) *Perspectives on Attitude Assessment: Surveys and their Alternatives*, Champaign, IL, Pendleton.

Burke, R. J., and Belcourt, M. L. (1974). Managerial role stress and coping responses, *Journal of Business Administration*, **5**, 55–68.

Campbell, D. T., and Stanley, J. C. (1963). *Experimental and quasi-experimental designs for research*, Chicago, Rand McNally.

Cook, T. D., and Campbell, D. T. (1979). *Quasi experimental: Design analysis issues for field settings*, Chicago, Rand McNally.

Cox, T. (1980). Repetitive work. In C. L. Cooper and R. Payne (eds.) *Current Concerns in Occupational Stress*, New York, Wiley.

Cox, T., Mackay, C. J., and Thirlway, M. A. (1978). Psychophysiological correlates of repetitive work. Report to Medical Research Council. Stress Research Report No. 11, Department of Psychology, University of Nottingham.

DeLongis, A., Coyne, J. C., Dakof, G., Folkman, S., and Lazarus, R. S. (1982). Relationship of daily hassles, uplifts and major life events to health status, *Health Psychology*, **1**, 119–36.

Feldman, R. E. (1976). Experimental and quasi-experimental field techniques: The protection of subjects. In H. W. Siraiko and L. A. Broeding (eds.) *Perspectives on Attitude Assessment: Surveys and their Alternatives*. Champaign, IL, Pendleton.

Fielding, J. E. (1984). Health promotion and disease prevention at the worksite. *Annual Review of Public Health*, **5**, 237–65.

Folger, R., and Belew, J. (1985). Nonreactive measurement: A focus for research on absenteeism and occupational stress. In L. L. Cummings and B. M. Staw (eds.) *Organizational Behavior*, Greenwich, Connecticut: JAI Press, Inc, Vol. 7.

Frankel, L. R. (1976). Restrictions to survey sampling–legal, practical, and ethical. In

H. W. Sinaiko and L. A. Broeding (eds.) *Perspectives on attitude assessment: Surveys and their alternatives*, Champaign, IL, Pendleton.

Frankenhaeuser, M., and Gardell, B. (1976). Underload and overload in working life: Outline of a multidisciplinary approach, *Journal of Human Stress*, **2**, 35–46.

French, J. R., Rodgers, R., and Cobb, S. (1974). Person-environment fit. In G. A. Coelho, H. Hamburg, and J. Adams (eds.) *Coping and adaptation*, New York, Basic Books.

Fried, Y., Rowland, K. M., Ferris, G. R. (1984). The physiological measurement of work stress: A critique, *Personnel Psychology*, **37**, 583–615.

Glass, D. C. (1977). *Behaviour Patterns, Stress, and Coronary Disease*, Hillsdale, NJ, Erlbaum.

Grossman, S. P. (1967). *A Textbook of Physiological Psychology*, New York, John Wiley and Sons.

Hoiberg, A. (1982). Occupational stress and illness incidence. *Journal of Occupational Medicine*, **24**, 445–51.

Indik, B., Seashore, S. E., and Slesinger, J. (1964). Demographic correlates of psychological strain, *Journal of Abnormal and Social Psychology*, **69**, 26–38.

Kahn, R. L., Wolfe, D. M., Quinn, R. P., Snoek, J. D., and Rosenthal, R. A. (1964). *Organizational Stress: Studies in Role Conflict and Ambiguity*, New York, Wiley.

Kanner, A. D., Coyne, J. C., Schaefer, C., and Lazarus, R. S. (1981). Comparison of two modes of stress measurement: Daily hassles and uplifts versus major life events. *Journal of Behavioural Medicine*, **4**, 1–39.

Kasl, S. (1980). The impact of retirement. In C. L. Cooper and R. Payne (eds.) *Current Concerns in Occupational Stress*, New York, Wiley, pp. 137–86.

Koch, J. L., Tung, R., Gmelch, W., and Swent, B. (1982). Job stress among school administrators: Factional dimensions and differential effect. *Journal of Applied Psychology*, **67**, 493–9.

Klinger, E. (1975). Consequences of commitment to and disengagement from incentives, *Psychological Review*, **82**, 1–25.

Klinger, E. (1977). *Meaning and void*, University of Minnesota Press.

Kraut, R. E., and McConahay, J. B. (1973). How being interviewed affects voting: An experiment, *Public Opinion Quarterly*, **36**, 398–406.

Lazarus, R. S., and DeLongis, A. (1983). Psychological stress and coping in aging, *American Psychologist*, **38**, 245–54.

Light, K. C. (1981). Cardiovascular responses to effortful active coping: Implications for the role of stress in hypertension development. *Psychophysiology*, **18**, 216–25.

Lyons, T. F. (1971). Role clarity, need for clarity, satisfaction, tension and withdrawal, *Organizational Behavior and Human Performance*, **6**, 99–110.

McGrath,. J. E. (1970). Settings, measures, and themes: An integrative review of some research on social-psychological factors in stress. In J. E. McGrath (ed.) *Social and Psychological Factors in Stress*, New York, Holt, Rinehart and Winston.

McGrath, J. E. (1976). Stress and behavior in organizations. In M. Dunnette (ed.) *Handbook of Industrial and Organizational Psychology*, Chicago, Rand McNally.

McGrath, J. E. (1982). Methodological problems in research on stress. In H. W. Krohne and L. Laux (eds.) *Achievement, Stress, and Anxiety*, Washington, Hemisphere.

MacKinnan, M. J. (1978). Role strain: An assessment of a measure and its invariance of factor structure across studies, *Journal of Applied Psychology*, **63**, 321–8.

Manenica, I. (1981). Physiological and work study assessment of physical workload. In E. N. Corlett and J. Richardson (eds.) *Stress, Work Design, and Productivity*, New York, Wiley.

Murphy, L. R. (1984). Occupational stress management: A review and appraisal, *Journal of Occupational Psychology*, **57**, 1–15.

Nicholson, N., Wall, T. D., and Lischeron, J. (1977). The predictability of absence and propensity to leave from employee's job satisfactions and attitudes towards influence in decision making. *Human Relations*, **30**, 499–514.

O'Hanlon, J. F. (1978). Performance and physiological reactions to monotony in simulated industrial inspection. Papers presented at the 19th International Congress of Applied Psychology in Munich, Germany.

Orne, M. T. (1962). On the social psychology of the psychological experiment: With particular reference to demand characteristics and their implications. *American Psychologist*, **17**, 776–83.

Rosen, R. H. (1984). The picture of health in the workplace, *Training and Development Journal*, **38**, 24–30.

Rosner, B., and Polk, B. F. (1979). The implications of blood pressure variability for clinical and screening purposes, *Journal of Chronic Diseases*, **32**, 451–61.

Rosner, B., and Polk, B. F. (1981). The instability of blood pressure variability over time. *Journal of Chronic Diseases*, **34**, 135–41.

Ruff, C. D., and Baltes, P. B. (1976). Value transition and adult development of women: The instrumentality sequence hypothesis. *Development Psychology*, **12**, 567–8.

Salancik, G. R., and Pfeffer, J. (1977). An examination of need-satisfaction models of job attitudes, *Administrative Science Quarterly*, **22**, 427–56.

Sallis, J. F., and Lichstein, K. L. (1979). The frontal electromyographic adaptation response: A potential source of confounding. *Biofeedback and Self-Regulation*, **4**, 337–9.

Selye, H. (1936). A syndrome produced by diverse nocuous agents, *Nature*, p. 138.

Selye, H. (1974). Stress without distress. Philadelphia, Lippincott.

Siddle, D. A. T., and Trupin, G. (1980). Measurement, quantification and analysis of cardiac activity. In I. Martin and P. H. Venables (eds.) *Techniques in Psychophysiology*, New York, Wiley.

Statland, B. E., Bokelund, H., and Winkel, D. (1974). Factors contributing to intra-individual variation of serum constituents: Effects of posture and tourniquet application on variation of serum constituents in healthy subjects, *Clinical Chemistry*, **20**, 1513–9.

Steers, R. M., and Mowday, R. T. (1981). Employee turnover and post-decision accommodation processes. In L. L. Cummings, and B. M. Staw (eds.) *Research in Organizational Behavior* (Vol. 3), Greenwich, CT, JAI Press.

Tung, R. L. (1980). Comparative analysis of the occupational stress profiles of male versus female administrators. *Journal of Vocational Behavior*, **17**, 344–55.

Ursin, H., and Ursin, R. (1979). Physiological indicators of mental workload. In N. Moray (ed.) *Mental workload: Its theory and measurement*, New York, Plenum.

Webb, E. J., Campbell, D. T., Schwartz, R. D., and Sechrest, L. (1966). *Unobtrusive measures: Nonreactive research in the social sciences*, Chicago, Rand McNally.

Webb, E. J., Campbell, D. T., Schwartz, R. D., Sechrest, L., and Grove, J. B. (1981). *Nonreactive Measures in the Social Science*, Boston: Houghton Mifflin.

Chapter 9

Issues in the Measurement of the Type A Behaviour Pattern

Lynda H. Powell

Department of Epidemiology & Public Health
School of Medicine,
Yale University

Epidemiologic research on the Type A–coronary heart disease (CHD) link has been conducted enthusiastically for the past fifteen years. In contrast to the late 1970s and early 1980s when positive findings for this link abounded, in the mid-1980s negative findings are more common. There now exists approximately equal numbers of studies that have found, and have failed to find, a prospective association between the Type A behaviour pattern (TABP) and hard CHD endpoints (Table 1).

At this juncture in Type A research, there is a danger of throwing the baby out with the bathwater. To avoid this, we must consider and control for plausible alternative explanations for negative findings. Heading the list of alternative explanations is problems in the measurement of the TABP. There is still confusion about what the behaviour pattern is, how to measure it across diverse population groups, and how to design studies that reduce the impact of these measurement problems.

The purpose of this chapter is to describe current approaches to Type A measurement and the common pitfalls that are associated with their use in epidemiologic research. Pertinent research will be reviewed in some detail, with an emphasis on those studies published within the last five years. It is hoped that this information will assist in the design of powerful prospective epidemiologic studies and will foster needed Type A assessment research.

THE TYPE A CONCEPTUALIZATION

An appreciation of the validity of a test depends upon a thorough understanding of the construct to be measured (Anastasi, 1982). Unlike other psychosocial risk factors which originated with a coherent conceptualization, the TABP was first isolated as a simple description of overt behaviours (Friedman and Rosenman, 1974). It was only through subsequent research that

Research Methods in Stress and Health Psychology. Edited by S. V. Kasl and C. L. Cooper.

Table 1: The predictive validity of Type A assessment instruments (1)

	Positive relationship			No relationship		
Measure	Study	Sample	Follow-up	Study	Sample	Follow-up
Structured Interview	Rosenman, Brand, Jenkins, et al. (1975)	3154 men in the WCGS, 39–59 yrs, 80% white-collar	8.5 years, incidence of MI, silent MI, angina			
Rosenman Structured Interview				Shekelle, Hulley, Neaton, et al. (1985)	3110 high-risk men in MRFIT, 35–57 yrs, 56% white-collar	8 years, coronary event; coronary death
Jenkins Activity Survey	Jenkins, Rosenman & Zyzanski (1974)	2750 men in the WCGS, 39–59 yrs, 80% white-collar	4 years, incidence of MI, silent MI, angina	Shekelle, Hulley, Neaton, et al. (1985)	12772 high-risk men in MRFIT, 35–57 yrs, 56% white-collar	6 to 8 years, new non-fatal MI or coronary death
	DeBacker, Kornitzer, Kittel, et al. (1983)	1958 men in Belgian Heart Study, 40–55 yrs	5 years, incidence of new fatal or non-fatal MI or sudden death	Case, Heller, Case et al. (1985)	516 male coronary patients in NYC, under 60 yrs, primarily blue-collar	2 years, coronary mortality: definite fatal and non-fatal recurrence
				Shekelle, Gale, Norusis et al. (in press)	2314 coronary patients in AMIS, 30–69 yrs, 71% blue-collar	3 years, incidence of definite MI, fatal MI

				Cohen and Reed (1985)	2187 men in Honolulu Heart Prog. 50–70 years, predom. blue-collar	9 years, definite MI, angina
				Dimsdale, Gilbert, Hutter et al., (1981)	189 symptomatic male angiography patients, 18–70 yrs. (50% white-collar)	1 year, new morbid event: hospitalization, MI, death
Framingham Type A Scale	Haynes, Feinleib & Kannel (1980)	1674 men & women in Framingham, 45–77 yrs.	8 years, MI, silent MI, angina			
Bortner Rating Scale	French-Belgian Collaborative group (1982)	3203 men in Belgium & France, 40–60 yrs	53–74 months, fatal & non-fatal MI, sudden death, angina	Koskenvuo, Kaprio et al. (1983)	23076 Finnish men, 35–64 yrs.	6 years, coronary death
Videotaped Structured Interview	Powell, Friedman, Fleischmann (in press)	862 male coronary patients, under 65 yrs, 50% white-collar	4.5 years, fatal and non-fatal recurrent MI			

(1) *Predictive validity defined as a prospective association between the Type A behaviour pattern and a hard CHD endpoint*

attempts were made to develop a conceptualization that fit this set of behaviours.

The use of such terms as Type A behaviour, Type A behaviour pattern, and Type A personality, illustrate the conceptual confusion that still exists. Perhaps the most popular Type A conceptualization assumes that it is a person-situation interaction. Type A behaviour is an action-emotion complex, exhibited by men and women so disposed, in the presence of appropriate environmental events (Friedman and Rosenman, 1974). This suggests that overt behaviour, people 'so disposed', and 'appropriate' environmental events are all parts of the TABP. That is, there are enduring trait-like characteristics within the person which interact with specific environmental events to produce the characteristic pattern of behaviour.

A framework that integrates fixed trait and interactional conceptualizations is cognitive social learning theory (Bandura, 1977). This theory assumes that a thorough understanding of behaviour requires an understanding of characteristic overt behaviours, behaviours in interaction with environmental demands, and underlying cognitions. If this framework is applied to the TABP, then overt behaviours, underlying cognitions, and specific environmental demands would be part of the behaviour pattern and, for purposes at hand, could be used as targets for assessment.

Most is known about characteristic overt Type A behaviours. They include drivenness, extremes of competitiveness, aggression, easily aroused irritabilities, work orientation, preoccupation with deadlines, and a chronic sense of time urgency. Type A individuals appear to be guarded, alert, and intense, with rapid and jerky body movements, tense facial and body musculature, and explosive speech.

Less is known about the characteristic environments that elicit Type A behaviour. It is assumed that they must present a challenge to the individual but there appears to be considerable variability in the kinds of events that individuals perceive as challenging (Krantz and Manuck, 1984).

Moreover, little is known about the psycholological underpinnings of individuals so disposed (Matthews, 1982). Early work by Glass (1977) suggested that need for control lay beneath the behaviour pattern, but current investigations suggest that enduring hostile attitudes, such as paranoia and cynicism (Williams, Barefoot, and Shekelle, 1985), or persistent feelings of low-esteem and insecurity (Friedman and Ulmer, 1984), are more basic motivational factors. The TABP does not appear to be related to achievement motivation, power motivation, or the absence of affiliation motives (Matthews and Saal, 1978). Some studies have suggested that it is independent of neurotic anxiety, depression, and symptom distress (Caffrey, 1968; Chesney, Black, Chadwick et al., 1981), while other studies have reported a connection with neuroticism and psychiatric morbidity, including emotional lability, instability, impulsiveness, dominance, tension, and daily stress (Bass, 1984; Haynes,

Levine, Scotch et al., 1978; Irvine, Lyle, and Allon, 1982; Lovallo and Pishkin, 1980).

A complete specification of the TABP is likely to be complex. But such complexity may be unnecessary for the task of measurement. Since most is known about overt Type A behaviours, they have been the most common targets of assessment.

In contrast to the complex conceptualization, the Type A operationalization is a simple dichotomy—either the individual has it (is Type A) or does not have it (is Type B). Varying degrees of Type A behaviour are collapsed within category. This rough categorical conceptualization emerged from early attempts to measure the TABP. It does not necessarily represent the best or most accurate way to evaluate individuals.

MEASURES OF THE TYPE A BEHAVIOUR PATTERN

Since 1960, the TABP has been measured with over twenty different instruments. Some have been shown to be valid and reliable in extensive psychometric research; others offer items that, at most, appear to have good face validity. One implication of the use of so many different measures of the TABP is operational imprecision and problems with construct validity. When a construct suffers from problems in construct validity, it is difficult to disentangle the extent to which findings apply to the construct itself or the specific operationalization of that construct (Cook and Campbell, 1979).

One way to reduce the ambiguity of research findings is to adopt minimum criteria for the acceptability of any Type A measure. Two criteria that have relevance for the TABP are construct and predictive validity: a Type A measure can be considered to be valid if it can be shown to be related to other validated measures of the TABP and if it can be shown to predict a hard CHD endpoint in prospective research. Use of measures that satisfy both these criteria insure that they reflect the coronary-prone aspects of Type A. Use of these criteria also serve to limit the practice of the ad hoc assembly of questionnaire items that appear to measure the TABP. (See Ruberman, Weinblatt, Goldberg et al., 1984 for an example of this).

Using these two criteria, five measures of the TABP can be considered to be valid—the Structured Interview (SI), the Jenkins Activity Survey (JAS), the Framingham Type A Scale (FTAB), the Bortner Rating Scale (BRS), and the Videotaped Structured Interview (VSI). A description of each of these instruments, including scale development, reliability, and validity will be provided. Reliability and validity will be defined in the following ways.

Test–retest reliability evaluates the error variance associated with random fluctuation of performance from one test session to another. It provides a measure of the extent to which scores can be generalized to different occasions. In observational measures, test–retest reliability applies to the subject (the consistency in subject behaviour observed by the same observer on two occasions) and the observer (the consistency in observer ratings of the same sample of behaviour on two occasions). In self-report measures, test–retest reliability applies to the subject only. Behaviours that are measured more than six months apart are apt to be cumulative and progressive rather than random (Anastasi, 1982). Thus, test–retest reliability will refer to measures taken less than six months apart.

Stability evaluates the consistency in subject behaviour over long intervals. Differences observed in people beyond six months can be assumed to reflect systematic changes (Nunnally, 1978). Thus, long-term stability will refer to retests of subjects taken six months or more from the original test.

Interjudge reliability evaluates error variance associated with different observers observing the same sample of behaviour. This type of reliability is meaningful for observational measures only.

Construct validity, as applied here, evaluates the relationship between a Type A measure and other standardized measures of the TABP.

Predictive validity, as applied here, evaluates the relationship between the Type A assessment and subsequent occurrence of a hard CHD endpoint.

A summary of the reliability and validity of the standard Type A measures is presented in Tables 1–6.

This section will conclude with a general discussion of the strengths and limitations of observational and self-report measures. Although this review will be limited to the five validated measures, it is important to keep in mind that other measures exist which offer promise as potentially valid measures of the TABP (e.g. the Gough Adjective Checklist (Gough and Heilburn, 1975); the Milwaukee Coronary-Prone Behavior Attitude Scale (Young and Barboriak, 1982).

The Structured Interview

The SI (Rosenman, Friedman, Straus et al., 1964a; Rosenman, Friedman, Straus et al., 1964b) was developed by cardiologists Ray Rosenman and Meyer Friedman for the purpose of determining the behaviour type of the 3500 men in the Western Collaborative Group Study (WCGS). During a face-to-face encounter, a trained interviewer asked subjects a series of questions about their degree of drive and ambition, past and present competitive, aggressive, and hostile feelings, job demands, impatience, and time consciousness. Concurrently, observations were made on characteristic speech and motor behaviours. Two questions were asked in a deliberately slow and hesitant manner for the purpose of providing subjects with the opportunity to interrupt, if they were so inclined. Detection of behaviour pattern A consisted of making a clinical judgement about whether a subject was in an active and continuous conflict with other people or with time. This judgement was based far more

Table 2: Subject test–retest reliability of measures of the Type A behaviour pattern (1)

Measure	Study	Sample	Weeks Apart	Reliability
Structured Interview				
Rosenman Structured Interview	Blumenthal, O'Toole, and Haney (1984)	60 men in North Carolina, mean age = 51 years	16	0.68: 4-level categories
Jenkins Activity Survey	Johnston and Shaper (1983)	British civil servants	17	0.79; 0.82
Framingham Type A Scale				
Bortner Rating Scale	Price (1979)	100 males	8	0.74
		53 females	8	0.72
	Johnston and Shaper (1983)	British civil servants	12	0.77
			17	0.80
	Bass (1984)	65 male angiography patients	16	0.84
		31 female angiography patients	16	0.84
Videotaped Structured Interview				

(1) *Subject test–retest reliability defined as two different samples of behaviour of the same subject assessed by the same judge less than 24 weeks apart.*

upon the emotional tone of the response than the content of the answer. Those who were judged to be in such conflict were categorized as Type A; those who were not were categorized as Type B. Finer distinctions into four categories of behaviour type (Type A1; A2; B3; B4) were originally made (Rosenman, Friedman, Straus et al., 1964a; 1970), but the finer distinctions did not enhance predictive capability and were measured with lower reliability. Later reports from the WCGS featured the simpler dichotomous categories only (Rosenman, Brand, Jenkins et al., 1975).

SI assessments were found to be stable over time. In the WCGS, 1064 subjects were rated once in 1960 and again twelve to twenty months later. A similar dichotomous assessment (i.e. Type A or Type B) was found in 80.4 per cent of these subjects, but stability dropped to 66.4 per cent when the

Table 3: Observer test–retest reliability for observational measures of the Type A behaviour pattern (1)

Measure	Study	Sample	Weeks Apart	Reliability
Structured Interview	Keith, Lown, and Stare, (1965)	100 male patients in Boston, 35–55 yrs.	12–72	74%: 2-level categories 57%: 4-level categories
Rosenman Structured Interview	Blumenthal, O'Toole, and Haney (1984)	60 men in North Carolina, mean age = 51 yrs.	16	0.68
Videotaped Structured Interview	Powell, Friedman, Thoresen, et al. (1984)	10 male coronary patients in the RCPP, under 65 yrs.	4	0.76

(1) *Observer test–retest reliability is defined as the agreement of the same judge observing the same interview on two different occasions less than 24 weeks apart.*

four-point system was used (Jenkins, Rosenman and Friedman, 1968). When only the extremes of the four-point system were evaluated (i.e. Type A1 and Type B4), stability increased to 98.4 per cent (Rosenman, Friedman, Straus et al., 1964b). Keith, Lown and Stare (1965) found stability in the dichotomous assessment in 74 per cent of the 100 subjects reinterviewed from three to eighteen months after the original interview. Interjudge reliability was found to be good when experts' judgements of dichotomous behaviour type were compared. Jenkins rerated twenty-five of Rosenman's WCGS classifications from audiotape and found 84 per cent agreement with dichotomous classifications, but agreement dropped to 64 per cent when the four-point rating scale was used (i.e. A1; A2; B3; B4) (Jenkins, Rosenman and Friedman, 1968). Agreement between Rosenman and two trained interviewers from the Coronary Prevention Program in Cleveland was reported to range between 80 and 84 per cent for the four-point categorical system (Friedman, Hellerstein, Eastwood et al., 1968).

Construct validity would ordinarily be evaluated by agreement with other validated measures. However, since the SI was developed by the originators of the Type A construct, it serves as the 'gold standard' against which other Type A measures are evaluated. The predictive validity of the SI was demonstrated in the WCGS (Rosenman, Brand, Jenkins et al., 1975). Subjects classified as Type A had over twice the rate of total CHD incidence over 8½ years (13.2 per 1000) as those classified as Type B (5.6 per 1000) ($p<0.001$). This differential held when endpoints were distilled into total myocardial infarction

Table 4: Stability of the Type A behaviour pattern (1)

Measure	Study	Sample	Weeks Apart	Stability
Structured Interview	Jenkins, Rosenman, and Friedman (1968)	1064 WCGS men	48–80	80.4%: 2-level categories 66.4%: 4-level categories
	Keith, Lown, and Stare (1968)	100 male patients in Boston, 35–55 yrs.	12–72	74%
Rosenman Structured Interview				
Jenkins Activity Survey	Jenkins, Zyzanski and Rosenman (1971)	WCGS men	52	0.66
	Johnston, and Shaper (1983)	British civil servants	34	0.79
Framingham Type A Scale	Matthews and Haynes (1986)	Framingham women, 45–54 yrs.	520	57–80%
Bortner Rating Scale	Johnston and Shaper (1983)	British civil servants	29	0.71
Videotaped Structured Interview	Powell and Fleischmann (in press)	Male coronary patients in the WCGS	78	0.61

(1) *Stability defined as relationship between two different samples of behaviour assessed 24 weeks or more apart.*

(MI) (Type A=10.4%, Type B=4.9%, $p<0.001$), symptomatic MI (Type A=6.9%, Type B=3.2%, $p<0.001$), unrecognized MI (Type A=3.6%, Type B=1.7%, $p<0.001$), or angina pectoris (Type A=2.7, Type B=1.1, $p<0.005$).

A question of considerable importance in current Type A research is the extent to which the SI, as originally conceived and administered by Rosenman and Friedman (Rosenman, Friedman, Straus et al., 1964a), is comparable to the current Rosenman SI (Rosenman, 1978) which is taught at SRI International and used in most of the SI-assessed Type A research studies. The original SI protocol '... allowed the interviewer to observe the all-important motor activities of the subject; to observe the intensity and quality of emotional change and overtones accompanying the intellectual response ... and to use facility, flexibility, and variability in approaching to a subject when such was needed to uncover or classify more accurately certain personality attributes ...' (Rosenman, Friedman, Straus et al., 1964a, p. 1). The Rosenman SI differs

Table 5: Interjudge reliability for interview measures of the Type A behaviour pattern (1)

Measure	Study	Sample	Judges	Reliability
Structured Interview	Jenkins, Rosenman & Friedman (1968)	25 WCGS men	2 experts	84%: 2-level 64%: 4-level
	Friedman, Hellerstein, Eastwood (1968)	Male coronary patients	1 expert 1 trained	80–84%: 4-level
Rosenman Structured Interview	Byrne, Rosenman, Schiller et al. (1985)	582 Australian male government workers	1 expert 1 trained	79%: 2-level 69%: 4-level
	Haynes, Feinleib, and Kannel (1980)	197 male aerospace employees	2 trained	77%: 2-level
		79 college males		78%: 2-level
		77 Framingham women		65%: 2-level
	Krantz, Durel, Davia et al. (1982)	88 angiography patients, primarily male	2 experts	80%: 4-level
	MacDougall, Dembroski, and Musante (1979)	149 male undergraduates	2 trained	89%: 2-level 78%: 4-level
		84 female undergraduates		84%: 2-level 70%: 4-level
	Menninger (1985)	149 women, 30–42 yrs.	2 trained	85%: 2-level (kappa = 0.775)
	Musante, MacDougall, Dembroski et al. (1983)	164 female undergraduates	2 experts	85%: 3-level (kappa = 0.69) 80%: 4-level (kappa = 0.62)
	Schmidt, Undeutsch, Dembroski et al. (1982)	212 German policemen	2 trained	98%: 2-level 72%: 4-level
Videotaped Structured Interview	Powell, Friedman, Thoresen et al. (1984)	40 male coronary patients	8 trained	0.79

(1) *Interjudge reliability defined as the average agreement among different judges observing the same subject.*

from this description in two ways. First, motor behaviours, considered critical to SI assessment, are de-emphasized. Classifications are made, instead, by relying primarily upon speech behaviour—most notably speed and volume of speech (Scherwitz, Berton and Leventhal, 1977; Schucker and Jacobs, 1977). Second, the SI protocol emphasized flexibility in the interviewer's approach to any particular subject as a way to promote involvement and more accurately detect personality attributes. But in the Rosenman SI the interview is administered in a highly standardized fashion, incorporating a rapid pace, predetermined emphasis on key words, and systematic attempts to challenge the subject (Rosenman, 1978).

The argument that the SI and the Rosenman SI are two different measures of the TABP has been further supported by reanalyses of interviews conducted using both classification systems. Scherwitz (1985) compared Rosenman SI interviews used in the MRFIT clinical trial (Multiple Risk Factor Intervention Trial Group, 1979) with those conducted in the WCGS and found that interviewer talk time was longer and interview length was shorter in MRFIT than in the WCGS. This resulted in less data on which to evaluate the behaviour type of the subject. Moreover, 74.4 per cent (2314 out of 3110) of the high-risk subjects in MRFIT were classified as Type A while only 52.5 per cent (1851 out of 3524) of the population-based subjects in the WCGS were so classified. The most serious difference between classifications made in these two trials was that the Rosenman SI classifications failed to predict total CHD or CHD mortality in 3524 high-risk men after a mean follow-up of 7.1 years (Shekelle, Hulley, Neaton et al., 1985). Because of the possible drift that has occurred in the administration, and perhaps the scoring, of these two interviews, this latter finding is difficult to interpret. To the extent that the Rosenman SI is considered to be the same as the SI used and validated in the WCGS, these results raise serious questions about the link between the TABP and coronary heart disease in high-risk subjects. Alternatively, if the differences between the instruments are significant enough to make the assumption that they are different procedures, then the failure of the MRFIT study would be more accurately explained by the use of an unvalidated Type A instrument.

At issue here is the implication of drift in the administration and scoring of the 'gold standard' for Type A measurement. Some of the interpretative problems could be resolved by conducting studies of the degree of concordance between the SI and the Rosenman SI. These have not been done and it is doubtful whether they could be done since the exact criteria used to make judgements in the WCGS were not well specified and variable across interviewers. Tables 1–6 present a summary of the validity and reliability of the Rosenman SI. It can be seen that more is known about the Rosenman SI than the other Type A measure. It is critical that the validity of these ratings as predictors of CHD endpoints be established.

Table 6: Construct validity of Type A assessment instruments (1)

Instrument	Study	Sample	Rosenman SI	JAS	FTAB	BRS	VSI
Structured Interview	Jenkins, Rosenman, and Friedman (1967)	WCGS men, prim white-collar		72%			
	Powell, Friedman, Thoresen et al. (1984)	RCPP male coronary patients					83.6%
Rosenman Structured Interview	Anderson and Waldron (1983)	suburban women		54% (r=.27)			
	Appels, Jenkins and Rosenman (1982)	Dutch males		73% (r=.63)			
	Byrne, Rosenman, Schiller et al. (1985)	Australian males		55%			
	Chesney, Black, Chadwick et al. (1981)	Lockheed male employees		.255	60% (r=.201)		
	Diamond, Schneiderman, Schwartz et al. (1984)	male undergraduates		63%			
	Haynes, Feinleib, and Kannel (1980)	aerospace men		60%			
		undergrad men		58%			
		Framingham women		52%			
	Kittel, Kornitzer, Zyzanski et al. (1978)	Belgian men		63–70%			
	MacDougall, Dembroski, and Musante (1979)	male undergraduates		74% (r=.30)	66% (r=.25)		
		female undergraduates		63% (r=.33)	67% (r = .39)		
	Matthews, Krantz, De-	white-collar		67%			

	ter (1984)	women				
	Menninger (1985)	employed women	50% (kappa=.027)	46% (kappa=−.02)		
	Musante, MacDougall, Dembroski et al. (1983)	female undergraduates	62%			
	Scherwitz, Berton, and Leventhal (1977)	male undergraduates	42% (r=.22)			
	Shekelle, Hulley, and Neaton (1985)	high-risk men	58%			
	Verhagen, Nass, Apples et al. (1980)	coronary patients	.50			
		healthy men	.62			
	Young and Barboriak (1982)	white-collar males	61%			
Jenkins Activity Survey	Byrne, Rosenman, Schiller et al. (1985)	Australian male govt workers		.53	.55	
	Haynes, Feinleib, and Kannel (1980)	aerospace men		.41		
		undergraduate men		.53		
	Herbertt and Innes (1982)	Australian undergrads			.33	
	Johnston and Shaper (1983)	British white-collar males			.70	
	Mayes, Sime, and Ganster (1984)	employed women			.56	
	Powell, Friedman, Thoresen et al. (1984)	RCPP males				.42
Framingham Type A Scale	Byrne, Rosenman, Schiller et al. (1985)	Australian male govt workers			.59	
	Powell, Friedman, Thoresen et al. (1984)	RCPP males				.52
Bortner Rating Scale						

(1) *Construct validity defined as the agreement of new Type A measure with a standard, validated Type A measure.*

The Jenkins Activity Survey

The Jenkins Activity Survey (Jenkins, Zyzanski, and Rosenman, 1979) is a 52-item computer-scored self-report questionnaire that was developed in the effort to duplicate the behaviour classifications made by the SI, and thereby simplify Type A measurement. It produces scores for a general Type A–B scale, and three Type A components—hard-driving (highly socialized but intense drives); speed and impatience (speed in eating, conversation, etc., impatience, strong temper); and job involvement (dedication to occupational activity). Scores are standardized to a mean of 0 and a standard deviation of 10, and the sign of the score (+ or −) signifies the behaviour type (+ = Type A; − = Type B). Items for the survey were assembled initially using questions from the SI or questions which were developed because they were consistent with Type A conceptual descriptions. These items were then subjected to a series of psychometric analyses spanning ten years, using data from the WCGS. A set of sixty-one items was found to discriminate between SI determined As and Bs using optimal scaling procedures (Jenkins, Rosenman, and Friedman, 1967). Discriminant analysis determined the best subset of these items that discrimintated between behaviour types, resulting in the 19–item AB scale. Then, all sixty-one items were subjected to factor analysis to determine underlying components (Jenkins, Zyzanski, and Rosenman, 1971).

The stability of the JAS AB score over one year was found to be 0.66, and this estimate did not change appreciably when stability over four years was assessed (Jenkins, Zyzanski, and Rosenman, 1971). More recently, Johnston and Shaper (1983) assessed the stability of the JAS AB score in a sample of male British civil servants over thirty-four weeks and found the correlation to be 0.79.

Since the JAS was the first questionnaire alternative to the SI, its validity as a measure of the Type A construct has been determined by studying its relationship to the SI. In 1965, 330 men from the WCGS were given the 61-item JAS and agreement between SI ratings made in 1960–61 and JAS categories derived from item analyses was 72.4 per cent (Jenkins, Rosenman, and Friedman, 1967). Subsequently, discriminant analysis was used to develop a global AB scale which was found to have 73 per cent agreement with SI classifications made in 1960 (Jenkins, Zyzanski, and Rosenman, 1971). JAS classifications became more accurate relative to the SI when only the extremes of the JAS distribution were examined. When agreement was tested for those individuals who scored beyond 1 standard deviation (SD) from the mean, it reached 91 per cent (score of 10 or more) and 88 per cent (score of −10 or less), but when agreement was tested in those individuals who scored above and below ½ SD, agreement dropped to 56 and 43 per cent, respectively (Jenkins, Zyzanski, and Rosenman, 1971).

The information on the relationship between the JAS AB scale and the

Rosenman SI is difficult to interpret. When considering adult males only, agreement has been reported to be as low as 34.3 per cent in Australian government workers (Byrne, Rosenman, Schiller et al., 1985) and as high as 70 per cent in Belgian factory workers (Kittel, Kornitzer, Zyzanski et al., 1978). Two American studies found moderate agreements of 67 per cent and 61 per cent (Matthews and Saal, 1978; Young and Barboriak, 1982, respectively), but a third study reported an extremely low correlation (r=0.255) (Chesney, Black, Chadwick et al., 1981). Studies on younger undergraduate males have found equally diverse relationships, ranging from a low of 42 per cent (Scherwitz, Berton, and Leventhal, 1977) to a high of 74 per cent (MacDougall, Dembroski and Musante, 1979). Sociodemographic differences that may be related to differing degrees of agreement are not readily apparent. What does seem clear is that earlier statements suggesting that the SI and the JAS are measuring different aspects of coronary-prone behaviour have been supported by later findings.

The predictive validity of the JAS was first observed in the WCGS. A sample of 2750 men were given the JAS and followed for four years to determine the occurrence of a CHD event (acute MI, silent MI, angina) (Jenkins, Rosenman, and Zyzanski, 1974). Cases had a JAS AB score of 1.70 while controls had a score of −0.6 (p<0.01). This relationship was not weakened when the total population was stratified by age or by different manifestations of CHD. Predictions were not, however, as strong as those made by the SI (Brand, Rosenman, Jenkins et al., unpublished manuscript). JAS scores also predicted recurrent coronary events (Jenkins, Zyzanski, and Rosenman, 1976). Of particular interest was the observation of a graded relationship between JAS scores and CHD following the grouping of subjects into tertiles according to their JAS score (<5, −5 to +5, >5). The predictive validity of the JAS was observed a second time in the Belgian Heart Disease Prevention Project where scores predicted CHD endpoints in a five-year follow-up of 2000 men (DeBacker, Kornitzer, Kittel et al., 1983). Again a graded relationship was found between JAS tertiles and incidence of acute MI events. However, the JAS failed to predict CHD endpoints in five other prospective studies in which the relationship was assessed (Case, Heller, Case et al., 1985; Cohen and Reed, 1985; Dimsdale, Gilbert, Hutter et al., 1981; Shekelle, Gale, Norusis, 1985; Shekelle, Hulley, Neaton et al., 1985).

The Framingham Type A Scale

The Framingham Type A Scale (Haynes, Levine, Scotch et al., 1978) is a ten-item self-report questionnaire which elicits information primarily about the self as hard-driving, achievement-oriented, and dominant, and about worries following a day of work. The FTAB was distilled from a 300-item questionnaire measuring five broad areas of psychosocial stress and strain in the Framingham cohort. A panel of three experts selected items which, in their opinion, measured the behaviour pattern. The list of items was submitted to item and factor analyses, and items with poor relationships to the total scale were dropped. All questions are scored on a range from 0 to 1 (1 meaning the complete presence of the trait), thus each question is given equal weight in the scale. Slightly different versions are available for employed persons, housewives, and students.

The stability of the FTAB scale has not been assessed in men, but in women, aged 45–54 years, concordance in individual items assessed ten years apart ranged from 57 to 80 per cent (Matthews and Haynes, 1986). No test–retest reliability data are available.

The construct validity of the FTAB has been examined by comparing scores to the SI and the JAS. For the purpose of comparisons with the SI, FTAB scores are dichotomized at the median of a distribution and scores in the upper end are labelled Type A. These classifications are then compared with SI classifications. Analyses using the Rosenman SI have resulted in approximately the same degree of agreement (58–67 per cent) across diverse samples including adult men and undergraduate men and women (Chesney, Black, Chadwick et al., 1981; Haynes, Feinleib, and Kannel, 1980). Correlations with the JAS on adult men have been reported to be 0.53 in two studies (Byrne, Rosenman, Schiller et al., 1985; Haynes, Feinleib and Kannel, 1980).

The predictive validity of the FTAB was observed in an eight-year follow-up of coronary incidence in 1674 men and women, ages 45–77, in the Framingham cohort (Haynes, Feinleib, and Kannel, 1980). Coronary incidence was defined as MI, coronary insufficiency syndrome, angina pectoris, and CHD death (sudden and non-sudden). In women, the CHD manifestation that was most strongly related to FTAB was angina, however in men all manifestations had about equal predictive potential.

The Bortner Rating Scale

The Bortner Rating Scale (Bortner, 1969) is a self-report scale which asks subjects to describe themselves using fourteen scales, each of which are overt behaviours or psychosocial traits scored in the SI, and each of which are written as polar opposites with Type A and Type B anchors (e.g. never late—casual about appointments; always rushed—never feels rushed; emphatic speech—slow, deliberate talker). The rationale behind the scale is that it may be possible for those overt behaviours observed by an interviewer during the SI to be observed by the subjects themselves. The Type A and Type B behaviours are separated by a 1½″ line, and subjects are instructued to mark a place on the continuum that most resembles where they see themselves. The Type A score is the length of the line from the Type B anchor to the point designated by the subject (to the nearest 1/16″), summed over all fourteen scales.

The stability of the BRS Type A score over twenty-nine weeks was observed to be 0.71 (Johnston and Shaper, 1983). Test–retest reliability ranged from 0.72 over eight weeks to 0.84 over sixteen weeks (Bass, 1984; Johnston and Shaper, 1983; Price, 1979).

The construct validity of the BRS has been supported in four studies by comparisons of it with the JAS (Byrne, Rosenman, Schiller et al., 1985; Herbertt and Innes, 1982; Johnston, and Shaper, 1983; Mayes, Sime, and Ganster, 1984). Correlations ranged from 0.33 in a sample of 233 Australian undergraduates (Herbertt and Innes, 1982) to 0.70 in 142 white-collar British men (Johnston and Shaper, 1983). The association in sixty-three women employees (0.56) was not appreciably different from that observed in 468 Australian males (0.55). No data on the relationship between the BRS and the SI have been reported. Predictive validity of the BRS was observed in the French-Belgian Collaborative Heart Study (French-Belgian Collaborative Group, 1982). A cohort of 2811 men in Belgium and France between forty and sixty years was followed for a period of between fifty-three and seventy-four months to determine CHD incidence defined as fatal and non-fatal MI, sudden death, and angina. In multivariate analysis, BRS Type A was a significant predictor of total coronary heart disease (including hard events and angina), and for hard events only (including fatal and non-fatal MI and sudden death). A subsequent prospective study of 23,076 Finnish men using a shortened version of the BRS (seven rather than fourteen items) failed to find an association between Type A and total coronary mortality in a six-year follow-up (Koskenvuo, Kaprio, Langinvainio et al., 1983).

The Videotaped Structured Interview

The Videotaped Structured Interview (Friedman and Powell, 1984; Friedman, Thoresen, Gill et al., 1982) is a refinement on the original SI, developed primarily for use as a measure of change in the TABP in the Recurrent Coronary Prevention Project (RCPP). Like the original SI, but unlike the Rosenman SI, it is conducted in a conversational manner and scores give equal weight to motor and speech psychomotor phenomena. Unlike both of the earlier SI versions, the VSI does not categorize subjects into a behaviour type. Instead, a continuous score is produced by adding the intensities (rated on a scale from 0 to 3) of each of thirty-five psychomotor indicators observed to be present.

The VSI score was found to be stable over eighteen months. In the RCPP, 135 subjects allocated to an untreated comparison group were interviewed twice, eighteen months apart by the same interviewer. The two scores were found to correlate 0.61 (Powell and Fleishmann, in press). Observer test–retest reliability was found to be 0.76 in a random sample of ten RCPP videotaped interviews which were rated twice by the same interviewers over one month (Powell, Friedman, Thoresen et al., 1984). No data are available on subject test–retest reliability. The interjudge reliability of the VSI, defined as the average agreement among eight newly trained raters in a random sample of forty subjects, was found to be 0.79 (Powell, Friedman, Thoresen et al., 1984).

The construct validity of the VSI was examined using RCPP data by comparing it to classifications made using the original SI and correlating scores with the JAS and the FTAB (Powell, Friedman, Thoresen et al., 1984). Agreement with the SI was determined using the videotapes of 135 subjects in the comparison groups of the RCPP. The cutpoint for A–B behaviour type using the VSI was designated to be the point on the scale that was two SDs above the mean score for Type Bs (so determined by previous clinical judgements). SI classifications were made by three newly trained interviewers using the audiotaped version of the videotape and the scoring technique employed by the WCGS. Agreement was found to be 83.6 per cent. Using the same sample of 135, the correlations between the VSI and the JAS AB scale were 0.42, and between the VSI and the FTAB were 0.52. Predictive validity of the VSI was observed using 339 male coronary patients in the RCPP control and comparison groups. The VSI score predicted incidence of recurrent infarction (fatal or non-fatal coronary events), after adjustment for nine standard risk factors ($p=0.003$) (Powell and Fleischmann, in press).

An important limitation of data on the VSI is that they have all come from one research study. Replication in a new sample is needed.

COMMENT: OBSERVATIONAL APPROACHES TO TYPE A ASSESSMENT

The strengths and limitations of the three observational measures of the TABP can be illustrated by way of comparison.

One point of comparison is the objectivity and standardization of the interview protocol. In form, an interview can range from a highly structured set of questions which is little more than an orally administered questionnaire, to one that is non-directive, where the intent is merely to provide a context within which the subject is free to talk about anything (Anastasi, 1982). On this continuum, the SI and the VSI are toward the non-directive end whereas the Rosenman SI is toward the structured end. Descriptions of the WCGS interview indicate that interviewers were trained to use 'facility, flexibility, and variability' in their approach to each subject (Rosenman, Friedman, Straus, et al., 1964a, p.1). In the VSI, subjects are similarly trained, the intent being to maximize subject involvement and permit the natural response style to emerge (Friedman and Powell, 1984). In contrast, the Rosenman SI employs a highly standardized protocol where the pace, emphasis on key words, and points of challenge are predetermined, regardless of the behaviour of the subject. The basic issue here is, as stated by Krantz and Manuck (1984), the trade-off between striving for tight experimental control by automating or standardizing stimuli versus maximizing subject involvement by making tasks more life-like or ecologically sound. Too much standardization could promote subject disengagement, suspiciousness, or lack of interest. Alternatively, flexibility in interviewer approach requires considerable interviewer skill, sensitivity, and in-depth training. Even with such training, the possibility exists that the way questions are formulated, or subtle expression of agreement or disagreement, influence subject response. A balance between standardization and flexibility is perhaps optimum.

A second point of comparison concerns the issue of the *elicitation* of Type A behaviours during the interview. The TABP is conceptualized as an action-emotion complex exhibited in the presence of appropriate environmental challenge (Friedman and Rosenman, 1974). This person-environment conceptualization is supported by laboratory research which compares the psychophysiologic responses to Type A and Type B subjects to a variety of physical and psychological stressors. In a review of thirty-seven of these studies, Krantz and Manuck (1984) reported that occasional differences between As and Bs occurred under non-challenge conditions, but approximately 70 per cent of these studies reported greater reactivity during challenge among Type A subjects on at least one of the several variables assessed. However, they note that large individual differences in reactivity exist because the effectiveness of psychosocial factors in arousing activation depends upon the individual's cognitive appraisal of those factors. Sex appears to be particularly important as a determinant of these appraisal processes (Frankenhaeuser, 1983; MacDougall, Dembroski, and Krantz, 1981; Manuck, Craft, and Gold, 1978).

In Type A interview assessment, emphasis is placed on the elicitation of Type A behaviour using direct behavioural tests. In all three interviews, questions are purposely drawn out to elicit impatience. The Rosenman SI protocol also instructs the interviewer to interrupt subjects in the middle of responses and insert meaningless questions at inopportune moments to arouse irritation. The problem with reliance on elicitation of behaviour concerns the possibility that important data will not be elicited due, perhaps, to systematic differences in appraisal. For example, the subject may perceive the situation to be contrived, regard it as silly, and thus not perform naturally (Nunnally, 1978). It is not known, in this case, whether the subject is not generally reactive (i.e. Type B) or simply not reactive to that particular stimulus. The alternative to elicitation is to make observations of more subtle Type A behaviours during casual conversation. This approach has been advocated by Friedman who includes not only speech, but also motor behaviour as sources of information (Friedman and Powell, 1984). Some tentative support for the non-challenge approach was provided by Guggisberg, Laederach, and Adler (1981) who found that the same speech indicators that discrimintate between As and Bs during the stress interview can be observed during a non-stress interview, and Dembroski, MacDougall, and Lushene (1979) who observed that behaviour during low-challenge conditions correlated with cardiovascular reactivity. Furthermore, Blumenthal, O'Toole, and Haney (1984) compared the stability and validity of interruptions when elicited and when naturally occurring during the interview and found that naturally occurring interruption was more reliable and more discriminating between Rosenman SI As and Bs than those elicited by the drawn-out questions.

At issue here is the extent to which it is possible to make observations of Type A behaviours in the absence of challenge. If it is demonstrated convincingly that this can be done, gains would include increased generalizability, especially by sex, and a more positive interview experience for both interviewer and subject.

The third and perhaps most important point of comparison among the observational approaches to Type A assessment is the use of clinical judgements to arrive at a category of behaviour type. Although most personality traits (Eysenck and Fulker, 1982) and risk factors are continuous, normally distributed variables, Type A behaviour, as measured by the SI and the Rosenman SI, is operationalized as a category of behaviour.

In 1981, the Review Panel on Coronary-Prone Behavior and Coronary Heart Disease (1981) recommended that the classification scheme used to assess the TABP be abandoned. Two types of problems are associated with behavioural categorizations. First, clinical judgements of risk are not well suited to large-scale research. Clinical judgements have the advantage of permitting flexibility in the use of any of a variety of cues deemed relevant. In the hands of experts this is an advantage, but it leads to problems when used with more inexperienced interviewers. Some of the problems with judgements that have particular relevance for Type A assessments are the halo effect where global judgements are highly influenced by a single favourable or unfavourable trait, the error of central tendency where judgements tend to be made toward the middle, and the tendency to look for confirmatory cues after hypotheses are already formed (Anastasi, 1982). These problems lead newly trained observers to see more Type A behaviour than experts.

The difficulties associated with teaching novices to make clinical judgements may prove to be one of the lessons learned in the MRFIT study. Despite excellent quality control procedures (The Multiple Risk Factor Intervention Trial Group, 1979), interviewers were found to vary in the percentage of subjects classified as Type A and in the validity with which their classifications predicted CHD (Scherwitz, 1985). Table 7 presents a summary of the prevalence of interview Type A behaviour as observed in a variety of studies. It can be seen that the range is wide—from a low of 32.3 per cent in 1965 to a high of 75 per cent in 1981.

A second problem with the classification of behaviour type is that it is methodologically imprecise. Categories preclude an investigation of the underlying structure of the TABP (Tasto, Chesney, and Chadwick, 1978), preclude an examination of the presence of a graded relationship, promote problems when subjects falling near the centre of the scale must be classified, and discard potentially useful variance (Mayes, Sime, and Ganster, 1984). One attempt to deal with the imprecision of the categorical score has been to make finer-grained judgements, but this makes the problem worse. In any investigation in which interjudge reliability was compared using two-level v. four-level classifications, the use of finer-grained analysis resulted in a drop of between 10 and 20 percentile points of agreement. This could be due to the fact that if there is an equal distribution of As and Bs in the population, there is approximately a 50 per cent chance that a random classification will be correct, but when a four-level classification system is used, this chance of being correct at random drops to 25 per cent.

Clinical judgements of behaviour type were needed in the early days of Type A research when it was difficult to specify the exact behaviours that were being used to make classifications. However, since that time, considerable work has been aimed at investigating individual behavioural components that make up the global Type A classification (Anderson and Waldron, 1983; Blumenthal, O'Toole, and Haney, 1984; Guggisberg, Laederach, and Adler, 1981; Lovallo and Pishkin, 1980; Scherwitz, Berton, and Leventhal, 1977; Scherwitz, McKelvain, Laman et al., 1983; Schucker and Jacobs, 1977) and CHD incidence (Powell and Thoresen, 1985). We may be at a point in observational assessment of the TABP where reliance on clinical judgements is no longer necessary.

COMMENT: SELF-REPORT APPROACHES TO TYPE A ASSESSMENT

Nunnally (1978) observed that even with the best efforts, interview ratings tend to have a low level of reliability and validity. This, combined with problems of cost and the effort involved in using interview measures of the TABP, has stimulated interest in the development of self-report questionnaires which would be quicker, less expensive, and more standardized.

In general, the self-report measures of the TABP assess competitive, hard-driving, and impatient components of Type A, but not anger and hostility. In particular, JAS-defined Type As can be characterized as vigorous achievement strivers who can be aggressive and competitive (Matthews, 1982). FTAB Type As are dissatisfied and uncomfortable with the competitive orientation and job pressures that their lives entail (Matthews, 1982). BRS Type As describe themselves and their behaviour as time-urgent,

Table 7: Prevalence of interview Type A behaviour

Population	Study	Sample	Location	Prevalence
North America	Chesney, Black, Chadwick et al. (1981)	male, skilled professional workers at Lockheed	California	75%
	Diamond, Schneiderman, Schwartz et al. (1984)	male undergraduates	Florida	65%
	Keith, Lown, and Stare (1965)	healthy males	Boston	32.3%
	MacDougall, Dembroski, and Musante (1979)	male undergraduates	Florida	55.7%
	Moss (1984)	male and female household probability sample	Michigan	42.6%
Outside North America	Byrne, Rosenman, Schiller et al. (1985)	male government workers	Australia	45.5%
	Appels, Jenkins, and Rosenman (1982)	males	The Netherlands	39.1%
	Schmidt, Undeutsch, Dembroski et al. (1982)	male policemen	Germany	57.5%
	Verhagen, Nass, Appels et al., (1980)	healthy men	The Netherlands	43%

High-risk Subjects	Blumenthal, Williams, Kong et al. (1978)	male & female angiography patients	North Carolina	59.9%
	Dembroski, MacDougall, Williams et al. (1985)	male & female angiography patients	North Carolina	62.6%
	Keith, Lown, and Stare (1965)	male coronary patients	Boston	47.4%
	Krantz, Durel, Davia et al. (1982)	angiography patients	Maryland	77.3%
	MacDougall, Dembroski, Dimsdale et al. (1985)	male angiography patients	Boston	76.0%
	The Multiple Risk Factor Intervention Trial Group (1979)	high-risk males	United States	74.4%
	Scherwitz, McKelvain, Laman et al. (1983)	angiography patients	Texas	70.0%
	Verhagen, Nass, Appels et al. (1980)	coronary patients	The Netherlands	59.5%
	Williams, Hanev, Lee et al. (1980)	male and female angiography patients	North Carolina	75.2%
Women	Anderson and Waldron (1983)	employed and non-employed women		69.9%
	Haynes, Feinleib and Kannel (1980)	Framingham women	Massachusetts	50.7%
	MacDougall, Dembroski, and Musante (1979)	female undergraduates	Florida	48.8%
	Menninger (1985)	employed women	Northeast US	45.0%
	Rosenman, and Friedman (1961)	healthy women	California	48.6%

impatient, hard-driving, and competitive. All questionnaire Type A scales appear to measure a stable characteristic, with stability correlations ranging from 0.7 to 0.8 over three to ten years 0.66 to 0.79 over 34 weeks to ten years (see Table 4).

Self-report measures of the TABP share three limitations. First, their validity as predictors of hard CHD endpoints has not been established for populations outside of the original, white-collar male population on which the construct was developed. Four studies investigated the prospective relationship between questionnaire Type A and subsequent occurrence of CHD in primarily blue-collar male populations (Case, Heller, Case et al., 1985; Cohen and Reed, 1985; Haynes, Feinleib, and Kannel, 1980; Shekelle, Gale, and Norusis, 1985), but not one reported an association (Table 1). Furthermore, Haynes, Feinleib, and Kannel (1980) studied the independent contribution of FTAB to CHD in women and found that it was independently related in working women. In housewives, tension—not FTAB—was an independent predictor. The most plausible explanation for this is that the emphasis on competitive, hard-driving behaviour as a response to work demands does not have relevance for the life-style of blue-collar men and housewives. It is possible that a more relevant measure of the TABP in blue-collar groups is one that relies more on strict behavioural indices (as measured by the interview) than indices which measure behaviours at and attitudes about work.

A second limitation of the Type A questionnaires is the potential bias associated with the reliance on self-reports. Major components of the TABP—impatience and irritability—are socially undesirable characteristics. The appeal of interview measures lies in their unobtrusive approach to assessment. It is difficult to make assessments of these characteristics using self-reports because Type A subjects may not be aware of or may not admit to them. In an investigation of self-descriptions of 378 employed males who were previously classified for behaviour type using the SI, Herman, Blumenthal, Black et al., (1981) found that those classified as Type A tended to describe themselves in socially desirable ways, including such adjectives as assertive, aggressive, outgoing, energetic, and autonomous, but not in less socially desirable ways, such as hostile, driven, or egocentric. The reluctance of Type As to admit to, or be aware of, negative traits makes the self-assessment of indices of anger and hostility difficult. If the less socially desirable characteristics are to be included in Type A self-report measures, social desirability bias must be taken into consideration.

A third limitation of self-reports concerns the transformation of continuous scales into behaviour categories. The JAS produces categories using a discriminant equation developed on WCGS data, and the FTAB produces categories by splitting population studies at the median. The generalizability of the JAS discriminant solution is questionable. In MRFIT, subjects classified as A2 by the Rosenman SI had an average JAS score in the Type B range (Shekelle, Hulley, Neaton et al., 1985), and in a sample of British white-collar men (Johnston and Shaper, 1983) and a sample of Australian male workers (Byrne, Rosenman, Schiller et al., 1985), the mean JAS score was in the Type B range. The median split used with the FTAB runs the risk of producing test–retest unreliability for subjects scoring toward the mean since classification could change depending upon the referent group. These problems, in addition to the loss of potentially valuable variance, raise questions about the advisability of this practice in cases other than to examine agreement with the categorical SI. Where questionnaire Type A is analyzed as a continuous variable, it is possible to investigate the extent to which increases in the amount of the TABP are related to increased risk of CHD.

The nature of the problems with Type A questionnaires provide some insight into research needs. In this regard, the BRS provides an example of a potentially valuable direction. The BRS is based upon the assumption that an individual can accurately self-observe his/her own psychomotor behaviour. The value of this assumption is that it eliminates the need for assessing the TABP as it occurs in the work context and presents a less costly alternative to the interview. The current form of the BRS may be criticized because it is not limited to overt behaviours and it de-emphasizes indices of anger and hostility. However the exact set of indices to be scored can be refined to include additional, or other, potentially important behaviours. Continued development of this approach to Type A questionnaire assessment may prove fruitful.

OVERLAP AMONG MEASURES OF THE TYPE A BEHAVIOUR PATTERN

Table 6 summarizes the overlap among Type A measures. Within observational methods, no studies have reported on the relationship between the SI and the Rosenman SI. This most likely reflects the assumption that these two interviews are the same. Agreement between the VSI and the SI was reported, in only one study, to be 83.4 per cent (Powell, Friedman, Thoresen, et al., 1984). However, this statistic is difficult to interpret since the exact method by which SI classifications were made in the WCGS is difficult to recapture and the dichotomization of a continuous scale (in this case, the VSI) into behaviour types is problematic, as discussed earlier. In one investigation, a continuous Type A interview score was created by adding ratings of Type A content and stylistics and was found to correlate 0.6 with the Rosenman SI classifications which were analyzed as a continuous variable (1=Type A; 2=Type B) (Mayes, Sime, and Ganster, 1984).

Within the self-report methods, interrelationships using correlations are easier to interpret. Table 6 shows that the average correlation reported between the JAS and the FTAB is 0.49, accounting for 24 per cent of mutual variance. The average correlation between the JAS and the BRS is 0.535, accounting for 29 per cent of mutual variance. The correlation between the

FTAB and BRS is 0.59, accounting for 35 per cent of mutual variance. The overlap within self-report methods is low; too low to assume that they are measuring the same thing. As best as can be determined, it may be lower than the overlap among interview measures.

Across methods, agreement is lower than within method. In general, behaviour and content are only weakly related. Jenkins, Rosenman, and Friedman (1967) observed 72 per cent agreement between the JAS and the SI in the white-collar male WCGS sample. Subsequent reports using the Rosenman SI indicate lower agreement in adult men, ranging from 54.8 per cent in Australian men (Byrne, Rosenman, Schiller et al., 1985) to 67 per cent in white-collar American men (Matthews, Krantz, Dembroski et al., 1982). Agreement in college men is approximately the same, with a range from 74 per cent (MacDougall, Dembroski, and Musante, 1979) to 42 per cent (Scherwitz, Berton, and Leventhal, 1977). In women, agreement drops to 63 per cent for college women (MacDougall, Dembroski and Musante, 1979) and a range of 49.7 to 52 per cent in adult women (Menninger, 1985; Haynes, Feinleib, and Kannel, 1980). Agreement between the Rosenman SI and the FTAB is slightly better than chance: 66 per cent in college men (MacDougall, Dembroski and Musante, 1979), 60 per cent in middle-aged men (Chesney, Black, Chadwick et al., 1981), 67 per cent in college women (MacDougall, Dembroski, and Musante, 1979) and 45.6 per cent in adult women (Menninger, 1985).

One limitation of these reports of percent agreement is the failure to use a kappa statistic (Fleiss, 1977), which corrects for chance associations. In the absence of a correction for chance, agreement between two dichotomous variables could easily appear to be spuriously high.

Both methods measure self-reported pressured drive, energy level, and competitiveness (Matthews, Krantz, Dembroski et al., 1982). What is unique to the SI is the assessment of speech stylistics (Matthews, Krantz, Dembroski et al., 1982) which are correlated with physiological responsivity (e.g. change in heart rate, skin temperature, skin conductance) (Mayes, Sime, and Ganster, 1984). What is unique to the JAS is self-reported time pressure (Matthews, Krantz, Dembroski, et al. 1982) which is correlated with self-reports of job strain (e.g. satisfaction, irritation, depression, physical symptoms) (Mayes, Sime, and Ganster, 1984).

In an excellent study of method bias in Type A assessment on a small number of employed women (N=63), Mayes, Sime, and Ganster (1984) reported that the average correlations among observational measures of the TABP (r=0.65) and the average correlations among self-report measures of the TABP (r=0.31) were higher than the correlations between Type A observational and self-report measures (r=0.13). When scales using different methods are intended to measure the same thing, higher correlations within methods than between methods are suggestive of method bias (Campbell and Fiske, 1959). Further supporting the possibility of method bias are reports indicating modest correlations between SI global ratings and behavioural ratings (Anderson and Waldron, 1983; Dembroski, MacDougall, Shields et al., 1978; Howland and Siegman, 1982; Matthews, Krantz, Dembroski et al., 1982; Scherwitz, Berton, and Leventhal, 1977; Schucker and Jacobs, 1977).

In general, these data suggest that observational and self-report measures of the TABP should not be considered substitutes for one another. A question of importance in this regard is the justifiability of labelling all of these different operationalizations "Type A." Consistent with the growing trend toward identifying pathogenic components, it may be advisable to label more precisely what these instruments are measuring. For example, Type A interview measures could be labelled 'behavioural hyperreactivity' scales while self-report measures could be labelled job strain or job pressure scales. This would allay problems of method bias and encourage research aimed at joint investigations of the relative contribution of these different measures to CHD endpoints.

POTENTIAL MEDIATORS OF THE TYPE A–CHD RELATIONSHIP

A critical analysis of existing Type A studies, and the development of powerful designs for new Type A studies, requires an understanding of factors which serve to weaken or condition the Type A–CHD link. Among the ways in which extraneous factors could mediate this relationship are: (a) they provide alternative explanations for results because they covary with both the TABP and CHD; (b) they reduce the accuracy with which the TABP can be assessed; and (c) they provide information about sub-groups in which the Type A–CHD link is most likely, or most unlikely, to occur. What follows is a review of some of the more common factors which have been reputed to mediate the Type A–CHD link.

Sex

The TABP was developed as a concept which reflected a pattern of behaviour characteristic of white-collar, employed men. It is possible, therefore, that studies conducted on women or on populations which are sex-mixed may fail to find a link because the TABP, or its operationalization, is not relevant for women.

In a recent review, Haynes (1984) concluded that the best assessment for the TABP in women has yet to be determined. Both interview and questionnaire methods have limitations. The stylistics of importance in the SI appear to be different for women than for men. Stylistics found to discriminate between global classifications in women feature speed (e.g. rate of speaking and answering, rapid motor pace) while those which discriminate in men feature volume (Anderson and Waldron, 1983; Smyth, Call, Hansell et al., 1978). Some Type A stylistics may be congruent with the social norm for women (e.g. interruptions), while others may be socially unacceptable (e.g. loud voice, competitiveness) (Haynes, 1984). Reliance on elicitation of stylistics, as is done with the Rosenman SI, may cause difficulties for women since they respond to challenge differently than men (MacDougall, Dembroski, and Krantz, 1981; MacDougall, Dembroski, and Musante, 1979). These limitations appear to create difficulties for raters. In Framingham, interjudge reliability for men was 77–78 per cent, but for women it dropped to 65 per cent (Haynes, Feinleib, and Kannel, 1980). Despite these limitations, SI defined Type A occurs with consistency in about 44–55 per cent of women (Haynes, Feinleib, and Kannel, 1980; MacDougall, Dembroski, and Krantz, 1981; Menninger, 1985; Rosenman, and Friedman, 1961; Smyth, Call, Hansell et al., 1978), with only one study finding a prevalence (68.8 per cent) comparable to that of recent studies in men (Anderson and Waldron, 1983). The only investigation of sex differences using the VSI found significantly lower scores for female coronary patients than for their male counterparts ($p=0.006$) (Powell and Fleischmann, in press).

Questionnaire items that discriminate SI classifications for women assess impatience and job involvement, in contrast to comparable analyses for WCGS men which found discriminating items to be anger, and competitiveness (Menninger, 1985). Questionnaire scores for women are lower than those for men (Haynes, Feinleib, and Kannel, 1980; MacDougall, Dembroski, Musante, 1979), but differences decrease when female samples are limited to working women (Haynes, Feinleib, and Kannel, 1980; Shekelle, Schoenberger, and Stamler, 1976). The only exception to this is one study of a high-risk population of men and women screened in Marseilles where women had significantly higher BRS scores and a significantly greater prevalence of Rosenman SI Type A1 classifications (Bernet, Drivet-Perrin, Blanc et al., 1982). JAS scores in women are influenced both by education and employment status, with higher scores associated with greater education and employment, especially professional employment (Davidson, Cooper, and Chamberlain, 1980; Lawler, Rixse, and Allen, 1983; Morell and Katkin, 1982; Shekelle, Schoenberger, and Stamler, 1976; Waldron, 1978).

Certainly, psychometric work on the assessment of the TABP in women is needed. In particular, validation of interview stylistics against hard CHD events is needed. When questionnaires are used with women who have a comparable work life to white-collar men, they appear to have comparable psychometric properties. This is especially true for women who are young enough to have been influenced by the women's movement. At present, only the FTAB has been validated as a predictor of CHD in women, and this validation is independent of other psychosocial risk factors only for the subgroup who are employed.

Age

To the extent that progressive changes in the TABP occur with age, and its pathogenic relevance coincides with these changes, a preponderance of subjects in a study who are at a specific benign age could weaken the Type A–CHD link.

In general, changes in the TABP by age can be observed only if the age range sampled is broad enough. In the WCGS entry data, there were 47.4 per cent SI Type As in the 39–49 age group and 57.6 per cent SI Type As in the 50–59 age group (Rosenman, Brand, Jenkins et al., 1975). The excess risk for Type A relative to Type B was 2.1 in both groups. In Framingham, there was a progressive decline in FTAB with age, grouped as 45–54, 55–64, and 65+ (women FTAB: 0.40, 0.39, 0.35; men FTAB 0.37, 0.32, 0.28, respectively) (Haynes, Levine, Scotch et al., 1978). Excess risk was observed at the 45–54 and 55–64 intervals, but not the 65+ interval (Haynes, Feinleib, and Kannel, 1980). Further support for a decline in FTAB with age was observed in a study of ninety women, ranging in age from 21–62 (Kelly and Houston, 1985), and a study of men in South Wales, ranging in age from 45 to 69 (Gallacher, Yarnell, Elwood et al., 1984). The JAS also was observed to decline with age in the Kelly and Houston sample (1985). One study, conducted in Marseilles, found no difference in the percentage of Rosenman SI Type A in men over (12.8%) and under (13.4%) 40, but significantly fewer Type As in women under age 40 (9.8%) compared to women over 40 (25.7%) (Bernet, Drivet-Perrin, Blanc et al., 1982). Keith, Lown, and Stare (1965) studied prevalence of SI Type A in coronary patients and found a greater proportion between the ages of 35 and 44 (65%) than between the ages of 45 and 49 years (37.5%). Prevalence studies of adults are difficult to interpret because of the problem of selection bias. Type As may suffer early deaths and thus account for the decreased prevalence with age in cross-sectional studies.

Studies of Type A in children, however, are not subject to this bias since they are not subject to coronary death at such an early age. In children, it appears that the TABP increases from pre-adolescence to adolescence. In the Bogalusa Heart Study, scores on the Hunter-Wolf Type A scale increased between pre-adolescence (ages 10–12) and adolescence (ages 13–17) (Mean scores: 64; 68.3, respectively) (Hunter, Wolf, Sklov et al., 1982). This finding was supported in the American-Hellenic Heart Study where classifications of Type A using the Miami Structured Interview for Children indicated that the prevalence of Type A in American and Greek pre-adolescents (ages 7–11 years) was 36.8 per cent and 39.3 per cent respectively, and in American and Greek adolescents (ages 12–16) was 57 per cent and 62 per cent respectively (Smith, Gerace, Christakis et al., 1985).

Although data are inconclusive about the relationship between the TABP and age during the middle adult years, what does seem apparent is that the time of increase in the TABP is the transition from childhood to adulthood—a time when the beginnings of coronary artery disease have been observed to occur. It is also possible that those Type As who survive to age sixty-five may be the hardy ones who are not at risk for CHD by virtue of their behaviour. Virtually no work has been done on Type A behaviour and CHD in the elderly.

Socio-economic status and education

Since all of the TABP measures were developed using white-collar male populations, their relevance for blue-collar and unemployed people must be determined.

The interview, with its focus on stylistics, may be least subject to influence by SES or education. In the WCGS, no differences in behaviour type by education were observed (48.4 per cent of those with high school or less and 50.9 per cent of those attending college were classified as Type A), but differences were evident when income was related to behaviour type (62.8 per cent of those making between $15,000 and $25,000 and 68.7 per cent of those making over $25,000 in 1960 were classified as Type A) (Rosenman, Friedman, Straus, et al., 1966). However, Keith, Lown and Stare (1965) observed a strong relationship between SI Type As and education with 38.2 per cent of those failing to graduate from college or high school and 67.7 per cent of those with college degrees being classified as Type A. Byrne, Rosenman, Schiller et al. (1985) found more Type A behaviour among Australian men educated to the tertiary level than among those educated at the high school or technical level.

The relationship between the FTAB and SES or education was not reported in Framingham, although the fact that their data were analyzed separately by SES suggests that a relationship may exist. The scale was a valid predictor for white-collar, but not for blue-collar men and was independently valid for employed women but not for housewives. FTAB was not related to education or SES in Australian men (Byrne, Rosenman, Schiller et al., 1985) and a modest relationship between FTAB and educational attainment was observed for employed women (Kelly and Houston, 1985). Associations are consistently positive between the JAS and education (Byrne, Rosenman, Schiller et al., 1985; Kelly and Houston, 1985; Zyzanski, 1978) and SES (Byrne, Rosenman, Schiller et al. 1985; Kelly and Houston, 1985) and between the BRS and education (Byrne, Rosenman, Schiller et al., 1985) and SES (Bass and Wade, 1982; Byrne, Rosenman, Schiller et al., 1985), particularly in the case of men.

The association between the TABP and indices of SES and education suggests the importance of controlling for these variables in studies of association. More importantly, with blue-collar populations, the Type A construct, or the way it is measured, appears to have limited applicability.

Research is needed to identify and measure Type A, or coronary-prone behaviour, in lower SES groups.

Urban–rural residence

Since the TABP is conceptualized as a response to an appropriately challenging environment, it is possible that in the absence of that challenge, it will not occur. Living in a fast-paced urban environment may very well present considerable challenge to individuals, relative to the slower-paced life of their rural counterparts. Thus, in rural individuals, the TABP would not occur with as much frequency or intensity and therefore the link to CHD in these subjects would be weakened.

There is limited evidence on this subject. However, what does exist suggests that some Type A behaviour exists in rural settings. Byrne, Rosenman, Schiller et al. (1985) investigated the differential prevalence of Type A in urban and rural Australian employed men. They found that when the Rosenman SI was used to classify subjects, significantly greater prevalence was observed in urban men (49.6 per cent) than in rural men (30.3 per cent) ($p<0.01$). However, no differences were observed when Type A was assessed using either the JAS (urban=−5.29; rural=−5.56) or the FTAB (urban=0.40; rural=0.58). In a case-control study of rural men in Israel, the JAS was found to discriminate strongly between CHD cases and healthy controls (cases = 2.01; controls = −2.18) ($p<0.001$) (Stockwell, Zyzanski, and Yodfat, 1985). The available data do not appear strong enough to consider residence to be a factor which would be a plausible mediator of the relationship between the TABP and CHD.

Employment status

If the TABP is a kind of stress that is a response to work demands, then individuals who are not employed outside of the home may not experience Type A behaviour. Inclusion of these people in studies of association would have the effect of weakening the relationship.

A comparison of the prevalence of SI-defined Type A in working women and housewives would provide the best test for this concern since the SI is less context specific than Type A questionnaires. However, no studies have reported on this relationship. In Framingham, at every age, working women scored significantly higher on FTAB than housewives (mean working women v. housewives=0.37 v. 0.29). Scores for working women were almost identical to scores for Framingham men (0.39) (Haynes, Feinleib, Levine et al., 1978). But, work pressures alone are not indicators of Type A behaviour. Wanting to work, but being unable to, also appears to promote the TABP. In a study of 558 men in South Wales, men who were disabled or looking for work had the highest FTAB scores, followed by employed men, with retired men having the lowest scores (Gallacher, Yarnell, Elwood et al., 1984). In a study of Type A in women, the JAS had the greatest agreement with the SI in employed women ($r=0.42$, $p<0.01$), relative to women who were not employed ($r=0.19$) or employed less than 35 hours per week ($r=0.21$) (Anderson and Waldron, 1983).

Employment status does appear to covary with the TABP. This relationship begs the question of how to assess coronary-prone behaviour in individuals who are not working. Data from Framingham sheds light on this issue. In housewives, FTAB and tension were highly related, were both associated on a univariate basis to eight-year cardiovascular incidence, and tension, but not FTAB, made an independent contribution. When tension was removed from the predictive equation, FTAB replaced it as an independent predictor. This suggests that behaviour does increase risk in housewives and that FTAB may not be the best operationalization of this behaviour.

Beta-blockade medication

The increased popularity of beta-blocking drugs in the treatment of angina, hypertension, arrhythmias, and as prophylaxis against coronary mortality following infarction has led to increasing numbers of individuals with symptoms of cardiovascular disease who are on these drugs and are also subjects in Type A studies. Beta-blockers block sympathetic arousal and may reduce the frequency of behaviours used to score the TABP during the SI. Alteration of the criteria used to create the SI Type A score could lead to misclassifications of subjects and a weakening of the relationship between Type A and CHD.

Although only a few studies have dealt with this issue, those that are available are consistent. Use of beta-blockers appears to dampen Type A stylistics. Krantz, Durel, Davia et al. (1982) compared the behaviour of eighty-eight angiography patients who were and were not taking beta-blockers. After adjusting for potential risk factors, they observed a decrease in loud/explosive voice, rapid/accelerated speech, and potential for hostility. Two studies from West Germany observed similar results. Subjects were randomly allocated to beta-blockade or diuretic medication and assessed using the Rosenman SI before and after four weeks of treatment. They observed a reduction in loud and explosive speech ($p=0.09$), rapid and accelerated speech ($p=0.001$), and response latency ($p=0.001$), but not in potential for hostility or competition (v. Eiff, Friedrich, Neus et al., 1982; Schneider, Fredleich, Neus, et al., 1983). In a study that was part of the RCPP, coronary patients who were and were not taking beta-blockers were compared on VSI scores. Although differences were non-significant, the trend was toward less Type A behaviour on the part of subjects taking beta-blockers (Powell and Fleischmann, in press). No studies have observed whether these behavioural changes were accompanied by changes in cognitions. Moreover, they did not determine the clinical significance of change in stylistics; that is, whether behavioural hyperreactivity as observed in the interview is a risk factor or simply a risk indicator.

This preliminary evidence is suggestive of the importance of controlling for beta-blockade medication when examining the relationship between SI determined Type A and cardiovascular endpoints.

CHD endpoints

Studies aimed at evaluating the Type A-CHD link have used a variety of CHD endpoints, including total CHD, angina, total myocardial infarction, fatal myocardial infarction, non-fatal myocardial infarction, sudden death, total coronary death, degree of coronary occlusion, and recurrent cardiac events. Epidemiologic evidence suggests that the link is stronger in some of these criteria than others.

More than half of the large-scale prospective epidemiologic studies of men that used the endpoint of total CHD (including angina, fatal MI, nonfatal MI, and sudden death) found a relationship (DeBacker, Kornitzer, Kittel et al., 1983; French-Belgian Collaborative Group, 1982; Friedman, Thoresen, Gill et al., 1984; Haynes, Feinleib, and Kannel, 1980), although some did not (Cohen and Reed, 1985; Dimsdale, Gilbert, Hutter et al., 1981; Shekelle, Hulley, Neaton et al., 1985). In the one study that examined women, the incidence of MI was so small that only total CHD (angina and fatal or non-fatal events) or angina alone (comprising 60 per cent of the events) was found to be predictive (Haynes, Feinleib, and Kannel, 1980).

Studies of coronary death are more negative. No relationship was found in one study investigating behaviour and coronary death as the first event (Koskenvuo, Kaprio, Langinvainio et al., 1983) or in studies observing coronary death following infarction (Case, Heller, Case et al., 1985; Friedman, Thoresen, Gill et al., 1984; Ragland, Brand and Rosenman, 1986). Relevant to this point is the recent finding from the RCPP that the effectiveness of change in Type A behaviour on reduction of risk of coronary death was mediated by cardiovascular risk status following the prior MI. Subjects at high risk, where the efficiency of the heart was decreased, were not protected following Type A modification, but those at low risk, who did not incur reduction in cardiac efficiency, underwent a significant reduction in coronary mortality (Powell, Friedman, Thoresen, et al., 1986). Behaviour has been shown to discriminate those who will incur a second cardiac event from those who will have only one event in three studies (Jenkins, Zyzanski, and Rosenman, 1976; Jenkins, Zyzanski, Rosenman et al., 1971; Friedman, Thoresen, Gill et al., 1986).

Behaviour may be related to CHD by two different disease processes—the long-term progression of coronary artery disease (Kaplan, Manuck, Clarkson et al., 1983), and cardiac arrhythmias resulting in sudden death (Lown, Verrier, and Corbalan, 1973; Lown, Verrier, and Rabinowitz, 1977). It is difficult to disentangle the contribution of behaviour to these two processes because they present problems in research design. The use of angina as an endpoint does not disentangle these two processes because angina could be a symptom either of obstruction or spasm. Autopsy studies present practical difficulties.

Angiography studies shed light on the strength of the connection between the TABP and coronary occlusion; however the results of fourteen of these studies conducted to date are inconclusive (Matthews and Haynes, 1986). When the TABP was assessed using the SI, an equal number of positive and no association studies was reported, and when the TABP was measured using the JAS or the BRS, no association was observed, with only one exception. Matthews and Haynes go on to note the variety of methodologic problems pervasive in angiography studies, including: (a) small sample sizes resulting in low power to find differences; (b) high prevalence of Type As, possibly resulting from disproportionate referral practices, weakening associations by incorporating non-representative homogeneity in the risk factor; and (c) the assessment of behaviour type at a time close in proximity to the invasive procedure when the patient is likely to be anxious and preoccupied.

It is likely that both processes may be implicated in the behaviour-CHD connection. Better controlled angiography studies and 24-hour holter monitoring could provide useful information.

There is preliminary evidence that the TABP is related to other cardiovascular endpoints, including stroke in men (Adler, MacRitchie, and Engle, 1971; Gianturco, Breslin, Heyman et al., 1974) and in women (Eaker, Feinleib, and Wolf, 1983), carotid artery atherosclerosis (Stevens, Turner, Rhodewalt et al., 1984), and peripheral vascular disease (Cottier, Adler, Vorkauf et al., 1983). An interesting new line of research, based upon the assumption that the TABP is a type of chronic stress, seeks to explore its relationship to disorders that are assumed to be stress related. Preliminary evidence exists for a relationship between the TABP and upper respiratory track infections (Stout and Bloom, 1982; Barton, Brautigan, Fogle et al., 1982), infectious mononucleosis (Barton and Hicks, 1985), and headaches (Hicks and Campbell, 1983; Woods, Morgan, Day et al., 1984), but not to diabetes (Robinson and Fuller, 1981). One limitation of these latter studies is that they are generally based upon small numbers of subjects and are not adequately controlled. This is, however, an untapped, but potentially important, line of research.

In summary, the relationship between behaviour and CHD is strongest when total CHD events are examined, including angina. The importance of angina as an endpoint was first observed by Keith, Lown and Stare (1965) who found that interview Type A was more prevalent among coronary patients with angina than with MI, and then by Jenkins, Zyzanski and Rosenman (1978) who reported that the personality characteristics associated with angina—impatience, irritability, competitiveness, and excessive effort—are more characteristic of the TABP than the characteristics associated with MI—self-control and hard work. More recent evidence suggests that the anger component of the TABP may be the link to angina (Smith, Follick and Korr, 1984). The inclusion of angina as an endpoint appears to be particularly important in studies of women.

NEW DIRECTIONS

The focus of this review has been on the strengths and limitations of standard measures of the TABP. Because each measure has limitations, new approaches, based upon new assumptions about the nature and measurement of coronary-prone behaviour, have been pursued. Three of these new approaches will be discussed.

Type A components

Interview and self-report measures of the TABP appear to be comprised of heterogeneous components that have only a moderate relationship to one another. Some researchers have suggested that not all of these components may be equally pathogenic and attempted to identify a substrate of behaviours responsible for the link to CHD.

Anger and hostility is one Type A component that offers promise for a pathogenic substrate. There is considerable conceptual ambiguity surrounding anger and hostility. Although often considered to be part of the same construct, they have been conceptualized by some to be distinct. Anger refers to an emotional state consisting of feelings varying in intensity from irritation to rage, and hostility refers to an attitudinal set, perhaps even a personality trait, which stems from an absence of trust in the basic goodness of others and centres around the belief that others are generally mean, selfish, and undependable (Williams, Barefoot, and Shekelle, 1985).

The connection between anger and hostility and cardiovascular outcomes was first identified in the area of hypertension, but considerable inconsistency in research findings has occurred since then (see Diamond, 1982 for an excellent review). More recently, indices of anger and hostility have been validated in prospective research as predictors of hard CHD endpoints. Matthews, Glass, Rosenman et al., (1977) scored ten responses to the SI of 186 cases and controls in the WCGS and found that seven components discriminated. Of the seven, the majority concerned anger and hostility. Building on this finding, Dembroski and colleagues, developed a component scoring system for the Rosenman SI (Dembroski, 1978) consisting of five stylistic scores and four self-report scores. (More recent publications have reported on seven stylistic scores and five factor scores (Dembroski, MacDougall, Williams et al., 1985; MacDougall, Dembroski, Dimsdale et al., 1985)). Support for the validity of these components comes primarily from studies of patients undergoing angiography. In general, findings suggest that one component—potential for hostility—predicts severity of occlusion in cases where global SI Type A does not (Dembroski, MacDougall, Williams et al., 1985; MacDougall, Dembroski, Dimsdale, 1985). In another line of research, hostility, as measured by the Cook-Medley Hostility Scale (Cook and Medley, 1954) was found to be a better predictor of coronary occlusion in angiography patients than SI Type A (Williams, Haney, Lee et al., 1980), and was related to coronary mortality in two long-term prospective studies (with twenty-five- and ten-year-follow-ups) (Barefoot, Dahlstrom, and Williams, 1983; Shekelle, Gale, Ostfeld et al., 1983). In a third line of research, indices of repressed anger predicted eight-year incidence of CHD in both men and women in Framingham (Haynes, Feinleib and Kannel, 1980).

While this research is provocative, psychometric studies are needed to determine exactly what these scales are measuring and how they are related to the global TABP. The Cook-Medley Hostility Scale appears to measure an enduring trait of ill-will and suspiciousness towards others. The stability coefficient in middle-aged men over four years was 0.84 (Shekelle, Gale, Ostfeld et al., 1983) and in medical students over one year was 0.85 (Barefoot, Dahlstrom, and Williams, 1983). This trait conceptualization could account for the 'person' in the person-situation conceptualization that is generally proposed. Correlations have been reported to be 0.57 with the Rosenman SI (Dembroski, MacDougall, Williams et al., 1985) and 0.18 with the VSI (Powell, Friedman, Thoresen et al., 1984). Conceptual integration is needed.

Potential for hostility is essentially a clinical judgement, although it is a less ambiguous than the term Type A behaviour. As such, all of the measurement problems associated with making subjective clinical judgements of Type A would similarly apply. Interjudge reliabilities have been reported to be high when experts (most commonly Dembroski and MacDougall) do the rating (agreement ranging from 0.74 to 0.84) (Dembroski, MacDougall, Williams, et al., 1985; MacDougall, Dembroski, Dimsdale, 1985; Musante, MacDougall, Dembroski, 1983). However, as with the global SI ratings, reliability drops when newly trained raters are used (agreement=0.61) (Diamond, Schneiderman, Schwartz et al., 1984). No information has been reported on the test–retest reliability of the score or its long-term stability. It correlates 0.57 with global SI and 0.37 with the Cook-Medley Hostility Scale (Dembroski, MacDougall, Williams et al., 1985). But the correlations with the SI may be inflated since Dembroski rated both the global category and the component scores. More importantly, this component is in need of validation in prospective research. Although it has been associated to coronary occlusion in some angiography studies, the design problems with these studies (as discussed earlier) makes these findings difficult to interpret.

The anger–expression scale used in Framingham has been subjected to few psychometric analyses. It appears to be distinct from FTAB (r=0.04) (Haynes, Levine, Scotch et al., 1978). Dembroski and colleagues currently score anger-in from the SI (Dembroski, MacDougall, Williams et al., 1985; MacDougall, Dembroski, Dimsdale et al., 1985). Although it too is unrelated to SI Type A (r=−0.07) (MacDougall, Dembroski, Dimsdale, 1985), its relationship to the Framingham Anger-Expression scale is not known, nor is its validity as a predictor of hard CHD endpoints.

Time urgency is the second major component of the TABP which offers some promise for an additional pathogenic substrate. Cannon (1915) first described the sympathetic adrenal-medullary stress response as the 'fight or flight' response. In Type A terms, this translates to the componence of hostility *and* time urgency. Time urgency appears to be comprised of heterogeneous characteristics which have some overlap with anger and hostility. Factor analyses of items measured on global Type A scales revealed clusters of such diverse items as speed of speech and behaviour, impatience, and irritation at waiting (Matthews, Glass, Rosenman et al., 1977).

Although a variety of instruments have been used to measure anger and hostility (Matthews, 1985), only a few exist with which to measure speed and impatience. The most studied measure is the JAS Speed and Impatience scale. It is significantly correlated to the Rosenman SI (r=0.233, p<0.001) (Byrne, Rosenman, Schiller et al., 1985) and to the VSI (r=0.31, p<0.001) (Powell, Friedman, Thoresen et al., 1984), and is significantly related to 4-level Rosenman SI classifications (p<0.01) (Chesney, Black, Chadwick et al., 1981). It is highly correlated with self-report measures of global Type A (r=0.52−0.60) (Byrne, Rosenman, Schiller et al., 1985; Mayes, Sime and Ganster, 1984). The Activity Scale of The Thurstone Temperament Schedule (Thurstone, 1953), which measures overall pace of activity in many facets of daily life, was found to have the highest correlation (r=0.31, p<0.001) with Rosenman SI of any of a variety of psychometric scales evaluated, including the Speed and Impatience scale from the JAS (Chesney, Black, Chadwick et al., 1981). Although there is no clinical rating similar to potential for hostility, individual behaviours including response latency, speed of speech, and interruptions can be scored from interview data. Dembroski and colleagues score a speed and impatience factor from interview content (Dembroski, 1978).

Two major prospective studies have reported that speed and impatience is predictive of hard CHD endpoints. In the Belgian Heart Disease Prevention Project, JAS Speed and Impatience was related to five-year incidence of CHD (DeBacker, Kornitzer, Kittel et al., 1983). In a fourteen-year follow-up of business and professional men from the twin cities, a higher score on the Thurstone Activity Scale was associated with greater incidence of CHD

(Brozek, Keys, and Blackburn, 1966). A measure of time anxiety was a significant discriminator between Dutch CHD cases and healthy controls (Verhazen, Nass, Appels et al., 1980). In two investigations, time urgency was significantly associated with cardiovascular arousal, independently of subject A–B classification (Delameter, Albrecht, Smith et al., 1986; Jennings, 1984). An unexpected and difficult to interpret finding in the angiography studies recently reported by the Dembroski group indicated that self-reported speed of activity and time pressure was significantly *inversely* related to indices of coronary occlusion, number of prior MIs and angina (Dembroski, MacDougall, Williams et al., 1985; MacDougall, Dembroski, Dimsdale, et al., 1985).

Although evidence linking impatience and time urgency to cardiovascular outcomes is inconsistent, it has been associated with hard CHD endpoints in two prospective epidemiologic investigations. Thus, when only the criterion of predictive validity is considered, impatience–time urgency is as valid a Type A component as anger-hostility. Studies suggesting that hostility is *the* key pathogenic component have compared it to global Type A—not to other Type A components. Thus a more accurate interpretation of the hostility findings is that hostility may be *a* key pathogenic component. More studies investigating time urgency, especially using the Thurstone Scale, are in order.

An alternative approach to the refinement of the Type A conceptualization has been to subdivide Type A traits into positive and negative attributes. This approach has been introduced by two different research teams. Friedman, Hall and Harris (1985) have suggested that the JAS Type As can be subdivided into repressed, tense, and illness-prone types or healthy, talkative, in control, and charismatic types. Leak and MaCarthy (1984) separated JAS items into a positive scale called Involvement, reflecting constructive ambition, assertiveness, and personal and social adjustment, and a negative scale called Drivenness, reflecting self-defeating interpersonal behaviour and anxiety.

Multivariate assessment of components

A new direction in assessment research on the TABP is to assume that the best predictions of CHD criteria come from assuming a multivariate, rather than a univariate, approach to the assessment of behaviour. This approach considers combinations of Type A behaviour and Type A components jointly.

Some investigations have assumed an additive approach to behavioural assessment. Jenkins, Zyzanski, and Rosenman (1971) studied WCGS men and observed that the JAS AB and hard-driving scales were relatively independent (r=0.34) but both able to discriminate prevalent CHD cases from controls. They then combined information from both sales and found that men who scored above the median on *both* scales had approximately twice the prevalence of CHD as those scoring below the median on both. Jenkins pursued this approach one step further in a second study (Jenkins, Zyzanski, Ryan et al., 1977) where the joint contribution of JAS AB and a measure of social insecurity on coronary occlusion was evaluated on ninety-five males undergoing angiography. Both scales predicted occlusion and were relatively uncorrelated. Of the men who scored above the median on both scales, 91 per cent had more than 50 per cent obstruction in two arteries relative to those who scored below the median on both, in which only 25 per cent had such obstruction. They then went on to investigate the possibility of an interactive relationship and found that the interaction term was not significant. Haynes, Feinleib, and Kannel (1980) reported that *both* FTAB and anger-out were independent predictors of CHD incidence in Framingham.

A more recent, but interesting finding along this line of research was reported by Dembroski and colleagues (Dembroski, MacDougall, Williams et al., 1985) who studied the relationship between hostility and coping style in patients undergoing angiography. They observed no correlation between potential for hostility and anger-in (r=0.00), but independent predictive potential for both the endpoints on number of prior MIs and coronary occlusion. Furthermore, they observed the presence of an interaction between them, suggesting that increases in potential for hostility were associated with increases in pathology only for patients who held their anger in. In a study of cardiovascular reactivity in sixty male undergraduates, an interactive relationship was also observed. Correlations between Rosenman SI, Framingham anger-in, Framingham anger-out, and systolic blood pressure changes were only observed in subjects who were high on hostility as measured by the Buss-Durkee Hostility Inventory. Potential for hostility, scored using the Dembroski components system, was correlated regardless of level of hostility (Diamond, Schneiderman, Schwartz, et al., 1984). The additive, but not the interactive, relationship was observed in a subsequent study of angiography patients (MacDougall, Dembroski, Dimsdale et al., 1985).

The potential importance of this interaction is that both an enduring style of appraisal and a characteristic style of coping with this appraisal may be important to the prediction of CHD endpoints.

Individual psychomotor stylistics

The measurement of individual psychomotor stylistics that occur during the interview presents an alternative to the use of clinical judgements of behaviour type or of psychological traits. The advantage of this approach is that it preserves the unobtrusiveness of observational assessment but reduces reliance on subjective judgement. A tension exists between validity and reliability. The more specific and well defined an indicator, the more reliably it can be assessed (Mischel, 1968), but in the process of this operationalization the meaning of the indicator could be altered. For this approach to provide an alternative to clinical judgements, it must be shown that individual stylistics can be identified that can be measured with good reliability and also be valid as predictors of hard CHD endpoints. There is more homogeneity within behavioural ratings than there is within content items (Anderson and Waldron, 1983) but variation within behavioural ratings still exists. Average interjudge reliabilities for sets of indicators ranging from 4 to 14 exceeded 0.65 (Anderson and Waldron, 1983; Blumenthal, O'Toole, and Haney, 1984; Guggisberg, Laederach, and Adler, 1981; Scherwitz, Berton, and Leventhal, 1977). Assessments of test–retest reliabilities of the observer (the same judge scoring the same interview on two occasions) were less common, but those that were conducted exceeded 0.75 (Powell and Thoresen, 1985; Schucker and Jacobs, 1977). The test–retest reliability of the subject (the persistence of the behaviour in a subject over time) was studied in only one investigation (Blumenthal, O'Toole, and Haney, 1984). Eleven behaviours observed twice, four months apart, revealed fair stability (mean = 0.45), but wide variability, in individual cases (range = 0.10 to 0.68).

Table 8 presents selected individual psychomotor stylistics and summaries of their reliability and validity. This table demonstrates that considerable variability exists among various indicators, with those requiring the most judgement being rated with the least reliability. What is most notable, however, is the presence of certain indicators that can be measured with excellent reliability and are also valid predictors of either global SI judgements or CHD endpoints. Some examples of these indicators include latency of response, emphasis in speech, emphatic content, and self-references.

Investigations which have measured individual indicators and combined these indicators into one score have achieved accurate predictions of recurrent MI (Powell and Thoresen, 1985) and have shown to be more reliable and valid than global Type A ratings (Mayes, Sime, and Ganster, 1984). More work in this area is needed.

SUMMARY AND IMPLICATIONS FOR FUTURE RESEARCH

The purpose of this review was to examine problems in the measurement of the TABP which could serve to confound the association between this risk factor and CHD. These problems can be summarized into three major points.

First, there is a need to establish criteria by which the integrity of Type A measures can be determined. A common practice in epidemiology is to assemble items from pre-existing data sets that appear to be valid indices of a psychosocial risk factor, and then use these items to study the relationship between the risk factor and disease endpoints. The assumption behind this practice is that face validity is sufficient to justify the relationship between the items and the risk factor. In Type A research, this practice has led to the publication of a large number of studies. But interpretations are difficult

Table 8: Reliability and validity of selected Type A psychomotor stylistics (1)

Indicator	Observer Reliability: Interjudge	Observer Reliability: Test–Retest	Subject Reliability: Test–Retest	Predictive Validity
speed of speech	r=.63, .65, .78 agree=90%		.58 (16 wks)	Rosenman SI
uneven speech	r=.49, .84		.26 (16 wks)	Rosenman SI
speech volume	r=.60, .65		.57 (16 wks)	Rosenman SI
interruptions	r=1.00		.64 (16 wks)	Rosenman SI
latency of response	r=.95, .98 agree=92%		.43 (16 wks)	Rosenamn SI, Bortner Rating Scale
emphasis in speech	r=.67, .84	r=.70 (4 wks)		Rosenman SI, Bortner Rating Scale, recurrent MI
talk time				Rosenman SI
plosive words	r=.50, .68, .90		.60 (16 wks)	Rosenman SI, Bortner Rating Scale
eye tension	r=.04	r=.74 (4 wks)		recurrent MI
demonstrative movement	r=.30	r=.60 (4 wks)		recurrent MI
hurried pace				Rosenman SI
emphatic content	r=.80	r=.71 (4 wks)		recurrent MI
self-references	r=.95	r=.91 (4 wks)		recurrent MI, coronary occlusion, systolic BP

(1) *Studies reviewed in this table are: Anderson & Waldron, 1983; Blumenthal, O'Toole & Haney, 1984; Guggisberg, Laederich & Adler, 1981; Lovallo & Pishkin, 1980; Powell & Thoresen, 1985; Scherwitz, Berton & Leventhal, 1977; Scherwitz, McKelvain, Laman et al., 1983; and Schucker & Jacobs, 1977.*

because generalizations about the construct cannot be separated from generalizations about the measurement of that construct. The approach in this review was to evaluate only those instruments for which construct and predictive validation has been reported. This insured that the instrument was measuring a coronary-prone part of the TABP. If standard criteria such as these were adopted by psychosocial researchers, psychometric studies of measures would be encouraged before studies of association, psychological underpinnings, or mechanisms were undertaken.

Second, this review has illustrated that all of the standard Type A measures have limitations. The most troublesome limitation, shared by observational and self-report measures, is the use of categorical assessment of behaviour type. This is a rudimentary and imprecise approach to a risk factor. Other major cardiovascular risk factors, including blood pressure, cholesterol, percent body fat, exercise activity, dietary cholesterol and fat intake are measured on precise, continuous scales. The failure to do so with the Type A risk factor stacks the cards against it. Some of the problems that have been discussed here include wide variations in estimates of the prevalence of Type A behaviour, difficulties in determining the behaviour type of the majority of subjects who fall in the centre of distributions, the reliance on less precise non-parametric statistics, and the loss of potentially important variance. A continuous conceptualization and operationalization is needed. We must begin to ask *how many* Type A characteristics one has, rather than whether one is Type A or Type B. This would permit the use of precise parametric statistics, including correlations, t-tests, analyses of variance, and regression, would reduce ambiguities associated with classification of people at the mid-range of the Type A scale, and would permit an empirical, not a subjective, determination of the point on the scale at which one's risk for CHD is increased.

The most important limitation of observational Type A measures exaggerates the problems associated with a categorical conceptualization. This is the use of subjective clinical judgements. The problems associated with clinical judgements apply not only to judgements of global Type A, but also to judgements of more specific constructs such as potential for hostility. A common design in epidemiologic research is to conduct long-term prospective studies on large numbers of subjects. Reliance on experts to determine the risk factor of interest in such designs is troublesome and costly. It would be less justifiable to raise this as an area of concern if alternatives were not available. However, there is considerable promise in the isolation of individual, molecular psychomotor behaviours that can be measured with excellent reliability and have excellent predictive validity. This approach offers an alternative to clinical judgements while still preserving the unobtrusiveness of observational assessment.

Large-scale epidemiologic research would ultimately be best served by the development of Type A questionnaires. However the main problem with existing questionnaires is that they are limited in their generalizability outside the white-collar male group on which they were normed. One direction is to isolate self-report items that predict CHD outcomes separately for sex, SES, and employment groups. Alternatively, It may be useful to develop items which are generalizable across these sociodemographic groups. The BRS is an example of this latter approach. Bortner hypothesized that if an observer could make observations of psychomotor behaviours in the subject, it was possible that the subject him/herself would also be an accurate observer. There is no compelling reason to believe that self-reports of discrete stylistics would be highly specific to particular sociodemographic groups or would be prone to social desirability bias. Unfortunately, the BRS is a combination of stylistics and trait-like generalizations. More development of this questionnaire may be in order.

A third point made in this review is that limitations of existing Type A instruments are not incorporated into designs of epidemiologic studies of association. For example, studies that include large numbers of lower SES groups, unemployed people, housewives, or subjects on beta-blocking drugs may fail to find hypothesized associations, not because the link is not there, but because of inadequacies in the measurement of the TABP among these groups. Furthermore, if the link to CHD is primarily through the promotion of arrhythmias in the absence of coronary obstruction, studies using angiography patients would be unable to detect this link. Finally, an assumption behind long-term studies of association is that the risk factor is stable over time. However, so few studies have assessed the long-term stability of measures of TABP that we simply cannot at this time make this assumption. Careful consideration must be made of issues such as these in the design of studies of association, and, more importantly, these issues should direct assessment research.

Limitations in the conceptualization and measurement of the TABP have already stimulated new directions. Many researchers are now looking for the key pathogenic components. This research direction can be construed from a measurement perspective. The idea that behaviour is related to CHD, and perhaps to other stress-related diseases, is alive and well. It is the reliance on self-perceptions of job stress, or on clinical judgements to determine behaviour type, that may be becoming outdated. Movement toward a more reliable assessment of an array of valid coronary-prone behaviours may be an important new direction for furthering our understanding of the behaviour–CHD link.

REFERENCES

Adler, R., MacRitchie, K., and Engel, G. (1971). Psychologic processes and ischemic stroke, *Psychosomatic Medicine*, **33**, 1–29.

Anastasi, A. (1982). *Psychological Testing, Fifth Edition*, MacMillan, New York.
Anderson, J. R., and Waldron, I. (1983). Behavioral and content components of the Structured Interview assessment of the Type A behaviour pattern in women, *Journal of Behavioral Medicine*, **6**, 123–34.
Appels, A., Jenkins, C. D., and Rosenman, R. H. (1982). Coronary-prone behaviour in the Netherlands: A cross-cultural validation study, *Journal of Behavioral Medicine*, **5**, 83–90.
Bandura, A. (1977). *Social Learning Theory*, Prentice-Hall, Englewood Cliffs.
Barefoot, J. C., Dahlstrom, W. G., and Williams, R. B. (1983). Hostility, CHD incidence, and total mortality: A 25-year follow-up study of 255 physicians, *Psychosomatic Medicine*, **45**, 59–63.
Barton, S., Brautigan, M., Fogle, G., Frietas, R., and Hicks, R. A. (1982). Type A–B behavior and the incidence of allergies in college students, *Psychological Reports*, **50**, 566.
Barton, S., and Hicks, R. A. (1985). Type A–B behavior and incidence of infectious mononucleosis in college students, *Psychological Reports*, **56**, 545–6.
Bass, C. (1984). Type A behaviour in patients with chest pain: Test-retest reliability and psychometric correlates of Bortner scale, *Journal of Psychosomatic Research*, **28**, 289–300.
Bass, C., and Wade, C. (1982). Type A behaviour: Not specifically pathogenic? *The Lancet*, Nov 20, 1147–50.
Bernet, A., Drivet-Perrin, J., Blanc, M. M., Ebagosti, A., Jouve, A. (1982). Type A behavior pattern in a screened female population, *Advances in Cardiology*, **29**, 96–105.
Blumenthal, J. A., O'Toole, L. C., and Haney, T. (1984). Behavioral assessment of the Type A behavior pattern, *Psychosomatic Medicine*, **46**, 415–23.
Blumenthal, J. A., Williams, R. B., Kong, Y., Schanberg, S. M., and Thompson, L. (1978). Type A behavior pattern and coronary atherosclerosis, *Circulation*, **58**, 634–39.
Bortner, R. W. (1969). A short rating scale as a potential measure of pattern A behavior, *Journal of Chronic Diseases*, **22**, 87–91.
Brand, R., Rosenman, R. H., Jenkins, C. D. et al. (unpublished manuscript). Comparison of coronary heart disease prediction in the Western Collaborative Group Study using the Standard Interview and the Jenkins Activity Survey assessments of the coronary-prone behavior pattern, University of California, Berkeley, CA.
Brozek, J., Keys, A., and Blackburn, H. (1966). Personality differences between potential coronary and non-coronary subjects, *Annals of the New York Academy of Science*, **134**, 1057–64.
Byrne, D. G., Rosenman, R. H., Schiller, E., and Chesney, M. A. (1985). Consistency and variation among instruments purporting to measure the Type A behavior pattern, *Psychosomatic Medicine*, **47**, 242–61.
Caffrey, B. (1968). Reliability and validity of personality and behavioral measures in a study of coronary heart disease, *Journal of Chronic Diseases*, **21**, 11–204.
Campbell, D. T., and Fiske, D. W. (1959). Convergent and discriminant validation by the multitrait-multimethod matrix, *Psychological Bulletin*, **56**, 81–105.
Cannon, W. B. (1915). *Bodily Changes in Pain, Hunger, Fear and Rage. An Account of Recent Researchers into the Function of Emotional Excitement*, D. Appleton and Co., New York.
Case, R. B., Heller, S. S., Case, N. B., Moss, A. J., and the Multicenter Post-Infarction Research Group (1985). Type A behavior and survival after acute myocardial infarction, *The New England Journal of Medicine*, **312**, 737–41.
Chesney, M. A., Black, G. W., Chadwick, J. H., and Rosenman, R. H. (1981).

Psychological correlates of the Type A behavior pattern, *Journal of Behavioral Medicine*, **4**, 217–29.

Cohen, J. B., and Reed, D. (1985). The Type A behavior pattern and coronary heart disease among Japanese men in Hawaii, *Journal of Behavioral Medicine*, **8**, 343–52.

Cook, T. D., and Campbell, D. T. (1979). *Quasi-Experimentation. Design and Analysis Issues for Field Settings*, Houghton Mifflin, Boston.

Cook, W. W., and Medley, D. M. (1954). Proposed hostility and pharisaic-virtue scales for the MMPI, *Journal of Applied Psychology*, **38**, 414–18.

Cottier, C., Adler, R., Vorkauf, H. et al., (1983). Pressured pattern or Type A behavior in patients with peripheral arteriovascular disease: Controlled retrospective exploratory study, *Psychosomatic Medicine*, **45**, 187–96.

Davidson, M. J., Cooper, C. L., and Chamberlain, D. (1980). Type A coronary-prone behavior and stress in senior female managers and administrators, *Journal of Occupational Medicine*, **22**, 801–5.

DeBacker, G., Kornitzer, M., Kittel, F., and Dramaix, M. (1983). Behavior, stress and psychosocial traits as risk factors, *Preventive Medicine*, **12**, 32–6.

Delamater, A. M., Albrecht, R., Smith, J., Strube, M. (1986). Cardiovascular correlates of Type A behavior components during social interaction, A paper presented to the 7th Annual Scientific Sessions of the Society of Behavioral Medicine, San Francisco, March.

Dembroski, T. M. (1978). Reliability and validity of methods used to assess coronary-prone behavior. In T. M. Dembroski, S. M. Weiss, J. L. Shields, S. G. Haynes, M. Feinleib (eds.) *Coronary-Prone Behavior*, Springer-Verlag, New York, pp. 95–106.

Dembroski, T. M., MacDougall, J. M., and Lushene, R. (1979). Interpersonal interaction and cardiovascular response in Type A subjects and coronary patients, *Journal of Human Stress*, **5**, 28–36.

Dembroski, T. M., MacDougall, J. M., Shields, J. L., Petitto, J., and Lushene, R. (1978). Components of the Type A coronary-prone behavior pattern and cardiovascular responses to psychomotor performance challenge, *Journal of Behavioral Medicine*, 159–76.

Dembroski, T. M., MacDougall, J. M., Williams, R. B., Haney, T. L., and Blumenthal, J. A. (1985). Components of Type A, hostility, and anger-in: Relationship to angiographic findings, *Psychosomatic Medicine*, **47**, 219–33.

Diamond, E. L. (1982). The role of anger and hostility in essential hypertension and coronary heart disease, *Psychological Bulletin*, **92**, 410–33.

Diamond, E. L., Schneiderman, N., Schwartz, D., Smith, J. C., Vorp, R., and DeCarlo Pasin, R. (1984). Harassment, hostility, and Type A as determinants of cardiovascular reactivity during competition, *Journal of Behavioral Medicine*, **7**, 171–89.

Dimsdale, J. E., Gilbert, J., Hutter, A. M., Hackett, T. P., and Block, P. C. (1981). Predicting cardiac morbidity based on risk factors and coronary angiographic findings, *The American Journal of Cardiology*, **47**, 73–6.

Eaker, E. D., Feinleib, M., and Wolf, P. (1983). Psychosocial factors and the ten-year incidence of cerebrovascular accident in the Framingham Heart Study, *American Heart Association Cardiovascular Disease Epidemiology Newsletter*, **33**, 54.

v. Eiff, A. W., Friedrich, G., Neus, H., Ruddel, H., and Schmieder, R. (1982). Effects of B-blockers on Type-A coronary-prone behaviour, *Klinische Wochenschrift*, **60**, 1315–6.

Eysenck, H. J., and Fulker, D. (1982). The components of Type A behavior and its genetic determinants, *Activitas Nervosa Superior* (Praha) Supplement, **3**, 111–25.

Fleiss, J. L. (1977). *Statistical Methods For Rates and Proportions* (2nd Edition), John Wiley, New York.

Frankenhaeuser, M. (1983). The sympathetic-adrenal and pituitary-adrenal response to challenge: Comparison between the sexes. In T. M. Dembroski, T. H. Schmidt, and G. Blumchen (eds.) *Biobehavioural Bases of Coronary Heart Disease*, Karger, Basel, Switzerland, pp. 91–105.

French-Belgian Collaborative Group (1982). Ischemic heart disease and psychological patterns. Prevalence and incidence studies in Belgium and France, *Advances in Cardiology*, **29**, 25–31.

Friedman, E. H., Hellerstein, H. K., Eastwood, G. L., and Jones, S. E. (1968). Behavior patterns and serum cholesterol in two groups of normal males, *The American Journal of the Medical Sciences*, **255**, 237–44.

Friedman, H. S., Hall, J. A., and Harris, M. J. (1985). Type A behavior, nonverbal expressive style and health, *Journal of Personality and Social Psychology*, **48**, 1299–315.

Friedman, M., and Powell, L. H. (1984). The diagnosis and quantitative assessment of Type A behavior: Introduction and description of the Videotaped Structured Interview, *Integrative Psychiatry*, July-August, 123–9.

Friedman, M., and Rosenman, R. H. (1974). *Type A Behavior and Your Heart*, Knopf, New York.

Friedman, M., Thoresen, C. E., Gill, J. J., Powell, L. H., Ulmer, D., Thompson, L., Price, V. A., Rabin, D. D., Breall, W. S., Dixon, T., Levy, R., and Bourg, E. (1984). Alteration of Type A behavior and reduction in cardiac recurrences in postmyocardial infarction patients, *American Heart Journal*, **108**, 237–48.

Friedman, M., Thoresen, C. E., Gill, J. J., Ulmer, D., Powell, L. H., Price, V. A., Brown, B., Thompson, L., Rabin, D. D., Breall, W. S., Bourg, E., Levy, R., and Dixon, T. (1986). Alteration of Type A behavior and its effect upon cardiac recurrences in post myocardial infarction subjects: Summary results of the Recurrent Coronary Prevention Project, *American Heart Journal*, **112**, 653–65.

Friedman, M., Thoresen, C. E., Gill, J. J., Ulmer, D., Thompson, L., Powell, L., Price, V., Elek, S. R., Rabin, D. D., Breall, W. S., Piaget, G., Dixon, T., Bourg, E., Levy, R. A., and Tasto, D. (1982). Feasibility of altering Type A behavior pattern after myocardial infarction. Recurrent Coronary Prevention Project Study: Methods, baseline results, and preliminary findings, *Circulation*, **66**, 83–92.

Friedman, M., and Ulmer, D. (1984). *Treating Type A Behavior and Your Heart*, Knopf, New York.

Gallacher, J. E. J., Yarnell, J. W. G., Elwood, P. C. and Phillips, K. M. (1984). Type A behaviour and heart disease prevalent in men in the Caerphilly study, *British Medical Journal*, **289**, 732–3.

Gianturco, D. T., Breslin, M. S., Heyman, A. et al. (1974). Personality patterns and life stress in ischemic cerebrovascular disease: Psychiatric findings, *Stroke*, **5**, 453–60.

Glass, D. C. (1977). Behavior Patterns, Stress and Coronary Disease, Erlbaum, Hillsdale, New Jersey.

Gough, H. H., and Heilburn, A. B. (1975). *The Adjective Checklist*, Consulting Psychologists Press, Palo Alto, California.

Guggisberg, R., Laederach, K., and Adler, R. (1981). Formal speech stylistics and Type A behavior in 38 subjects during nonstress interviews, *Psychotherapy and Psychosomatics*, **36**, 86–91.

Haynes, S. G. (1984). Type A behavior, employment status, and coronary heart disease in women, *Behavioral Medicine Update*, **6**, 11–15.

Haynes, S. G., Feinleib, M., and Kannel, W. B. (1980). The relationship of psychosocial factors to coronary heart disease in the Framingham study. III. Eight-year incidence of coronary heart disease, *American Journal of Epidemiology*, **111**, 37–58.

Haynes, S. G., Feinleib, M., Levine, S., Scotch, N., and Kannel, W. B. (1978). The relationship of psychosocial factors to coronary heart disease in the Framingham study. II. Prevalence of coronary heart disease, *American Journal of Epidemiology*, **107**, 384–402.

Haynes, S. G., Levine, S., Scotch, N., Feinleib, M., and Kannel, W. B. (1978). The relationship of psychosocial factors to coronary heart disease in the Framingham study. I. Methods and risk factors, *American Journal of Epidemiology*, **107**, 362–83.

Herbertt, R. M., and Innes, J. M. (1982). Type A coronary-prone behavior pattern, self-consciousness, and self-monitoring: A questionnaire study, *Perceptual and Motor Skills*, **55**, 471–8.

Herman, S., Blumenthal, J. A., Black, G. M., and Chesney, M. A. (1981). Self-ratings of Type A (coronary prone) adults: Do Type A's know they are Type A's?, *Psychosomatic Medicine*, **43**, 405–13.

Hicks, R. A., and Campbell, J. (1983). Type A–B behavior and self-estimates of the frequency of headaches in college students, *Psychological Reports*, **52**, 912.

Howland, E. W., and Siegman, A. W. (1982). Toward the automated measurement of the Type A behavior pattern, *Journal of Behavioral Medicine*, **5**, 37–54.

Hunter, S., MacD., J. M., Wolf, T. M., Sklov, M. C., Webber, L. S., Watcon, R. M., and Berenson, G. S. (1982). Type A coronary-prone behavior pattern and cardiovascular risk factor variables in children and adolescents: The Bogalusa Heart Study, *Journal of Chronic Diseases*, **35**, 613–21.

Irvine, J., Lyle, R. C., and Allon, R. (1982). Type A personality as psychopathology: Personality correlates and an abbreviated scoring system, *Journal of Psychosomatic Research*, **26**, 183–9.

Jenkins, C. D., Rosenman, R. H., and Friedman, M. (1967). Development of an objective psychological test for the determination of the coronary-prone behavior pattern in employed men, *Journal of Chronic Diseases*, **20**, 371–9.

Jenkins, C. D., Rosenman, R. H., and Friedman, M. (1968). Replicability of rating the coronary-prone behaviour pattern, *British Journal of Preventive and Social Medicine*, **22**, 16–22.

Jenkins, C. D., Rosenman, R. H., and Zyzanski, S. J. (1974). Prediction of clinical coronary heart disease by a test for the coronary-prone behavior pattern, *The New England Journal of Medicine*, **290**, 1271–5.

Jenkins, C. D., Zyzanski, S. J., and Rosenman, R. H. (1971). Progress toward validation of a computer-scored test for the Type A coronary-prone behavior pattern, *Psychosomatic Medicine*, **33**, 193–202.

Jenkins, C. D., Zyzanski, S. J., and Rosenman, R. H. (1976). Risk of new myocardial infarction in middle-aged men with manifest coronary heart disease, *Circulation*, **53**, 342–7.

Jenkins, C. D., Zyzanski, S. J., and Rosenman, R. H. (1978). Coronary-prone behavior: One pattern or several?, *Psychosomatic Medicine*, **40**, 25–43.

Jenkins, C. D., Zyzanski, S. J., and Rosenman, R. H. (1979). *The Jenkins Activity Survey for Health Prediction*, The Psychological Corporation, New York.

Jenkins, C. D., Zyzanski, S. J., Ryan, T. J., Flessas, A., and Tannenbaum, S. I. (1977). Social insecurity and coronary-prone Type A responses as identifiers of severe atherosclerosis, *Journal of Consulting and Clinical Psychology*, **45**, 1060–7.

Jenkins, C. D., Zyzanski, S. J., Rosenman, R. H., and Cleveland, G. L. (1971).

Association of coronary-prone behavior scores with recurrence of coronary heart disease, *Journal of Chronic Diseases*, **24**, 601–11.

Jennings, J. R. (1984). Cardiovascular reactions and impatience in Type A and B college students, *Psychosomatic Medicine*, **46**, 424–40.

Johnston, D. W., and Shaper, A. G. (1983). Type A behaviour in British men: Reliability and intercorrelation of two measures, *Journal of Chronic Diseases*, **36**, 203–7.

Kaplan, J. R., Manuck, S. B., Clarkson, T. B., Lusso, F. M., Taub, D. B., and Miller, E. W. (1983). Social stress and atherosclerosis in normocholesterolemic monkeys, *Science*, **200**, 733–5.

Keith, R. A., Lown, B., and Stare, F. J. (1965). Coronary heart disease and behavior patterns: An examination of method, *Psychosomatic Medicine*, **27**, 424–34.

Kelly, K. E., and Houston, B. K. (1985). Type A behavior in employed women: Relation to work, marital, and leisure variables, social support, stress, tension, and health, *Journal of Personality and Social Psychology*, **48**, 1067–79.

Kittel, F., Kornitzer, M., Zyzanski, S. J., Jenkins, C. D., Rustin, R. M., and Degre, C. (1978). Two methods of assessing the Type A coronary-prone behaviour pattern in Belgium, *Journal of Chronic Diseases*, **31**, 147–55.

Koskenvuo, M., Kaprio, J., Langinvainio, H., and Romo, M. (1983). Mortality in relation to coronary-prone behavior; a six year follow-up of the Bortner scale in middle-aged Finnish men, *Activas Nervosa Superior*, **25**, 107–9.

Krantz, D. S., Durel, L. A., Davia, J. E., Shaffer, R. T., Arabian, J. M., Dembroski, T. M., and MacDougall, J. M. (1982). Propranolol medication among coronary patients: Relationship to Type A behavior and cardiovascular response, *Journal of Human Stress*, **8**, 4–12.

Krantz, D. S., and Manuck, S. B. (1984). Acute psychophysiologic reactivity and risk of cardiovascular disease: A review and methodologic critique, *Psychological Bulletin*, **96**, 435–64.

Lawler, K. A., Rixse, A., and Allen, M. T. (1983). Type A behavior and psychophysiological responses in adult women, *Psychophysiology*, **20**, 343–50.

Leak, G. K., and McCarthy, K. (1984). Relationship between Type A behavior subscales and measures of positive mental health, *Journal of Clinical Psychology*, **40**, 1406–8.

Lovallo, W. R., and Pishkin, V. (1980). Type A behavior, self-involvement, autonomic activity, and the traits of neuroticism and extraversion, *Psychosomatic Medicine*, **42**, 329–41.

Lown, B., Verrier, R., and Corbalan, R. (1973). Psychologic stress and threshold for repetitive ventricular response, *Science*, **182**, 834–6.

Lown, B., Verrier, R. L., and Rabinowitz, S. H. (1977). Neural and psychologic mechanisms and the problem of sudden death, *American Journal of Cardiology*, **39**, 890–902.

MacDougall, J. M., Dembroski, T. M., Dimsdale, J. E., and Hackett, T. P. (1985). Components of Type A, hostility, and anger-in: Further relationships to angiographic findings, *Health Psychology*, **4**, 137–52.

MacDougall, J. M., Dembroski, T. M., and Krantz, D. S. (1981). Effects of types of challenge on pressor and heart rate responbses in Type A and B women, *Psychophysiology*, **18**, 1–9.

MacDougall, J. M., Dembroski, T. M., and Musante, L. (1979). The structured interview and questionnaire methods of assessing coronary-prone behavior in male and female college students, *Journal of Behavioral Medicine*, **2**, 71–82.

Manuck, S. B., Craft, S. J., and Gold, K. J. (1978). Coronary-prone behavior pattern and cardiovascular response, *Psychophysiology*, **15**, 403–11.

Matthews, K. A. (1982). Psychological perspectives in the Type A behavior pattern, *Psychological Bulletin*, **91**, 293–323.

Matthews, K. A. (1985). Assessment of Type A behavior, anger, and hostility in epidemiological studies of cardiovascular disease. In A. M. Ostfeld, and E. D. Eaker (eds.) *Measuring Psychosocial Variables in Epidemiologic Studies of Cardiovascular Disease*, NIH Publication No. 85–2270, US Department of Health and Human Services, March, 1985, pp. 153–83.

Matthews, K. A., Glass, D. C., Rosenman, R. H., and Bortner, R. W. (1977). Competitive drive, pattern A, and coronary heart disease: A further analysis of some data from the Western Collaborative Group Study, *Journal of Chronic Diseases*, **30**, 489–98.

Matthews, K. A., and Haynes, S. G. (1986). Type A behavior pattern and coronary risk: Update and critical evaluation, *American Journal of Epidemiology*, **6**, 923–60.

Matthews, K. A., Krantz, D., Dembroski, T., and MacDougall, J. (1982). Unique and common variance in structured interview and Jenkins Activity Survey measures of Type A behavior pattern, *Journal of Personality and Social Psychology*, **42**, 303–13.

Matthews, K. A., and Saal, F. E. (1978). Relationship of the Type A coronary-prone behavior pattern to achievement, power, and affiliation motives, *Psychosomatic Medicine*, **40**, 631–6.

Mayes, B. T., Sime, W. E., and Ganster, D. C. (1984). Convergent validity of Type A behavior pattern scales and their ability to predict physiological responsiveness in a sample of female public employees, *Journal of Behavioral Medicine*, **7**, 83–108.

Menninger, J. C. (1985). The validity of Type A behavior scales for employed women, *Journal of Chronic Diseases*, **38**, 375–83.

Mischel, W. (1968). *Personality and Assessment*, Wiley, New York.

Morell, M. A., and Katkin, E. S. (1982). Jenkins Activity Survey scores among women of different occupations, *Journal of Consulting and Clinical Psychology*, **50**, 588–9.

Moss, G. E. (1984). The sociodemographic distribution of Type A behavior in population sample, *Psychosomatic Medicine*, **46**, 85.

The Multiple Risk Factor Intervention Trial Group (1979). The MRFIT behavior pattern study. I. Study design, procedures, and reproducibility of behavior pattern judgements, *Journal of Chronic Diseases*, **32**, 293–305.

Musante, L., MacDougall, J. M., Dembroski, T. M., Van Horn, A. E. (1983). Component analysis of the Type A coronary prone behavior pattern in male and female college students, *Journal of Personality and Social Psychology*, **45**, 1104–17.

Nunnally, J. C. (1978). *Psychometric Theory, Second Edition*, McGraw-Hill, New York.

Powell, L. H., and Fleischmann, N. (in press). The predictive validity of the Videotaped Structured Interview: A test for diagnosing Type A behavior, *American Journal of Epidemiology*.

Powell, L. H., Friedman, M., Thoresen, C. E., Gill, J. J., and Ulmer, D. K. (1984). Can the Type A behavior pattern be altered after myocardial infarction? A second year report from the Recurrent Coronary Prevention Project, *Psychosomatic Medicine*, **46**, 293–313.

Powell, L. H., Friedman, M., Thoresen, C. E., Gill, J. J., and Ulmer, D. K. (1986). Survival in high- and low-risk coronary patients following behavioral counseling. A paper presented to the 26th Annual Conference on Cardiovascular Disease Epidemiology, San Francisco, March.

Powell, L. H., and Thoresen, C. E. (1985). Behavioral and physiologic determinants of long-term prognosis after myocardial infarction, *Journal of Chronic Diseases*, **38**, 253–63.

Price, K. P. (1979). Reliability of assessment of coronary-prone behaviour with special reference to the Bortner rating scale, *Journal of Psychosomatic Research*, **23**, 45–7.

Ragland, D. R., Brand, R. J., and Rosenman, R. H. (1986). Type A behavior pattern and CHD mortality among 257 cases in the Western Collaborative Group Study, a paper presented to the 26th Annual Conference on Cardiovascular Disease Epidemiology, San Francisco, March.

Review Panel on Coronary-Prone Behavior and Coronary Heart Disease (1981). Coronary-prone behavior and coronary heart disease: A critical review, *Circulation*, **63**, 1199–215.

Robinson, N., and Fuller, J. H. (1981). Type A (coronary prone) behaviour in diabetics, *The Lancet*, August 8, 314.

Rosenman, R. H. (1978). The interview method of assessment of the coronary-prone behavior pattern. In T. M. Dembroski, S. M. Weiss, J. L. Shields, S. G. Haynes, M. Feinleib (eds.) *Coronary-prone behavior*, Springer-Verlag, New York, pp. 55–69.

Rosenman, R. H., Brand, R. J., Jenkins, C. D., Friedman, M., Straus, R., and Wurm, M. (1975). Coronary heart disease in the Western Collaborative Group Study: Final follow-up experience of 8½ years, *Journal of the American Medical Association*, 233, 872–7.

Rosenman, R. H., and Friedman, M. (1961). Association of specific behavior pattern in women with blood and cardiovascular findings, *Circulation*, **24**, 1173–84.

Rosenman, R. H., Friedman, M., Straus, R., Jenkins, C. D., Zyzanski, S. J., and Wurm, M. (1970). Coronary heart disease in the Western Collaborative Group Study. A follow-up experience of 4½ years, *Journal of Chronic Diseases*, **23**, 173–90.

Rosenman, R. H., Friedman, M., Straus, R., Wurm, M., Jenkins, C. D., and Messinger, H. B. (1966). Coronary heart disease in the Western Collaborative Group Study. A follow-up experience of two years, *Journal of the American Medical Association*, **195**, 130–6.

Rosenman, R. H., Friedman, M., Straus, R., Wurm, M., Kositchek, R., Hahn, W., and Werthessen, N. T. (1964a). A predictive study of coronary heart disease: Appendix, *Journal of the Amercian Medical Associations*, **189**, 1–4.

Rosenman, R. H., Friedman, M., Straus, R., Wurm, M., Kositchek, R., Hahn, W., and Werthessen, N. T. (1964b). A predictive study of coronary heart disease, *Journal of the American Medical Association*, **189**, 113–24.

Ruberman, W., Weinblatt, E., Goldberg, J. D., and Chaudhary, B. S. (1984). Psychosocial influences on mortality after myocardial infarction, *New England Journal of Medicine*, **311**, 552–95.

Scherwitz, L. (1985). The Type A behavior pattern and coronary heart disease: Issues and problems, a paper presented to the Sixth Annual Scientific Sessions of the Society of Behavioral Medicine, New Orleans.

Scherwitz, L., Berton, K., and Leventhal, H. (1977). Type A assessment and interaction in the behavior pattern interview, *Psychosomatic Medicine*, **39**, 229–40.

Scherwitz, L., McKelvain, R., Laman, C., Patterson, J., Dutton, L., Yusim, S., Lester, J., Kraft, I., Rochelle, D., and Leachman, R. (1983). Type A behavior, self-involvement, and coronary atherosclerosis, *Psychosomatic Medicine*, **45**, 47–57.

Schmidt, T. H., Undeutsch, K., Dembroski, T. M., Langosch, W., Neus, H., and Ruddel, H. (1982). Coronary prone behavior and cardiovascular reactions during the German version of the Type A interview and during a quiz, *Activitas Nervosa Superior*, Supplement 3(pt. 2), 241–51.

Schmieder, R., Friedrich, G., Neus, H., et al. (1983). The influence of beta-blockers on cardiovascular reactivity and type A behavior pattern in hypertensives, *Psychosomatic Medicine*, **45**, 417–23.

Shekelle, R., Gale, M., Norusis, M., for the Aspirin Myocardial Infarction Study Research Group. (1985). Type A score (Jenkins Activity Survey) and risk of recurrent coronary heart disease in the Aspirin Myocardial Infarction Study, *American Journal of Cardiology*, **56**, 221–25.

Shekelle, R. B., Gale, M., Ostfeld, A. M., and Paul, O. (1983). Hostility, risk of coronary heart disease, and mortality, *Psychosomatic Medicine*, **45**, 109–14.

Shekelle, R. B., Hulley, S. B., Neaton, J. D., Billings, J. H., Borhani, N. O., Gerace, T. A., Jacobs, D. R., Lasser, N. L., Milltemark, M. B., and Stamler, J. for the Multiple Risk Factor Intervention Trial Research Group (1985). The MRFIT behavior pattern study. II. Type A behavior and incidence of coronary heart disease, *American Journal of Epidemiology*, **122**, 559–70.

Shekelle, R. B., Schoenberger, J. A., and Stamler, J. (1976). Correlates of the JAS Type A behavior pattern score, *Journal of Chronic Disease*, **29**, 381–394.

Shucker, B., and Jacobs, D. R. (1977). Assessment of behavioral risk for coronary disease by voice characteristics, *Psychosomatic Medicine*, **39**, 219–28.

Smith, T. W., Follick, M. J., and Koor, K. S. (1984). Anger, neuroticism, Type A behaviour and the experience of angina, *British Journal of Medical Psychology*, **57**, 249–52.

Smith, J. C., Gerace, T. A., Christakis, G., and Kafatos, A. (1985). Cross-cultural validity of the Miami Structured Interview-1 for Type A in children: The American-Hellenic Heart Study, *Journal of Chronic Diseases*, **38**, 793–9.

Smyth, K., Call, J., Hansell, S., Sparacino, J., Strodbeck, F. L. (1978). Type A behaviour and hypertension among inner-city black women, *Nursing Research*, **27**, 30–5.

Stevens, J. H., Turner, C. W., Rhodewalt, F., and Talbot, S. (1984). The Type A behavior pattern and carotid artery atherosclerosis, *Psychosomatic Medicine*, **46**, 105–113.

Stockwell, N., Zyzanski, S. J., and Yodfat, Y. (1985). Type A behaviour in two ethnic rural communities of males in Israel with and without coronary heart disease, *Social Science in Medicine*, **20**, 331–4.

Stout, C. W., and Bloom, L. J. (1982). Type A behavior and upper respiratory infections, *Journal of Human Stress*, June 4–7.

Tasto, D. L., Chesney, M. A., and Chadwick, J. H. (1978). Multi-dimensional analysis of coronary-prone behavior. In T. M. Dembroski, S. M. Weiss, J. L. Shields, S. G. Haynes, M. Feinleib (eds.) *Coronary-Prone Behavior*, Springer-Verlag, New York, pp. 107–18.

Thurstone, L. L. (1953). *Thurstone Temperment Schedule*, Science Research Associates, Chicago.

Verhagen, F., Nass, C., Appels, A., van Bastelaer,, A., and Winnubst, J. (1980). Cross-validation of the A/B typology in the Netherlands, *Psychotherapy and Psychosomatics*, **34**, 178–86.

Waldron, I. (1978). The coronary-prone behavior pattern, blood pressure, and socioeconomic status in women, *Journal of Psychosomatic Research*, **22**, 79–87.

Williams, R. B., Barefoot, J. C., and Shekelle, R. B. (1985). The health consequences of hostility. In M. A. Chesney and R. H. Rosenman (eds.) *Anger and Hostility in Cardiovascular and Behavioral Disorders*, Hemisphere, Washington, pp. 173–85.

Williams, R. B., Haney, T. L., Lee, K. L., Kong, Y., Blumenthal, J. A., and Whalen, R. E. (1980). Type A behavior, hostility, and coronary atherosclerosis, *Psychosomatic Medicine*, **42**, 539–49.

Woods, P. J., Morgan, B. T., Day, B. W., Jefferson, T., and Harris, C. (1984). Findings on a relationship between Type A behavior and headaches, *Journal of Behavioral Medicine*, **7**, 277–86.

Young, L. D., and Barboriak, J. J. (1982). Reliability of a brief scale for assessment of coronary-prone behavior and standard measures of Type A behavior, *Perceptual and Motor Skills*, **55**, 1039–42.

Zyzanski, S. J. (1978). Coronary-prone behavior pattern and coronary heart disease: Epidemiological evidence. In T. M. Dembroski, S. M. Weiss, J. L. Shields, S. G. Haynes, and M. Feinleib (eds.) *Coronary-Prone Behavior*, Springer-Verlag, New York, pp. 25–40.

Chapter 10

Measurement of Coping

Frances Cohen, Ph.D

Graduate Program in Health Psychology
University of California, San Francisco

Coping is increasingly implicated as an important factor influencing recovery from illness and surgery and mediating the relationship between stress and illness outcomes (Cohen, 1979; Cohen and Lazarus, 1979, 1983; Elliott and Eisdorfer, 1982; Jenkins, 1979). However, researchers wanting to measure coping often despair at the lack of consensus about how to measure it. The aim of this chapter is to review current measures of coping and to provide a framework within which they can be evaluated. To set the stage, a number of key issues concerning coping assessment are first discussed. For an introduction to other issues in the coping field see Lazarus and Folkman (1984), Lazarus (1966), Coelho, Hamburg, and Adams (1974), and Cohen and Lazarus (1979, 1983).

Because of the vast array of studies purporting to measure coping, this chapter will not be exhaustive in its review. For other reviews of coping measures sees Moos and Billings (1982), Haan (1982), and Moos (1974). This chapter will focus only on assessment of individual coping strategies measured from interviews or self-report questionnaires, thereby excluding coping ratings derived from case materials (e.g. Haan, 1963, 1969, 1977; Vaillant, 1976, 1977). It will for the most part include only coping measures that have been used in more than one study, thus eliminating the numerous unique coping measures utilized only once.

GENERAL ISSUES

Definition of coping

Coping is defined here as 'efforts, both action-oriented and intrapsychic, to manage (that is, master, tolerate, reduce, minimize) environmental and internal demands, and conflicts among them, which tax or exceed a person's resources' (Cohen and Lazarus, 1979, p. 219). Coping can occur in anticipation of a stressful confrontation or in reaction to a present or past

Research Methods in Stress and Health Psychology. Edited by S. V. Kasl and C. L. Cooper.

situation. This definition is intended to be broad, including within it both 'defences' and 'coping' strategies that other investigators have studied separately (e.g. Haan, 1963, 1969, 1977; Kroeber, 1963). Thus 'coping' and 'coping processes' refer to any efforts to manage demands, including processes that others might label as defences.

Functions of coping

Coping may serve one of two functions: problem-solving or emotion-regulation (Hamburg, Coelho, and Adams, 1974; Lazarus, 1975). Problem-solving functions involve dealing with internal or environmental demands that create threat, such as studying for an exam or confronting a noisy neighbour. Emotion-regulating functions involve efforts to modify the distress that accompanies threat—for example, by denying that the threat exists or by drinking to excess. Folkman and Lazarus' (1980) Ways of Coping scale and Billings and Moos' (1981) coping scheme can be used to differentiate problem-focused and emotion-focused coping. Pearlin and Schooler (1978) consider three functions of coping, making a separate distinction between modes that control the meaning of the situation and those that control the emotional response itself (see also Moos and Billings, 1982). Numerous researchers who have developed their own coping instruments have used the distinction between problem-focused coping and emotion-focused coping to guide their scale development. However, the distinction is not always easy to make, since a similar behaviour can serve several functions. Folkman, Lazarus, Dunkel-Schetter, DeLongis, and Gruen (1986) recently suggested that one may need to know the context before being able to distinguish which function a coping strategy serves. Most people use both types of strategies simultaneously. In Folkman and Lazarus' (1980) study of a community sample of middle-aged men and women, they found that both modes were used in 98 per cent of the episodes.

Modes of coping

Modes of coping represent broad categories of strategies that vary in certain structural properties. Five modes of coping can be identified: information-seeking, direct action, inhibition of action, intrapsychic processes, and turning to others for support (Cohen and Lazarus, 1979, 1983). Information-seeking involves trying to learn more about the situation and about what can be done to deal with it. Direct actions include any concrete behavioural act, such as building a fence, taking tranquilizers, or confronting a friend about a problem that is interfering with the friendship. Inhibition of action involves *not* doing something, such as inhibiting movement to avoid the pain of walking or refraining from striking out though provoked. Intrapsychic processes involve ways of reappraising the situation, for example by denying the threat or distracting oneself, and include those processes that traditionally are called defences. Turning to others for support is also a mode of coping that may enhance one's feelings of well-being or one's efforts to deal with unexpected events. Coping scales vary in terms of how many of these modes are assessed. Some tap only intrapsychic processes (e.g. Gleser and Ihilevich, 1969) or a limited number of modes (e.g. Stone and Neale, 1984).

Outcomes of coping

Some researchers confuse the study of coping modes with the outcomes of coping, thus labelling as 'copers' those who show little emotional distress or decreased physiological response. This is a special problem in the animal literature, where it appears to be the dominant view (e.g. Ursin, 1980). This creates conceptual confusion and assumes a simplistic relationship between coping and outcome. Coping can have effects in three domains: psychological, social, and physiological. Psychological outcomes include emotional reactions (e.g. how depressed or anxious one is), general well-being, and performance on tasks. Social outcomes studied include changes in interpersonal relationships and in the ability to fulfill social roles. Physiological outcomes run the gamut from short-term physiological reactions (autonomic nervous system, hormonal, immunological, and neuroregulator changes) to long-term health changes (e.g. development of coronary heart disease). Since a particular coping mode can have different effects on psychological, social, and physiological outcomes, it is important to keep these concepts separate and study their interrelationships.

Adaptiveness of coping

Researchers, health practitioners, and the public want to know which coping modes are most adaptive, but that question cannot be simply answered. The adaptiveness of coping depends on three factors: (a) the domain of outcome studied; (b) the point in time; and (c) the context (Cohen and Lazarus, 1979). The stress literature is filled with numerous cases in which a particular coping mode may have a positive influence on outcomes in one domain of functioning and a negative influence in another (e.g. Gal and Lazarus, 1975; Katz, Weiner, Gallagher, and Hellman, 1970). A value judgement is involved in determining which outcome is most important. Short-run and long-run outcomes may also be quite different. For example, denial defences have been found to be associated with decreased mortality in the coronary care unit (Hackett, Cassem, and Wishnie, 1968) but also with decreased compliance with medical treatment one year later (Croog, Shapiro, and Levine, 1971). A meta-analysis of twenty-six studies that examined avoidant v. vigilant coping strategies in relation to measures of physical adaptation concluded that avoidant strategies resulted in better adaptation when short-run outcomes were examined, whereas vigilant strategies were associated with better outcomes when long-run outcomes were studied (Mullen and Suls, 1982).

The context must also be considered when assessing adaptiveness. A particular strategy may be adaptive in one situation but not in another. Denial-like forms of coping may reduce complications of surgery for patients facing elective hernia or gall bladder operations (Cohen and Lazarus, 1973) but may be maladaptive for patients facing life-threatening open-heart surgery, where this form of coping is associated with increased risk of post-operative delirium (Layne and Yudofsky, 1971). The expression of emotion may exacerbate symptoms for patients suffering from irreversible diffuse obstructive pulmonary syndromes (Dudley, Verhey, Masuda, Martin, and Holmes, 1969) but is associated with longer survival for patients with cancer (e.g. Derogatis, Abeloff, and Melisaratos, 1979). Further, different coping strategies may be effective for dealing with acute as compared to chronic stressors.

MEASUREMENT ISSUES

Coping measures differ in a number of important ways which will be outlined and discussed here. There are no simple answers as to which approaches are most fruitful. An investigator's choice of a coping measure will be guided by his or her theoretical assumptions and conceptual model as well as by the type of stress situation to be studied and the psychometric and predictive properties of the measure.

Dispositional (trait) v. episodic approaches

Coping can be assessed either as a disposition, trait or style, or as an episodic indicator (Averill and Opton, 1968; Cohen and Lazarus, 1973, 1979). Coping *dispositions* refer to tendencies of an individual to use a particular type of coping across a variety of stressful encounters. The person's tendency to use one or another coping mode is assessed by a questionnaire or projective measure and this test behaviour is considered as an indicator of the type of coping behaviour the individual would use in a stressful situation under study. For example, Andrew (1967, 1970) used a sentence-completion test to measure the tendency of a person to use 'coping' (sensitizing) or 'avoiding' strategies. Responses to these sentence stems were scored and used as a measure of whether subjects would be utilizing avoiding or coping strategies in response to a forthcoming surgical operation. The repression–sensitization scale developed by Byrne (1961, 1964) measures a similar dimension—the tendency to avoid or seek out threatening information—using true–false questions from the Minnesota Multiphasic Personality Inventory (MMPI).

Other investigators have measured coping processes or *episodic* coping, that is, the strategies individuals actually use in coping with a particular situation. Cohen and Lazarus (1973) interviewed patients pre-operatively and rated whether they sought or avoided information about their illness and forthcoming operation. As another example, other researchers have interviewed parents during their child's terminal illness and evaluated the defences those patients were using and the successfulness of those defences (Wolff, Friedman, Hofer, and Mason, 1964). However, the dispositional approach has been criticized for assuming consistency in coping behaviour (Cohen and Lazarus, 1979). There is little evidence of consistency in mode of coping from one situation to another, and only weak or non-significant relationships have been found between measures of coping dispositions and actual coping behaviour observed (Austin, 1974; Cohen and Lazarus, 1973; Hoffman, 1970; Kaloupek, White, and Wong, 1984). Thus coping dispositions do not seem to be predictive of how individuals actually cope in stressful situations.

Further, it appears incorrect to assume that individuals use the same coping strategies in dealing with all aspects of a particular situation. There is now considerable evidence that different modes of coping are used in dealing with different sub-areas of a stressful situation, and at different stages in a stressful encounter. For example, Cohen, Reese, Kaplan, and Riggio (1986) found that different coping modes were used in dealing with the pain of rheumatoid arthritis as compared to those used in dealing with the threats to self-esteem brought on by the disease. Different modes were used to deal with other specific stresses associated with arthritis such as mobility problems and difficulties with self-care (Cohen, Riggio, Reese, and Kaplan, in preparation). Further, several research studies have shown that there may be changes in individual coping modes during different periods of a stressful life situation (e.g. Folkman and Lazarus, 1985; Hofer, Wolff, Friedman, and Mason, 1972a, b). Horowitz (1976) and Parkes (1972) describe how individuals oscillate between denial and intrusive modes in reaction to stressful life events such as bereavement. Mages and Mendelsohn (1979) outline different demands and strategies found in the various stages of cancer, arguing that such coping should be seen as a developmental process.

It thus seems clear that a dispositional measure of coping will not be able to characterize the array of coping strategies used in dealing with a complex stressful event. However, to the extent that dispositional coping measures tap general dimensions of personality, rather than tendencies to cope in a particular way, they may be meaningfully related to health-relevant outcomes and show good predictive validity.

Dimensions of coping tapped

The choice of a coping measure depends on whether or not it taps the dimensions the investigator thinks are important theoretically or the literature shows are

Table 1: Types of Coping Dimensions Assessed by Commonly Used Measures

---

I. Trait measures
  A. Unidimensional schemes
    1. Repression–Sensitization
      a. Byrne (1961) Repression–Sensitization Scale
      b. Epstein and Fenz (1967) modified Repression–Sensitization Scale
      c. Rorschach Index of Repressive Style (Gardner, Holzman, Klein, Linton, and Spence, 1959; Levine and Spivack, 1964)
      d. Weinberger, Schwartz, and Davidson (1979) Repressive Style Index
    2. Goldstein (1959) Coping-Avoidance Sentence Completion Test (Andrew, 1967, 1970)
  B. Multidimensional Schemes
    1. Defense Mechanism Inventory (Gleser and Ihilevich, 1969)
      a. Turning Against Object
      b. Projection
      c. Principalization
      d. Turning Against Self
      e. Reversal
    2. Joffe and Naditch (1977) Coping-defence measure:
      a. coping cf. defence mechanism scale
      b. coping modes
        (1) objectivity
        (2) intellectuality
        (3) logical analysis
        (4) concentration
        (5) tolerance of ambiguity
        (6) empathy
        (7) regression in service of the ego
        (8) sublimation
        (9) substitution
        (10) suppression
      c. defence mechanisms
        (1) isolation
        (2) intellectualization
        (3) rationalization
        (4) denial
        (5) doubt
        (6) projection
        (7) regression
        (8) displacement
        (9) reaction formation
        (10) repression
      d. categories of coping and defence
        (1) controlled coping
        (2) expressive coping
        (3) structured defence
        (4) primitive defence

II. Episodic measures
    A. Unidimensional schemes
        1. Cohen Avoidance-vigilance interview (Cohen and Lazarus, 1973)
        2. Hackett and Cassem (1974) Denial Scale (Shaw, Cohen, Doyle, and Palesky, 1985)
    B. Multidimensional schemes
        1. Folkman and Lazarus (1980) Ways of Coping Scale
            a. Functions of coping
                (1) emotion-focused
                (2) problem-focused
            b. Eight coping factors (Folkman, Lazarus, Dunkel-Schetter, DeLongis, and Gruen, 1986)
                (1) confrontive coping
                (2) distancing
                (3) self-control
                (4) seeking social support
                (5) accepting responsibility
                (6) escape/avoidance
                (7) planful problem-solving
                (8) positive reappraisal
        2. Billings and Moos (1984)
            a. appraisal-focused (logical analysis)
            b. problem-focused
                (1) information-seeking
                (2) problem-solving
            c. emotion-focused
                (1) affective regulation
                (2) emotional discharge
        3. Cohen, Reese, Kaplan, and Riggio (1986) assessment of coping modes
            a. direct actions
            b. inhibition of action
            c. information seeking
            d. intrapsychic processes
            e. turning to others for support
III. Cross-dimensional schemes
    A. Coping flexibility (Cohen, Riggio, Reese, and Kaplan, in preparation; Kemeny, 1985)

---

empirically relevant. However, coping instruments vary widely in the dimensions they tap; there is no consensus about which dimensions are most useful, or the level of generality required. To illustrate the scope of the problem, Table 1 presents a list of coping dimensions assessed by some commonly used instruments. Some measure only one dimension of coping, the most common being repression–sensitization or avoidance–vigilance, that is, one's tendency to be sensitized to or avoid threatening information. Other coping measures assess multiple dimensions such as the eight factors measured in Folkman and Lazarus' Ways of Coping. A few assessment techniques are cross-dimensional, combining coping assessments across several categories in order to provide a conceptually different measure, e.g. that of coping flexibility.

The variety of dimensions listed in Table 1 is not exhaustive and is provided as background for understanding the number of different conceptualizations found in the literature. Moos and Billings (1982) have tried to incorporate a number of these dimensions into a conceptual scheme that emphasizes their similarity.

Situation-specific measures v. scales with broad applicability

Some coping scales aim for wide applicability (e.g. Folkman and Lazarus, 1980; Billings and Moos, 1981) while others are designed to measure coping in a particular context only (e.g. Weisman and Worden, 1976–7). For example, the Ways of Coping (Lazarus and Folkman, 1984) can be used to assess coping in any stressful encounter since it contains general coping items (e.g. 'stood my ground and fought for what I wanted'; 'took it out on other people'; 'I changed something about myself'). Use of this check-list yields general types of strategies but not the very specific coping responses that can be elicited in situation-specific structured coping interviews (e.g. 'applied heat packs to alleviate my pain', 'thought about others whose disease was so bad they had to stay in bed', 'hid my cane in a closet before the interview so no one would know I needed it'; Cohen et al., 1986). The situation-specific measures provide a richer portrait of how people cope and may be essential for understanding coping in situations of serious illness, where the specific strategies used vary depending on disease and treatment parameters. Some investigators have added items to the Ways of Coping in order to assess coping more accurately in a particular illness context (e.g. Nakell, 1985). Others have dropped items, questioning their appropriateness (e.g. Bachrach and Zautra, 1985). The choice of a scale thus depends on the type of situation studied, the level of generality desired, the researcher's goals, and whether consistency of coping across situations is a research question to be tested.

Interview v. self-report checklists

How can one best assess how an individual is coping in a particular situation? There are problems with just asking people how they are coping: each person may interpret the question differently, some do not know, others may forget, while others may try to present the best picture or be influenced by already knowing the outcome. Clinical evidence suggests that people may be more aware of the coping strategies they are struggling to use, or ones that are problematic, than they are of strategies they are successfully using or that have resolved the situation (Horowitz and Wilner, 1980). People may also be unaware of particular strategies that they use (e.g. seeking social support) if the strategies dovetail with life routines (e.g. daily phone calls to friends).

Nevertheless, self-report can yield important information, and studies have shown significant relationships between self-reported coping and adaptational outcomes (Lazarus and Folkman, 1984). Shrauger and Osberg (1981) suggest that self-assessments of behaviours are at least as predictive of outcomes as are other assessment methods.

An alternative to self-report is a structured interview that asks questions about how people are dealing with a situation, and what they think and feel about it. The interview responses are not taken at face value; detailed criteria are used to evaluate what the person says and to make a clinical rating about how the person is actually coping. This approach has been used extensively by Cohen and her colleagues (e.g. Cohen, 1975; Cohen and Lazarus, 1973; Cohen et al., 1986; LaMontagne, 1982; Shaw, 1984; see also Hitchcock, 1982) with good predictive validity and interrater reliability. Hackett and Cassem's (1984) Denial Interview is another example of this assessment approach (see also Shaw, Cohen, Doyle, and Palesky, 1985). However, interview methods are time-consuming and may not be feasible for some investigators.

Retrospective assessments v. coping 'as it happens'

Similar problems plague retrospective accounts of coping as those described above for self-report check-lists. If it is possible, the best solution is to assess coping 'as it happens', that is, while the person is anticipating or confronting the stressor (e.g. Cohen and Lazarus, 1973; Folkman and Lazarus, 1985; Kaloupek et al., 1984; Stone and Neale, 1984). If coping is assessed in regards to a past stressor, it may be most fruitful to examine quite recent stressors (Folkman et al., 1986, assessed coping with stressors that have occurred in the last week rather than stressors that took place during the previous month, as they had done in earlier studies).

REVIEW OF TRAIT COPING MEASURES

Repression–sensitization

Interest in the dimension of repression–sensitization grew out of the perceptual defence literature in which it was shown that some people defended against threatening stimuli (i.e. had slower reaction time to emotional words than to neutral words) while others displayed perceptual vigilance (i.e. had faster response times to emotional words than to neutral ones). This type of dimension was also represented in psychodynamic writings as a dichotomy between the defensive processes of repression and isolation (Schafer, 1954). Basically, the concept represents avoidant v. vigilant/approach ways of dealing with threatening, anxiety-evoking cues. Numerous scales have been developed to measure the concept of repression–sensitization (Byrne, 1961;

Byrne, Barry, and Nelson, 1963; Epstein and Fenz, 1967; and Weinberger, Schwartz, and Davidson, 1979), and the closely related concepts of repression–isolation (Gardner, Holzman, Klein, Linton, and Spence, 1959; Levine and Spivack, 1964), avoidance-coping (Andrew, 1970; Goldstein, 1959), and denial-intellectualization (Lazarus and Alfert, 1964).

Although the theoretical basis of these various dimensions appears to be similar, research reveals low or non-significant correlations among them (Cohen and Lazarus, 1973; Levine and Spivack, 1964; Silver, 1970). Even similar scoring techniques (e.g. for rating repressive style from the Rorschach) showed correlations of only 0.54 with each other (Levine and Spivack, 1964). The problem of low correlations between similarly-named measures plagues the coping field in general, and no definitive studies have yet indicated which may be the best measure of the concept of repression–sensitization.

The most commonly used measure is the Byrne Repression–Sensitization (R–S) Scale although it has come under considerable attack (e.g. Chabot, 1973; Golin, Herron, Lakota, and Reineck, 1967; Lazarus, Averill, and Opton, 1974; Lefcourt, 1966). The most serious problem has been the 0.9 correlation between R–S Scale and the Taylor Manifest Anxiety Scale, leading many to conclude that R–S measures nothing but manifest anxiety. Lefcourt (1966) argues that it is a measure of attitudes toward emotional expression.

Bell and Byrne (1978) review evidence of the predictive validity of the R–S scale. They also argue that some of the high correlation between the Taylor Manifest Anxiety Scale and the R–S is due to overlapping items. However, the correlation between the scales after common items are omitted is still 0.76. Bell and Byrne conclude that the R–S scale is a useful measure of something and that research to date shows results that are consistent with the broad notion of what repression–sensitization should mean. They feel that the name generates productive research and 'that a construct by any other name does not predict as sweetly' (p. 476).

Weinberger, Schwartz, and Davidson (1979) Repressive Style Measure

Weinberger and his colleagues developed a method for measuring repressive style that would differentiate those people who report no emotional distress in a stressful situation because they are experiencing low levels of anxiety ('low anxious') from those who are actually repressing anxious feelings ('true repressors'). Sensitizers report high levels of distress. They used both the Taylor Manifest Anxiety Scale (TMAS) (which correlates 0.9 with Byrne's R–S Scale) and the Marlowe-Crowne Social Desirability Scale (SD) to classify subjects. 'True repressors' were viewed as those who would be low on the TMAS and high on SD, whereas the 'low anxious' were thought to be those with low scores on both the TMAS and SD. Weinberger et al. (1979) found significant differences between these two groups on self-report, physiological, and behavioural measures, with true repressors showing poorer performance on cognitive tasks and greater discrepancy between physiological reactions to stress and their report of emotional distress. These findings were recently replicated by Asendorpf and Scherer (1983). This scale has also shown good predictive validity in two studies with coronary heart disease patients (Shaw et al., 1985; Shaw, Cohen, Fishman-Rosen, Murphy, Stertzer, Clark, and Myler, in press), and in a variety of other studies (Weinberger, 1985).

However, the construct validity of this measure of repressive style has never been clearly established. Shaw (1985) did not find a relationship between this classification and scores on Hackett and Cassem's (1974) Denial Scale. Although the measure is intriguing and shows good predictive validity, it is not clear why 'true repressors' would necessarily be high, and 'low anxious' necessarily low, on the social desirability dimension. Further work is needed to establish what this scale is actually measuring. However, it is quite promising in its ability to predict discrepancies between psychological and physiological measures.

Defense Mechanism Inventory

The Defense Mechanism Inventory (DMI) was developed by Gleser and Ihilevich (1969) to measure defensive modes of ego functioning. It is a forced choice test that measures the relative intensity of five major clusters of ego defence mechanisms: (a) turning against object (i.e. identification with the aggressor, regression, and displacement); (b) projection; (c) principalization (i.e. intellectualization, rationalization, and isolation of affect); (d) turning against self (i.e. masochism and autosadism); and (e) reversal (i.e. denial, undoing, reaction formation, repression, and negation).

The DMI presents ten short stories dealing with different conflict areas, and questions ask what the person would actually do in the situation and the thoughts, fantasies and feelings the story evokes. Although there is some evidence for the predictive and construct validity of the instrument (Cooper and Kline, 1982; Gleser and Sacks, 1973; Walsh, 1972), questions have been raised about its content validity and reliability (Juni, 1982; Weissman, Ritter and Gordon, 1971). A multitrait-multimethod approach comparing the DMI to two other similarly named scales found a lack of convergent and discriminant validity (Vickers and Hervig, 1981). Similar problems were found when the DMI was compared to the Blacky Defense Preference Inventory (Massong, Dickson, and Ritzler, 1982). Further a factor-analytic study concluded that three factors are measured by the DMI: turning attention outward, turning attention inward, and turning against self (Woodrow, 1973). Juni and Masling (1980) suggest scoring the DMI on a single continuum, with one end representing defences that facilitate the expression of aggression and the other end with defences that inhibit acting out. Juni (1982) later reformulated this into a composite measure which includes only four of the subscales combined in the following way: turning against object + projection − principalization − reversal of affect. Inhibition and internalization of frustration are at one end of the scale and acting out and externalization of frustration at the other.

The scale has also been criticized because of its ipsative scoring which makes it difficult to interpret correlations between the DMI and other scales to determine construct validity (Cooper and Kline, 1982). Woodrow (1973) developed a version that uses a normative rating scale format.

Joffe and Naditch (1977) Coping-Defence Scales

Joffe and Naditch developed a paper and pencil measure of coping and defence using empirically derived scales. These were constructed by selecting California Psychological Inventory and MMPI items that predicted interviewer ratings of coping and defence ego mechanisms made according to the conceptual schema developed by Haan (1963, 1969, 1977). Haan's framework differentiates coping from defence processes on the basis of congruence with reality, rationality, flexibility of response, and other value-laden criteria. Joffe and Naditch derived three ways to score their scale: (a) summing coping and defence items separately; (b) scoring for controlled coping, expressive coping, structured defence, and primitive defence; and (c) scoring on each of the twenty ego mechanisms described by Haan (see Table 1). However, not all of the twenty ego mechanisms could be measured accurately for both sexes. The Joffe and Naditch scale has been used in a few studies (Joffe and Bast, 1978; Vickers, Conway, and Haight, 1983; Vickers, Hervig, Rahe, and Rosenman, 1981) with some evidence of predictive validity. However, a study that utilized a multitrait-multimethod approach to compare the Joffe and Naditch scale with the Defense Mechanism Inventory and Schutz's (1967) Coping Operations Preference Enquiry found poor convergent and discriminant validity (Vickers and Hervig, 1981). These results are hard to evaluate since the validity of each of these scales is open to question.

Coping with life strains

Pearlin and Schooler (1978) used a survey questionnaire to measure the stresses of living that arise from four social roles—marriage partner, household economic manager, parent, and co-worker—and the types of coping strategies used in response. This is a trait measure of coping since it asks how people usually coped rather than how they actually coped in a specific encounter. They factor analyzed the coping responses in each of the four areas (see also Fleishman, 1984, for a similar factor analysis), producing six factors of marital coping (self-reliance v. advice seeking, controlled reflectiveness v. emotional discharge, positive comparison, negotiation, self-assertion v. passive forbearance, selective ignoring), five of parental coping (selective ignoring, non-punitiveness v. reliance on discipline, self-reliance v. advice-seeking, positive comparisons, exercise of potency v. helpless resignation), four in the household economic area (devaluation of money, selective ignoring, positive comparisons, optimistic faith), and four concerning occupation (substitution of rewards, positive comparisons, optimistic action, and selective ignoring). Pearlin and Schooler evaluated the efficacy of these coping behaviours and found that coping modes varied among different sociodemographic groups. Those highly educated, affluent, and of the male sex made greater use of effective strategies. They also found coping to be most effective in dealing with problems of marriage and parenting, and least effective in the occupational arena.

Pearlin and Schooler's work has been influential in the coping field, both in its conceptualization of functions of coping, its focus on chronic life strains, and its provocative results. However, their measure is limited to the four stress areas outlined above. Further, because they focus on persistent life strains, that is, those that subjects were *not* able to resolve, the measure cannot be used to measure coping in response to acute stressful situations. It also probably excludes the types of coping responses that may be effective in altering stressful episodes.

REVIEW OF EPISODIC COPING MEASURES

Avoidance–vigilance

Cohen and Lazarus (1973) developed a structured interview for assessing avoidance–vigilance in surgical patients, using a detailed set of criteria to judge the degree to which patients were using avoidant or vigilant coping strategies. The interview asks questions about the person's emotional state; knowledge about the illness, operation, and post-operative course; what other information the person wanted to know, and so on. Ratings are made on a 10-point scale. This interview has been used in other studies of surgical patients and a version for angioplasty patients has been developed (Shaw, 1984). The interrater reliability of ratings has been high, averaging around 0.9 (Cohen, 1975; Cohen and Lazarus, 1973; LaMontagne, 1982; Shaw, 1984). Cohen and Lazarus (1973) found that this episodic coping measure was a better predictor of recovery from surgery outcomes than were two dispositional coping instruments (the Epstein and Fenz, 1967, modified Repression–Sensitization scale; and Andrew's, 1970, Sentence–Completion Test) measuring the same dimension.

Hackett and Cassem's Denial Scale

Hackett and Cassem (1974) developed an interview to assess denial in myocardial infarction patients. They define denial as a 'multifaceted behavioral complex' (p. 95) and their interview taps indirect and direct manifestations of denial in present and past situations. Thus their measure is not truly an episodic measure, since it also evaluates past indicators of denial. The Hackett and Cassem measure has been criticized for lumping together a variety of 'denial-like' coping mechanisms—such as minimization, avoidance, nonchalance, and delay in seeking treatment—thereby overextending the meaning of denial (Cohen and Lazarus, 1979; Lazarus, 1983). However, this measure is the most commonly used measure of denial in heart disease patients (e.g. Dimsdale and Hackett, 1982; Soloff, 1980; Stern, Pascale, and Ackerman, 1977) and has been validated with clinician ratings (Froese, Vasquez, Cassem, and Hackett, 1973).

The original Hackett and Cassem interview is semi-structured, which can lead to wide variability in the information collected. The scoring criteria are somewhat vague. Very little systematic work has been done assessing the reliability and validity of the scale. Recently Shaw et al. (1985) systematized the interview and rating criteria to make them less subject to individual variation. These authors developed a structured interview schedule and a detailed scoring manual that provided a more elaborate description of how situations would be coded. An independent rater scored a subsample of the interview tapes, and an interrater reliability of 0.82 was found. Shaw et al. (1985) found that denial was associated with less information gain from the cardiac rehabilitation program.

Despite the predictive validity of the scale, there still is question about what constructs the denial interview is assessing. For example, Shaw (1985) reports no significant associations between the denial rating and the Byrne R–S scale or the Weinberger et al. (1979) index of repressive style. However, this may just reflect the lack of congruence usually found between trait and episodic measures of coping.

Ways of Coping

The Ways of Coping scale was originally developed as a check-list of sixty-eight items that described a broad range of cognitive and behavioural strategies (Folkman and Lazarus, 1980). It was intended for use as an episodic measure. Subjects responded in terms of a specified stressful situation, for example, a stressful situation that had happened over the last month, and checked off those strategies they had used to deal with it. Folkman and Lazarus revised the scale subsequently by deleting or rewording redundant or unclear items, adding items, and changing the response format to a 4-point Likert scale (Folkman et al., 1986; see Lazarus and Folkman, 1984, for a copy of the revised 67-item version). In the revised version subjects indicate to what extent they used each of the strategies in dealing with the situation being described.

The Ways of Coping scale has been factor analyzed using four different data sets, the latter two utilizing the revised Ways of Coping (Aldwin, Folkman, Schaefer, Coyne, and Lazarus, 1980; Vitaliano, Russo, Carr, Maiuro, and Becker, 1985; Folkman and Lazarus, 1985; Folkman et al., 1986). Four different factor structures have been derived, each with somewhat different factors. The most recent factor analysis (Folkman et al., 1986) produced the following eight factors: (a) confrontive coping; (b) distancing; (c) self-control; (d) seeking social support; (e) accepting responsibility; (f) escape/avoidance; (g) planful problem-solving; and (h) positive appraisal. Five of these factors are similar to ones derived from the earlier factor analyses although each analysis contributed unique factors which may be influenced by the subject population (e.g. college students cf. middle-aged adults) or the situation being studied (Folkman et al., 1986).

Modified versions of the Ways of Coping have been used in a number of different studies (e.g. Baum, Fleming, and Singer, 1983; McCrae, 1984; Nakell, 1985; Parkes, 1984). However, there is not yet any standard way to score this instrument. Some investigators use a large number of distinct mechanisms for analysis while others use only a few broad categories (e.g. emotion-focused v. problem-focused).

Billings and Moos coping measures

Billings and Moos (1981) developed a 19-item check-list with a yes/no format to assess how people cope with a recent stressful event. The items were grouped into three coping method categories—active-cognitive, active-behavioural, and avoidance—as well as according to the emotion-focused v. problem-focused distinction. Their classification of some of the coping items can be questioned (e.g. they consider 'prepared for the worst' to be an avoidance strategy). Their results revealed that coping attenuated the relationship between negative life events and measures of personal functioning.

Billings and Moos (1984) revised their earlier coping procedure in a study of depressed patients. Respondents described their response to a recent stressful event by rating the frequency of use (on a 4-point scale) of thirty-two different possible coping responses. Using preliminary item analyses, they classified strategies into the conceptual categories they had described in earlier work (Moos and Billings, 1982): (a) appraisal-focused coping (logical analysis); (b) problem-focused coping (information-seeking, problem-solving); and (c) emotion-focused coping (affective regulation, emotional discharge). This apparently reduced the scale to twenty-eight items. Billings and Moos found these coping indices were significantly related to outcome measures of functioning. There was no evidence that coping had stress-attenuation or buffering effects.

It is hard to evaluate these measures since they have not been widely used. The coping dimensions they outline have influenced other researchers' classification of coping responses (e.g. Kaloupek et al., 1984).

Other coping measures

This review of coping measures has focused on measures used in more than one study. Space limitations prevent discussion of other coping measures that may nonetheless be of interest. For example, Miller and Mangan (1983) developed a trait measure to classify individuals as 'blunters' or 'monitors' (another attempt to measure a repression–sensitization strategy) based on their responses to four hypothetical situations. Stone and Neale (1984) present subjects with eight abstract coping categories and ask subjects to specify whether they did anything that fit those categories with respect to the daily problems of living they reported. The categories are: distraction, situation redefinition, direct action, catharsis, acceptance, social support, relaxation, and religion.

REVIEW OF CROSS-DIMENSIONAL COPING MEASURES

Coping flexibility

Recently there has been interest in developing new ways of categorizing coping that do not merely look at coping modes. It may not be important whether individuals utilize one coping strategy rather than another, but whether they can draw on very different ones adaptively depending on the requirements of the situation (Cohen, Horowitz, Lazarus, Moos, Robins, Rose, and Rutter, 1982). Unfortunately we do not yet have a good way of assessing coping flexibility. Cohen and her colleagues (Cohen et al., in preparation; Kemeny, 1985) assessed coping flexibility in studies of arthritis and herpes patients. In the study of arthritis patients, subjects' inverview responses were coded in each of five stressor areas for the subject's use of five modes of coping (direct actions, inhibition of action, information seeking, intrapsychic processes, and turning to others for support). Two coping flexibility measures were determined: the number of different coping modes used within a stress area (e.g. in dealing with mobility problems) and the number used across the five stress areas studied. However, the coping flexibility measure was significantly correlated with ratings of the stressfulness of each stress area and also with indicators of emotional distress. Thus rather than being a measure of flexibility, the measure may indicate that in highly stressful situations more coping strategies may be required, or that individuals may use many methods because they cannot find a few that are effective.

Kemeny (1985) interviewed genital herpes patients monthly and assessed coping in response to two stressful situations of the previous month. Coping was rated on eleven different coping modes. Coping flexibility was measured by determining the number of different modes used across both situations. Kemeny also found coping flexibility scores associated with measures of life stress and anxiety. Further, her results showed that coping flexibility did not interact with stress in predicting recurrence rate or immunological change as had been originally hypothesized.

A more adequate measure of coping repertoire is needed. The number of strategies used does not really measure what is available. Further, although it may be good to have a large repertoire, the best idea may be to choose the most appropriate strategy for each situation. How to measure that may require looking both at the nature of the situation and the types of strategies used.

CONCLUSIONS

This chapter has discussed a number of issues relevant to the evaluation of coping, and has reviewed commonly used trait and episodic measures. The reader expecting a conclusion about the best scales will unfortunately be disappointed. Not enough is known about the construct validity of any of the coping measures reviewed. The distressing fact is that similarly named measures show low correlations with each other, and not enough validity information is available to suggest the best measure of each concept. Further, in terms of content validity, we do not know enough about what coping dimensions are most important to include nor what level of generality is required. Existing coping check-lists have been criticized for not including enough coping items, or for including too many that are irrelevant. More work is needed to evaluate the relative advantages and disadvantages of brief versus lengthy check-lists.

The choice of a unidimensional or multidimensional scale is still a perplexing question. The unidimensional measures do not reflect the vast array of strategies people use in dealing with life stressors. And yet they have remained popular because they have good predictive validity and are intuitively appealing. Further, since there is no consensus about which dimensions to include in multidimensional scales, their use has not led to comparability in instruments which would make it possible to make comparative evaluations.

A considerable conceptual and empirical effort is needed to bring clarity to this area. Various conceptual frameworks have been suggested for classifying coping (e.g. Haan, 1977; Lazarus and Folkman, 1984; Moos and Billings, 1982; Pearlin and Schooler, 1978) but no one can agree on which is best. Further these different conceptual schemes have not been pitted against each other empirically to see which is the best predictor of outcome. Pitting similarly named coping scales against each other in predicting outcome would also be quite useful. For unidimensional traits such as repression–sensitization, episodic measures of coping seem to be better predictors than trait measures, but this type of question has never been examined with multidimensional instruments.

The choice of a coping instrument will depend on the type of situation to be studied, the researcher's goals and conceptual framework, the level of generality desired, and the degree to which it taps the dimensions of coping the investigator thinks are most important. If more investigators use more than one coping scale at a time, and evaluate their validity, we will be better able to judge in the future which measures are most useful.

REFERENCES

Aldwin, C., Folkman, S., Schaefer, C., Coyne, J. C., and Lazarus, R. S. (1980, September). Ways of coping: A process measure, Paper presented at meetings of the American Psychological Association, Montreal.

Andrew, J. M. (1967). Coping styles, stress-relevant learning, and recovery from surgery. Unpublished doctoral dissertation, University of California, Los Angeles.

Andrew, J. M. (1970). Recovery from surgery, with and without preparatory instruction, for three coping styles, *J. Pers. Soc. Psychol.*, **15**, 223–6.

Asendorpf, J. B., and Scherer, K. R. (1983). The discrepant repressor: Differentiation between low anxiety, high anxiety, and repression of anxiety by autonomic-facial-verbal patterns of behavior, *J. Pers. Soc. Psychol.*, **45**, 1334–46.

Austin, S. H. (1974). Coping and psychological stress in pregnancy, labor, and delivery, with 'natural childbirth' and 'medicated' patients. Unpublished doctoral dissertation, University of California, Berkeley.

Averill, J. R., and Opton, E. M., Jr. (1968). Psychophysiological assessment: Rationale and problems. In P. McReynolds (ed.) *Advances in Psychological Assessment*, Vol. 1, Science and Behavior Books, Palo Alto, pp. 265–88.

Bachrach, K. M., and Zautra, A. J. (1985). Coping with a community stressor: The threat of a hazardous waste facility, *J. Health Soc. Behav.*, **26**, 127–41.

Baum, A., Fleming, R., and Singer, J. E. (1983). Coping with victimization by technological disaster, *J. Soc. Issue*, **39**, 117–38.

Bell, P. A., and Byrne, D. (1978). Repression–sensitization. In H. London and J. E. Exner (eds.) *Dimensions of Personality*, John Wiley, New York, pp. 449–85.

Billings, A., and Moos, R. (1981). The role of coping responses and social resources in attenuating the stress of life events, *J. Behav. Med.*, **4**, 139–57.

Billings, A. G., and Moos, R.H. (1984). Coping, stress, and social resources among adults with unipolar depression, *J. Pers. Soc. Psychol.*, **46**, 877–91.

Byrne, D. (1961). The repression–sensitization scale: Rationale, reliability, and validity, *J. Pers.*, **29**, 334–49.

Byrne, D. (1964). Repression–sensitization as a dimension of personality. In B. A. Maher (ed.) *Progress in Experimental Personality Research*, Vol. 1 Academic Press, New York, pp. 170–220.

Byrne, D., Barry, J., and Nelson, D. (1963). Relation of the revised repression–sensitization scale to measures of self-description, *Psychol. Reports*, **13**, 323–34.

Chabot, J. A. (1973). Repression–sensitization: A critique of some neglected variables in the literature, *Psychol. Bull.*, **80**, 122–9.

Coelho, G. V., Hamburg, D. A., and Adams, J. E. (eds.) (1974). *Coping and Adaptation*, Basic Books, New York.

Cohen, F. (1975). Psychological preparation, coping, and recovery from surgery. Unpublished doctoral dissertation, University of California, Berkeley.

Cohen, F. (1979). Personality, stress, and the development of physical illness. In G. C. Stone, F. Cohen, N. E. Adler, and Associates *Health Psychology—A Handbook: Theories, Applications, and Challenges of a Psychological Approach to the Health Care System*, Jossey-Bass, San Francisco, pp. 77–111.

Cohen, F., and Lazarus, R. S. (1973). Active coping processes, coping dispositions, and recovery from surgery, *Psychosom. Med.*, **35**, 375–89.

Cohen, F., and Lazarus, R. S. (1979). Coping with the stresses of illness. In G. C. Stone, F. Cohen, N. E. Adler, and Associates *Health Psychology—A Handbook: Theories, Applications, and Challenges of a Psychological Approach to the Health Care System*, Jossey-Bass, San Francisco, pp. 217–54.

Cohen, F., Horowitz, M., Lazarus, R., Moos, R., Robins, L. N., Rose, R., and Rutter, M. (1982). Panel report on psychosocial assets and modifiers of stress. In G. R. Elliott and C. Eisdorfer (eds.) *Stress and Human Health*, Springer, New York, pp. 147–88.

Cohen, F., and Lazarus, R. S. (1983). Coping and adaptation in health and illness. In D. Mechanic (ed.) *Handbook of Health, Health Care, and the Health Professions*, Free Press, New York, pp. 608–35.

Cohen, F., Reese, L. B., Kaplan, G. A., and Riggio, R. E. (1986). Coping with the stresses of arthritis. In R. W. Moskowitz and M. R. Haug (eds.) *Arthritis and the Elderly*, Springer, New York, pp. 47–56.

Cohen, F., Riggio, R. E., Reese, L. B., and Kaplan, G. A. (in preparation). Coping modes of elderly rheumatoid arthritis patients.

Cooper, C., and Kline, P. (1982). A validation of the Defense Mechanism Inventory, *Br. J. Med. Psychol.*, **55**, 209–14.

Croog, S. H., Shapiro, D. S., and Levine, S. (1971). Denial among male heart patients: An empirical study, *Psychosom. Med.*, **33**, 385–97.

Derogatis, L. R., Abeloff, M. D., and Melisaratos, N. (1979). Psychological coping mechanisms and survival time in metastatic breast cancer, *JAMA*, **242**, 1504–8.

Dimsdale, J. E., and Hackett, T. P. (1982). Effect of denial on cardiac health and psychological assessment, *Am. J. Psychiatry*, **139**, 1477–80.

Dudley, D. L., Verhey, J. W., Masuda, M., Martin, C. J., and Holmes, T. H. (1969). Long-term adjustment, prognosis, and death in irreversible diffuse obstructive pulmonary syndromes, *Psychosom. Med.*, **31**, 310–25.

Elliott, G. R., and Eisdorfer, C. (eds.) (1982). *Stress and Human Health*, Springer, New York.

Epstein, S., and Fenz, W. D. (1967). The detection of areas of emotional stress through variations in perceptual threshold and physiological arousal, *J. Exp. Res. Pers.*, **2**, 191–9.

Fleishman, J. A. (1984). Personality characteristics and coping patterns, *J. Health Soc. Behav.*, **25**, 229–44.

Folkman, S., and Lazarus, R. S. (1980). An analysis of coping in a middle-aged community sample, *J. Health Soc. Behav.*, **21**, 219–39.

Folkman, S., and Lazarus, R. S. (1985). If it changes it must be a process: Study of emotion and coping during three stages of a college exam, *J. Pers. Soc. Psychol.*, **48**, 150–70.

Folkman, S., Lazarus, R. S., Dunkel-Schetter, C., DeLongis, A., and Gruen, R. J. (1986). The dynamics of a stressful encounter: Cognitive appraisal, coping, and encounter outcomes, *J. Pers. Soc. Psychol.*, **50**, 992–1003.

Froese, A. P., Vasquez, E., Cassem, N. H., and Hackett, T. P. (1973). Validation of anxiety, depression and denial scales in a coronary care unit, *J. Psychosom. Res.*, **18**, 137–41.

Gal, R., and Lazarus, R. S. (1975). The role of activity in anticipating and confronting stressful situations, *J. Human Stress*, **1(4)**, 4–20.

Gardner, R. W., Holzman, P. S., Klein, G. S., Linton, H. B., and Spence, D. P. (1959). Cognitive control: A study of individual consistencies in cognitive behavior, *Psychol. Issues*, **1** (Whole no. 4).

Gleser, G. C., and Ihilevich, D. (1969). An objective instrument for measuring defense mechanisms, *J. Consult. Clin. Psych.*, **33**, 51–60.

Gleser, G., and Sacks, M. (1973). Ego defenses and reaction to stress: A validation study of the Defense Mechanisms Inventory, *J. Consult. Clin. Psych.*, **40**, 181–7.

Goldstein, M. J. (1959). The relationship between coping and avoiding behaviour and response to fear-arousing propaganda, *J. Abnorm. Soc. Psychol.*, **58**, 247–52.

Golin, S., Herron, E. O., Lakota, R., and Reineck, L. (1967). Factor analytic study of the manifest anxiety, extraversion, and repression–sensitization scale, *J. Consult. Psychol.*, **31**, 564–69.

Haan, N. (1963). Proposed model of ego functioning: Coping and defense mechanisms in relationship to IQ change, *Psychol. Monogr.*, **77** (8, Whole no. 571).

Haan, N. (1969). A tripartite model of ego functioning: Values and clinical research applications, *J. Nerv. Ment. Dis.*, **148**, 14–30.

Haan, N. (1977). *Coping and Defending: Processes of Self-Environment Organization*, Academic Press, New York.

Haan, N. (1982). The assessment of coping, defenses, and stress. In L. Goldberger and S. Breznitz (eds.) *Handbook of Stress: Theoretical and Clinical Aspects*, Free Press, New York, pp. 254–69.

Hackett, T. P., Cassem, N. H., and Wishnie, H. A. (1968). The coronary-care unit: An appraisal of its psychologic hazards, *N. Engl. J. Med.*, **279**, 1365–70.

Hackett, T., and Cassem, N. (1974). Development of a quantitative rating scale to assess denial, *J. Psychosom. Res.*, **18**, 93–100.

Hamburg, D. A., Coelho, G. V., and Adams, J. E. (1974). Coping and adaptation: Steps toward a synthesis of biological and social perspectives. In G. V. Coelho, D. A. Hamburg, and J. E. Adams (eds.) *Coping and Adaptation*, Basic Books, New York, pp. 403–40.

Hitchcock, L. S. (1982). Improving recovery from surgery: The interaction of preoperative interventions, coping processes, and personality variables. Unpublished doctoral dissertation, University of Texas, Austin.

Hofer, M. A., Wolff, C. T., Friedman, S. B., and Mason, J. W. (1972a). A psychoendocrine study of bereavement: Part 1. 17-hydroxycorticosteroid excretion rates of parents following death of their children from leukemia, *Psychosom. Med.*, **34**, 481–91.

Hofer, M. A., Wolff, C. T., Friedman, S. B., and Mason, J. W. (1972b). A psychoendocrine study of bereavement: Part 2. Observations on the process of mourning in relation to adrenocortical function, *Psychosom. Med.*, **34**, 492–504.

Hoffman, H. E. (1970). Use of avoidance and vigilance by repressors and sensitizers, *J. Consult. Clin. Psych.*, **34**, 91–6.

Horowitz, M. J. (1976). *Stress Response Syndromes*, Aronson, New York.

Horowitz, M. J., and Wilner, N. (1980). Life events, stress, and coping. In L. Poon (ed.) *Aging in the 1980's: Selected Contemporary Issues*, American Psychological Association, Washington, D.C., pp. 363–70.

Jenkins, C. D. (1979). Psychosocial modifiers of response to stress, *J. Human Stress*, **5(4)**, 3–15.

Joffe, P. E., and Naditch, M. (1977). Paper and pencil measures of coping and defense processes. In N. Haan (ed.) *Coping and Defending: Processes of Self-Environment Organization*, Academic Press, New York, pp. 280–297.

Joffe, P. E., and Bast, B. A. (1978). Coping and defense in relation to accommodation among a sample of blind men, *J. Nerv. Ment. Dis.*, **166**, 537–52.

Juni, S. (1982). The composite measure of the Defense Mechanism Inventory, *J. Res. Pers.*, **16**, 193–200.

Juni, S., and Masling, J. (1980). Reaction to aggression and the defense mechanism inventory, *J. Pers. Assess.*, **44**, 484–6.

Kaloupek, D. G., White, H., and Wong, M. (1984). Multiple assessment of coping strategies used by volunteer blood donors: Implications for preparatory training, *J. Behav. Med.*, **7**, 35–60.

Katz, J. L., Weiner, H., Gallagher, T. G., and Hellman, L. (1970). Stress, distress, and ego defenses, *Arch. Gen. Psychiatry*, **23**, 131–42.

Kemeny, M. E. (1985). Psychological and immunological predictors of genital herpes recurrence. Unpublished doctoral dissertation, University of California, San Francisco.

Kroeber, T. C. (1963). The coping functions of ego mechanism. In R. W. White (ed.) *The Study of Lives*, Prentice-Hall, Englewood Cliffs, New Jersey, pp. 178–98.

LaMontagne, L. L. (1982). Children's locus of control beliefs as predictors of their preoperative coping behavior. Unpublished doctoral dissertation, University of California, San Francisco.

Layne, O. L., Jr., and Yudofsky, S. C. (1971). Postoperative psychosis in cardiotomy patients, *N. Engl. J. Med.*, **284**, 518–20.

Lazarus, R. S. (1966). *Psychological Stress and the Coping Process*, McGraw-Hill, New York.

Lazarus, R. S. (1975). The self-regulation of emotion. In L. Levi (ed.) *Emotions—Their Parameters and Measurement*, Raven Press, New York, pp. 47–67.

Lazarus, R. S. (1983). The costs and benefits of denial. In S. Breznitz (ed.) *Denial of Stress*, International University Press, New York, pp. 1–30.

Lazarus, R. S., and Alfert, E. (1964). The short-circuiting of threat by experimentally altering cognitive appraisal, *J. Abnorm. Soc. Psychol.*, **69**, 195–205.

Lazarus, R. S., Averill, J. R., and Opton, E. M. Jr. (1974). The psychology of coping: Issues of research and assessment. In G. V. Coelho, D. A. Hamburg, and J. E. Adams (eds.) *Coping and Adaptation*, Basic Books, New York, pp. 207–232.

Lazarus, R. S., and Folkman, S. (1984). *Stress, Appraisal and Coping*, Springer, New York.

Lefcourt, H. M. (1966). Repression–sensitization: A measure of the evaluation of emotional expression, *J. Consult. Psychol.*, **30**, 444–9.

Levine, M., and Spivack, G. (1964). *The Rorschach Index of Repressive Style*, Thomas, Springfield, Illinois.

McCrae, R. R. (1984). Situational determinants of coping responses: Loss, threat, and challenge, *J. Pers. Soc. Psychol.*, **46**, 919–28.

Mages, N. L., and Mendelsohn, G. A. (1979). Effects of cancer on patients' lives: A personological approach. In G. C. Stone, F. Cohen, N. E. Adler, and Associates *Health Psychology—A Handbook: Theories, Applications, and Challenges of a Psychological Approach to the Health Care System*, Jossey-Bass, San Francisco, pp. 255–84.

Massong, S. R., Dickson, A. L., and Ritzler, B. A. (1982). A correlational comparison of Defense Mechanism measures: The Defense Mechanism Inventory and the Blacky Defense Preference Inventory, *J. Pers. Assess.*, **46**, 477–80.

Miller, S. M., and Mangan, C. E. (1983). Interacting effects of information and coping style in adapting to gynecologic stress: Should the doctor tell all?, *J. Pers. Soc. Psychol.*, **45**, 223–36.

Moos, R. H. (1974). Psychological techniques in the assessment of adaptive behavior. In G. V. Coelho, D. A. Hamburg, and J. E. Adams (eds.) *Coping and Adaptation*, Basic Books, New York, pp. 334–97.

Moos, R. H., and Billings, A. G. (1982) Conceptualizing and measuring coping resources and processes. In L. Goldberger and S. Breznitz (eds.) *Handbook of Stress: Theoretical and Clinical Aspects*, Free Press, New York, pp. 212–30.

Mullen, B., and Suls, J. (1982). The effectiveness of attention and rejection as coping styles: A meta-analysis of temporal differences, *J. Psychosom. Res.*, **26**, 43–9.

Nakell, L. (1985). Family adaptation to the stress of having a premature baby cared for in the intensive care nursery. Unpublished doctoral dissertation, University of California, San Francisco.

Parkes, C. M. (1972). *Bereavement: Studies of Grief in Adult Life*, International Universities Press, New York.

Parkes, K. R. (1984). Locus of control, cognitive appraisal, and coping in stressful episodes, *J. Pers. Soc. Psychol.*, **46**, 655–68.

Pearlin, L., and Schooler, C. (1978). The structure of coping, *J. Health Soc. Behav.*, **19**, 2–21.

Schafer, R. (1954). *Psychoanalytic Interpretation in Rorschach Testing: Theory and Application*, Grune and Stratton, New York.

Schutz, W. C. (1967). *The FIRO Scales Manual*, Consulting Psychologists Press, Palo Alto.

Shaw, R. E. (1984). The impact of coping, anxiety and social support on information, medical and rehabilitation outcomes in patients undergoing coronary angioplasty. Unpublished doctoral dissertation, University of California, San Francisco.

Shaw, R. E. (1985). Personal communication.

Shaw, R. E., Cohen, F., Doyle, B., and Palesky, J. (1985). The impact of denial and repressive style on information gain and rehabilitation outcomes in myocardial infarction patients, *Psychosom. Med.*, **47**, 262–73.

Shaw, R. E., Cohen, F., Fishman-Rosen, J., Murphy, M. C., Stertzer, S. H., Clark, D. A., and Myler, R. K. (in press). Psychological predictors of psychosocial and medical outcomes in patients undergoing coronary angioplasty, *Psychosom. Med.*

Shrauger, J. S., and Osberg, T. M. (1981). The relative accuracy of self-predictions and judgments by others in psychological assessment, *Psychol. Bull.*, **90**, 322–51.

Silver, M. J. (1970). Hypnotizability as a function of adaptive regression, repression, and mood. Unpublished doctoral dissertation, Boston University.

Soloff, P. H. (1980). Effects of denial of mood, compliance, and quality of functioning after cardiovascular rehabilitation, *Gen. Hosp. Psychiatry*, **2**, 134–40.

Stern, M. J., Pascale, L., and Ackerman, A. (1977). Life adjustment post myocardial infarction: Determining predictive variables, *Arch. Intern. Med.*, **137**, 1680–5.

Stone, A. A., and Neale, J. M. (1984). New measure of daily coping: Development and preliminary results, *J. Pers. Soc. Psychol.*, **46**, 892–906.

Ursin, H. (1980). Personality, activation, and somatic health: A new psychosomatic theory. In S. Levine and H. Ursin (eds.) *Coping and Health*, Plenum, New York, pp. 259–79.

Vaillant, G. E. (1976). Natural history of male psychological health: V. The relation of choice of ego mechanisms of defense to adult adjustment, *Arch. Gen. Psychiatry*, **33**, 535–45.

Vaillant, G. E. (1977). *Adaptation to Life*, Little Brown, Boston.

Vickers, R. R., and Hervig, L. K. (1981). Comparison of three psychological defense mechanism questionnaires, *J. Pers. Assess.*, **45**, 630–8.

Vickers, R. R., Hervig, L. K., Rahe, R. H., and Rosenman, R. H. (1981). Type A behavior pattern and coping and defense, *Psychosom. Med.*, **43**, 381–96.

Vickers, R. R., Conway, T. L., and Haight, M. A. (1983). Association between Levenson's dimensions of locus of control and measures of coping and defense mechanisms, *Psychol. Reports*, **52**, 323–33.

Vitaliano, P. P., Russo, J., Carr, J. E., Maiuro, R. D., and Becker, J. (1985). The Ways of Coping Checklist: Revision and psychometric properties, *Multiv. Be. R.*, **20**, 3–26.

Walsh, J. A. (1972). Defense Mechanism Inventory. In O. K. Buros (ed.) *The Seventh Mental Measurements Yearbook*, Vol. 1, Gryphon Press, Highland Park, New Jersey, pp. 63–4.

Weinberger, D. A. (1985). Summary of recent research and current plans. Unpublished manuscript, Stanford University, Palo Alto.

Weinberger, D. A., Schwartz, G. E., and Davidson, J. R. (1979). Low anxious, high anxious and repressive coping styles: Psychometric patterns and behavioral physiological responses to stress, *J. Abnorm. Psychol.*, **88**, 369–80.

Weissman, H. N., Ritter, K., and Gordon, R. M. (1971). Reliability study of the Defense Mechanism Inventory, *Psychol. Reports*, **29**, 1237–8.

Weisman, A. D., and Worden, J. W. (1976–7). The existential plight in cancer: Significance of the first 100 days, *Int. J. Psychiatry Med.*, **7**, 1–15.

Wolff, C. T., Friedman, S. G., Hofer, M. A., and Mason, J. W. (1964). Relationship between psychological defenses and mean urinary 17-hydroxycorticosteroid excretion rates: I. A predictive study of parents of fatally ill children, *Psychosom. Med.*, **26**, 576–91.

Woodrow, J. Z. (1973). A factor analysis and revision of the Defense Mechanism Inventory. Unpublished doctoral dissertation, Ohio University.

Chapter 11

Methodologies in Stress and Health: Past Difficulties, Present Dilemmas, Future Directions

Stan V. Kasl

Visiting Professor of Epidemiology of the University of London

INTRODUCTION

Human research on stress and health represents an exquisite blend of characteristics which conspire to make the investigator's task ... well, uh ... a stressful one: demands certainly exceed resources and response capabilities. The investigator's distress is easily reduced by emotional support from colleagues and by various coping strategies, including denial, selective ignoring, and positive comparisons. However, the many problems remain, persist, continue.

In this overview chapter, I wish to assess the current situation. The comments which follow represent a continuation of my own strong interest in the methodology of stress and health research (Kasl, 1978, 1981, 1982, 1983, 1984a, b, c, 1985, 1986). I have also benefited immensely from reading the various excellent contributions to this volume. However, my editorializing, indebted though it is to these separate contributions, is not meant to speak in a summary fashion for a multiplicity of authors. Rather, I speak for myself and in the process may be distorting or misinterpreting their ideas and insights, or using them in ways with which they might not agree.

THE CHALLENGING FEATURES OF STRESS AND HEALTH RESEARCH

One can recognize several characteristics of human research on stress and health which make this a formidable area of investigation. The orientation is invariably aetiological—to establish cause–effect relationships—rather than merely descriptive. Often, the goal is to study both the process and the disease outcome, since linkages between psychosocial risk factors and biomedical outcomes are mysterious and hard to understand without some hints of the

Research Methods in Stress and Health Psychology. Edited by S. V. Kasl and C. L. Cooper.

processes involved. And the aetiological dynamics are, as all evidence so far indicates, invariably quite complex so that a rich array of variables needs to be assessed and reassessed one or more times. At the same time, investigators work under considerable constraints. Random assignment to exposures of interest or to suspected risk factors is generally not feasible and we need to make the most of quasi-experimental designs. Translating real-life stressful experiences into experimental laboratory manipulations is difficult: the meaning of the laboratory exposure and its brief duration will lead to poor analogues of limited external validity. (Experimental animal research, by revealing the great importance for outcomes of very minor variations in design, suggests the difficulty of extrapolating to the human condition). Measurement of crucial variables runs into the most fundamental problems of assessment bias and confounding. And all of this is wrapped in a conceptual mantle, stress 'theory', regarding which the very basic questions of scientific usefulness all still remain to be answered.

RAISING INVESTIGATORS' CONSCIOUSNESS REGARDING METHODOLOGICAL SOPHISTICATION

Methodological weaknesses of studies of stress and health of the recent past can be, logically, attributed to several (not mutually exclusive) causes: (a) ignorance of specific methodological weaknesses and pitfalls; (b) low standards of methodological rigour for stress research; (c) absence of superior solutions to particular problems; (d) the inevitability of trade-offs, that is, a change in methodology lessens some problems and increases others; (e) a close linkage between quality of methodology and amount of resources consumed by such methodology.

I have listed these possible reasons in order of what I consider to be their increasing importance. Thus, particularly low levels of methodological training and skills among investigators in the stress and health area would not seem to be a powerful or plausible explanation. (However, to the extent that this is a popular area of research which has attracted investigators who were originally trained for different areas of research, one may suspect that this issue is not altogether negligible.) Similarly, low standards of methodological rigour would also seem to be a minor and rather jaundiced explanation. However, there is a real issue here. The sheer volume of studies which has been generated by cross-sectional retrospective designs, in which only self-reports of independent, intervening, and outcome variables are correlated to each other, is so enormous that they have created their own standard of 'acceptable' methodology. Journal editors (presumably quite aware of methodological limitations) may be reluctant to put a moratorium on a methodology which was 'acceptable' only yesterday. However, a meta-analysis of such a body of research would reveal the futility of adding to a large body of research another finding about which the same host of questions, reservations, and alternate explanations must be raised as about all the previous ones.

The other three possible reasons for methodological inadequacies of current stress and health research all relate to the same point: better designs are more a function of resources available to the investigator and less a reflection of his/her level of methodological sophistication. Furthermore, for a given level of resources, many designs may represent a considered choice of strengthening some aspects of the design and giving up on others, rather than a failure to find the one optimal design. The sheer absence of methodologically superior solutions, when considered independently of resources and trade-offs, is likely to be a relatively rare explanation for poorer quality of research methodology.

Overall, it would seem that an increased sensitivity to the limitations of pay-off which accrues from methodologically flawed studies of stress and health should, in turn, increase investigators' resolve to commit more resources to contemplated future research designs.

NECESSARY INGREDIENTS OF SATISFACTORY METHODOLOGIES AND THE ORGANIZATION OF THIS VOLUME

The chapters selected for this volume reflect the conviction that there are several components of satisfactory research methodology in stress and health studies, and that these must all come together: (a) the adequacy of the design of the study, which in quasi-experimental research essentially means: what data are collected from (or about) what subjects at what time; (b) the adequacy of the conceptualization and operationalization of the study variables; (c) the adequacy of data analysis, both from the perspective of ruling out alternate explanations as well as the perspective of testing a particular causal or conceptual model; (d) the adequacy of the theoretical formulation regarding the aetiological dynamics of the stress–disease process.

The five methodological chapters illuminate issues of design and measurement, and design and data analysis. Both of these themes are seen as closely linked to the need to have an explicit formulation of the specific processes which might be involved in the specific stress–disease connection under study. Such a formulation would inform issues of design, assessment, and analysis. This is not a call for a broad 'stress theory' which would be, in some sense, tested by the study. Rather, it is much more a reminder of the need for a 'best guess' formulation of the processes involved so that study design decisions can be made rationally and optimally. The epidemiological perspective illuminates more richly the processes involving the outcome, while the social psychology/health psychology perspective throws better light on the processes involving the independent variable. The two disciplinary perspectives need to be brought into closer collaboration.

The other five chapters are more narrowly focused on issues of conceptualization and measurement of specific areas of central concern to stress and health investigators. Two chapters deal with stressors arising out of the two fundamental roles of human beings: work and the family. The former is as richly researched as the latter is neglected. Thus the Pearlin and Turner chapter is primarily conceptual, opening up theoretical issues with respect to sources of family stress and the special dynamics of the stress processes in the family settings. A crucial unfinished business is the absence of formulations of the differential processes: when outside stressors impact negatively on the family v. when the family remains unaffected and, instead, buffers the effects of the outside stressors. The Bhagat and Bailey chapter, on the other hand, builds upon an enormous empirical literature. Here, the need is to provide wise commentary on this literature and to suggest methodological (primarily assessment) improvements for the future. The study of the work–family interface remains an often mentioned, much neglected recommendation. Two other chapters deal with social support and coping, two conceptual domains which together cover most of the territory represented by processes intervening (or theorized to intervene) between exposure to stressors and disease outcomes. The juxtaposition of these two chapters brings on the stark realization that there is a substantial overlap in the basic formulations and in the proposed typologies (of types of social support, of different coping behaviours). A unified theory covering both would be of benefit to both sides, leading to greater clarity and comprehensiveness of formulations; much overall economy of theory and measurement could also be achieved. Finally, a chapter on Behaviour Type A is included. This remains a fascinating case history of the evolution of a psychosocial risk factor. It occupies an uncertain position between personality traits and environmentally based concepts. Its many operationalizations, its somewhat nebulous (and drifting) conceptual boundaries, and the mixture of positive and negative evidence, all continue to illuminate fundamental methodological issues in stress and health research.

USEFULNESS OF THE STRESS CONCEPT AND LINKED FORMULATIONS

The likelihood that 'stress' will fade away from our vocabulary is as good as are the chances that the state will wither away in communist Russia. Nevertheless, a periodic review of the impediments created by the dominant stress formulation is useful.

There are two crucial components of the stress-theoretic formulation with which we need to be concerned. One posits the existence of a unique state of the organism (state of stress) which has identifiable characteristics and which, no matter what specific environmental exposures or what disease outcomes are involved, represents the one common pathway linking diverse exposures to diverse disease outcomes. The second component of the formulation represents a frank commitment to the subjective nature of stress. There are actually two versions of this. One assumes that the stress state is linked to the subjective perception (interpretation, appraisal) of the environmental exposure, not its objective characteristics. The second, stronger version, adds the experiential aspects to the subjective perceptions: 'a stressor is not a stressor until it is experienced as such.'

To be sure, various stress-theoretic formulations have other elements in them as well. Furthermore, different investigators embrace these formulations with varying degrees of enthusiasm or reluctance. Nevertheless, these are central ideas influencing much of our thinking about stress and how to study it.

It is somewhat of a surprise to realize that the above formulation brings together two diametrically opposite assumptions: one presupposes the universality of the common pathway, state of stress, while the other emphasizes the idiosyncracy of the reaction. Even more surprising is the realization that these formulations have been treated as a sacred meta-theory handed down to us from above, not as a set of constructions of reality which need constant empirical support for their continued existence.

I believe that a thorough review of the evidence accumulated thus far would lead to two conclusions: (a) There is every indication that the linkages between environmental exposures and disease outcomes consist of innumerable specific aetiologic processes. The specific nature of these linkages, not surprisingly, depends on the characteristics of the exposure and the set of risk factors (translated into a specific disease-development set of stages or steps) for the particular disease. The assumption of a common pathway is quite difficult to sustain and, at best, represents a gratuitous assumption of dubious verifiability; (b) It has been impossible to identify and agree upon a criterion or, more appropriately, a set of criteria for identifying the presence of the state of stress and then calibrating its intensity and duration. All classes of indicators which have been proposed—performance decrements, experienced distress, biological reactivity of one sort or another, and so on—have their own large set of other determinants and the unique additional contribution of stress is difficult to pin down. The behaviour of these indicators over time is an additional problem: the duration of the stress state does not confidently translate into a corresponding duration of reactivity of one or another of the criterial variables. Behind it all, of course, is a logical difficulty: we don't know how to get out of the bind of deciding that a variable is an inappropriate indicator of stress v. that the stress state is not present.

These conclusions, if justifiable, strike at the heart of the stress-theoretic formulation. This naturally leads to the question: what benefits can we expect if we discard the stress-theoretic formulations? The comments which follow are frankly speculative. Furthermore, the reader must remember that they are meant to apply *only* to that part of the total domain of stress research which is concerned with the aetiological role of stress in disease.

LIVING WITHOUT THE STRESS CONCEPT

The most general answer regarding anticipated benefits is that we will begin our next study with fewer preconceptions about the dynamics we will encounter and about the ways we should study them. For example, we are less likely to believe that the study of the *phenomenology* of the stress process (experience) leads to findings which illuminate the steps in the *aetiology* of a disease. We will be less committed to the dogma that the effects of the objectively defined environmental exposure are strictly mediated by subjective perceptions and appraisals. We will be more interested in analyzing the details of the environmental exposure since it will be this analysis, not some *a priori* general stress theoretic formulation, that should dictate our choice of what variables to include and when to schedule data collections.

It is likely that abandoning the stress perspective will lead to a better set of priorities for our research. Our primary goal should be to identify linkages between exposure to an environmental condition, identified as clearly as possible by objective parameters, and adverse health outcomes. We should design our studies, and conduct our analyses, to optimize our chances of demonstrating that such linkages represent, in fact, cause–effect relationships. Additional effort used to design the study (such as additional data collection or data analysis) should be in the service of this primary goal, e.g. eliminate self-selection biases, pin down more precisely the pathogenic component of the exposure. Two other goals should also have high priority: (a) identify variables which explain additional variance in the adverse health outcomes and which, thereby, indicate differential vulnerability to the environmental explosure; and (b) provide information on the possible underlying mechanisms involved in the overall association.

There is no inherent necessity, when we give up the stress concept, to give up even a single well-formulated testable proposition. For example, it is still highly desirable to examine the hypothesis that the amount of felt distress, generated by the environmental exposure, contributes to the likelihood of an adverse health outcome. Whether distress is an epiphenomenon, or plays an aetiological role, has considerable implications for our concepts of coping and social support. Conceptual developments in both these areas have been heavily influenced by general formulations about the stress state and are thus prominently concerned with managing distress. However, in those exposure–disease linkages in which distress is found to have no aetiological role, coping and social support which reduce distress will not lower the risk of disease. Here, presumably only coping and supportive behaviours which reduce the demands of the environmental exposure have a chance of reducing risk of disease.

ISSUES THAT PERSIST: SOME RECOMMENDATIONS

In this section I wish to comment on a few methodological issues which have occupied the centre stage of stress and health research for some time. Some of these may be seen as 'problems': we need to work on them and possible solutions seem to exist. Other issues may be seen as 'dilemmas': no particular solutions seem to exist now but we do not wish to forget about them altogether. (Relabelling insoluble problems as dilemmas brings about a certain amount of relief.)

Objective v. subjective measures of environmental exposures

There is increasing consensus that the *objective* identification and assessment of the environmental exposure (the stimulus condition, the independent variable), which is examined as a risk factor for some disease outcome, provides considerable advantages to the investigator: the true independent variable can be identified with greater certainty, and thus also the environmental modification that might prove effective. Moreover, the variables which relate to exposure status can be studied more easily and, in general, cause–effect interpretations are facilitated. However, the notion persists that objective measures of environmental exposure are inappropriate or unnecessary, given the subjective nature of stress. This notion is incorrect since it ignores the variety of measures that can actually be utilized: (a) objective measures of exposure; (b) additional objective characteristics of the situation and of the individuals exposed, so that sub-types of exposure can be generated; (c) objective characteristics of individuals that may be moderator variables; (d) measures of traits and dispositions, also potential moderators; (e) self-reports of exposure, devoid of evaluations and reactions; (f) evaluations and appraisals of exposure; and (g) affective reactions to exposure (bothered, concerned, distressed, etc.). Exclusive reliance on the last two types creates many methodological problems.

The main point of this list of measures is that we can go a long way in measuring the (possibly) idiosyncratic meaning of a stressor before we need to resort to subjective appraisals and affective reactions, variables that are perilously close to some of the outcome variables of usual interest. The inclusion of trait and dispositional measures is particularly useful (viz. Pearlin's research on objective status inequality in marriage and the disposition toward status advancement): they are not 'objective' measures, generally, but they tap a class of variables unlikely to be confused with early stages of outcome, while providing us with a handle on individual differences in impact. Neutral self-reports of exposure are also promising but neglected measures. Frequently, an investigator does not have an objective measure of exposure and relies on the subject to provide data on it. The self-report is intended as a substitute for objective data, not as a way of getting at appraisals or reactions. If one avoids global judgements ('How demanding is your job?') and distress-laden descriptions ('How often are you upset by ... ?') and tries to state the exposure in precise language ('How many times during a work day are you talking to an important client and another client interrupts with a telephone call?'), one may improve on existing measures considerably. The solution, of course, is only a partial one: an anxious person, for example, may overstate (consciously or unconsciously) the frequency of some events, no matter how neutrally and concretely they are described.

It remains true that the specific nature of exposure one studies must be allowed to influence the choice of measures. For example, in the study of sudden, unexpected, quickly-ending, overwhelming disasters, such as the Mexico City earthquake, the need for subjective descriptors appears minimal. On the other hand, if one is studying the differential impact of having moved to two different retirement settings, using only the objective characterization of exposure is likely to defect very little impact. Such voluntary moves involve powerful self-selection with a long prior history of plans, intentions and aspirations, and the meaning of the exposure must be sought in some relational construct which links the actual environmental characteristics to all the intentions and aspirations.

Relying only on subjective measures of exposure

As indicated above, this is not a recommended procedure since data on objective exposure and on the linkage between objective and subjective exposure provide crucial information. However, when only subjective measures of exposure are used, certain other features of the study may compensate for this weakness. They include: (a) strong designs, often of the 'natural experiment' variety, where self-selection factors may be minimal and subjects are comparable on many other dimensions; (b) separation of independent and dependent variables from each other (i) in time (longitudinal and prospective data) and (ii) by distinctly different methodologies; and (c) use of stable (trait) marker variables in order to keep track of persistent influences on measurement, on exposure, and on outcomes.

To illustrate: reports of 'feeling tired and exhausted at the end of the day', assessed in men free of coronary heart disease, may predict the development of myocardial infarction and sudden death during a five-year follow-up period. When this holds up after adjustment for known biomedical risk factors, and provided the symptom data are not collected during the prodromal period, we have some faith that a risk factor of potential aetiological significance has been identified. We do not know: (a) to what objective environmental exposure, if any, it is linked; (b) what modification, in some exposure or in the risk factor itself, would reduce the risk of disease; and (c) how it may link up to some stable trait such as neuroticism. But it represents a worthwhile aetiological lead. The situation quickly deteriorates when, for example, the dependent variable is angina, where diagnosis is linked to symptom reporting. Or even worse is the situation when the dependent variable is something like 'burnout' at work or a depressive episode, where both methodological and conceptual overlap exist and the separation in time counts for little. In a retrospective, cross-sectional design, the separation in assessment counts for little if the presence of disease leads to pain, distress, disability, anxiety about future, and 'search for meaning' (a subjective reconstruction of disease aetiology along lay terms).

Developing new specific concepts and measures

The conclusion that the linkages between environmental exposures and disease outcomes are likely to consist of different, quite specific aetiological processes, if correct, calls for a corresponding conceptual and operational specificity of coping and supportive behaviours. An analogy may be helpful here in advancing the argument. Rotter's concept of locus of control (internal v. external orientation), and the associated measure, were quickly recognized by investigators in the health field as too broad and unworkable for understanding health relevant behaviours. The more specific health locus of control scale was developed, but its usefulness, too, has been extremely limited, even allowing for its further fractionation into several separate dimensions. We are undoubtedly now moving toward even more specific scales, such as locus of control for compliance with medications, for acquiring and for maintaining health habits (exercise, smoking cessation), for participating in screening for early detection of disease, and so on.

With respect to coping and social support, we have inherited broad, 'all purpose' instruments which are likely to need similar fractionation when used in health research. After all, different stressors have their specific demands (which may change over time) and it makes sense that if coping and social supports are going to modify the demands, then the behaviours assessed should be demand-specific. Similarly, if the pathway to a particular disease involves specific risk factors and specific steps in diagnosis, treatment, and recovery, then coping and social support should be linked to such pathways. One exception to this argument is the area of felt distress: to the extent that the phenomenology of distress is non-specific (independent of course), to that extent measures of coping and support directed at distress management would not need to be cause-specific.

The suggested direction of greater specificity is not without its disadvantages. It will lead to a great proliferation of measures, each of which is incompletely developed and validated. However, the alternative of continuing to use measures that don't do much for us is not very attractive, either. The suggested direction also raises basic questions of how to formulate issues of validity for these concepts; that is, it seems to give up on broad notions of construct validity and drives us toward narrower notions of specific criterion validity. The reader will note that the chapters on social support and coping raise the issue of construct validity for the different measures discussed, but in fact do not spell out the nomological network in which the construct validity of these measures should be embedded. I assume this is because none exists as yet.

Recognizing limitations of 'superior' methodologies

Recommendations about how to do something better have a way of becoming rigid dicta which then blind us to the remaining limitations. Thus the emphasis on objective assessments of exposure status (such as in the work setting) may drive us to use trivial or irrelevant measures, since these are the only ones we were able to develop under the pressure of this recommendation. Measuring exposure objectively and selecting exposures which appear 'beyond control' may make us forget that problems of self-selection into exposure still remain. For example, the Three Mile Island accident was 'beyond control' of the residents around, but we find that we can't study the impact unless we take into consideration whether people did or did not leave the area. But this is a profoundly confounding self-selection variable. Similarly, permanent plant closing may be 'beyond control' of the former workers there, but if we calibrate the dose of this exposure by length of the ensuing unemployment, we have introduced another powerful self-selection variable. With respect to the recommendation to use prospective, longitudinal designs, the chapter by Kessler is a particularly good reminder of the failure of such a design to solve all the problems we may encounter.

SOME ISSUES FOR THE FUTURE

This will be idiosyncratic and incomple listing of some of the issues raised by an overview of the contents of this volume. The research domain of stress and health is both amorphous and diverse; no conceptual framework is possible for organizing the evidence so that one could then reveal the gaps and the neglected areas.

At the broad programmatic level, we need considerable clarification of the methodology of psychosocial epidemiology so that processes and outcomes can be studied together. Our process variables, ideally, need to be sensitive to both the antecedent stressor and the consequent health outcome. At present, they tend to link up with one or other but not both. We need to be more sensitive to the crossing of levels of observation when we work both with psychosocial and biological variables. We may need to give up, for the moment, the idea that we can identify pairs of biological and psychosocial indicators that will track isomorphically through the stressor–reaction–adaptation–outcome experience. And we need much more thought about the scheduling of data collection contacts: this bears both on the issue of variable time span of sensitivity of the different indicators, as well as the issue of detecting the order in which events and processes evolve.

Another needed programmatic area of research is the explicit and directed study of biases and distortions in self-report measures (e.g. recall of past events, descriptions of present life circumstances, self-assessments of distress, etc.) in relation to: (a) state of exposure to a stressor; (b) presence of disease or some psychosocial outcome; and (c) stable traits and response tendencies. At present, our research practices (and our reviews of the literature) are based on very fragmentary knowledge and very personal inclinations to be optimistic or pessimistic about such issues.

With respect to specific content areas, a few suggestions can also be offered. Certainly the Beehr and O'Hara chapter strongly suggests the need for a major reorientation of the stress reduction studies if they are to become relevant to the stress–disease literature: (a) they need to address the issue of modifying the work environment, the stressor exposures; and (b) those that work with distress modification will need to link that distress to the work settings, rather than working with non-specific distress of undetermined origin. In the occupational stress literature, we need to take the rich set of available measures which are subjective assessments of the various work stressor dimensions, and to begin to develop commensurate objective indicators. In the process, it may become necessary to develop many more occupation-specific indicators. And for the area of coping, a number of agenda items could be listed: we need measures that do not require introspective insights but only call for descriptions of behaviours. The need is to develop measures which can be given prospectively, and the development of more specific measures, linked to specific demands, may facilitate this. Since coping tends to be so often confounded both with stressor severity and quality of outcome, we need to see if our conceptualizations or our methodologies (or both) are at fault. A neglected area of new measurement is the concept of anticipatory coping, i.e. managing one's life in a way so as to reduce chances of exposure to stressors; this might include coping which improves one's skills and abilities.

REFERENCES

Kasl, S. V. (1978). Stress at work: Epidemiological contributions to the study of work stress. In Cooper, C. L., and Payne, R. (Eds.) *Stress at Work*, New York, Wiley, 3–48.

Kasl, S. V. (1981). The challenge of studying the disease effects of stressful work conditions (editorial). *Amer. J. Pub. Health*, **71**, 682–4.

Kasl, S. V. (1982). Strategies of research on economic instability and health. *Psychol. Med.*, **12**, 637–49.

Kasl, S. V. (1983). Pursuing the link between stressful life experiences and disease: A time for re-appraisal. In Cooper, C. L. (ed.), *Stress Research: Issues for the Eighties*, Chichester, J. Wiley & Sons, Ltd., pp. 79–102.

Kasl, S. V. (1984a). Chronic life stress and health. In A. Steptoe, and A. Mathews, (eds.) *Health Care and Human Behaviour*, London, Academic Press, Inc., Ltd., pp. 41–75.

Kasl, S. V. (1984b) Stress and health. *Ann. Rev. Pub. Health*, **5**, 318–41.

Kasl, S. V. (1984c) When to welcome a new measure (editorial). *Amer. J. Pub. Health*, **74**, 106–8.

Kasl, S. V. (1985) Environmental exposure and disease: an epidemiological perspective on some methodological issues in health psychology and behavioral medicine. In J. E. Singer, and A. Baum, (eds.) *Advances in Environmental Psychology, Vol. 5: Methods and Environmental Psychology*, Hillsdale, N. J., L. Erlbaum Assoc., pp. 119–46.

Kasl, S. V. (1986). Stress and disease in the workplace: A methodological commentary on the accumulated evidence. In M. F. Cataldo, and T. J. Coates, (eds.), *Health Promotion in Industry: A Behavioral Medicine Perspective*, New York, Wiley, pp. 30–50.

Index